GLOBAL SURGERY AND ANAESTHESIA

A SHORT GUIDE TO MEANINGFUL INVOLVEMENT

LESLEY HUNT

Global Anaesthesia, Surgery & Obstetric Collaboration

Published by GASOC Publishing

Global Anaesthesia Surgery and Obstetric Collaboration 15130421

Accounting for Good CIC, 2 Geordie Ridley Place, Upper Precinct Court, Blaydon, England NE21 5BT

Website: www.gasocuk.co.uk

Print ISBN: 978-1-9193283-0-0

eBook ISBN: 978-1-9193283-1-7

Editor: Paul Mayhew (developmental and copy editing)

All proceeds from the sale of this book support GASOC's work—encouraging responsible and impactful involvement in global surgery and empowering members in LMICs.

For permissions and enquiries: gasocdirectors@gmail.com

Cover image: Sherbro Island ferry, Sierra Leone. Photo: author's own.

FOREWORD

Lesley Hunt is a consultant colorectal and general surgeon in Sheffield, whose career has been distinguished by her commitment to both surgical excellence and global collaboration. Over the past decade she has trained and mentored local surgeons in Sierra Leone, and supported the growth of indigenous trainers, while developing curricula that meet the realities of low-resource health systems. More recently, she has contributed to training programs in Ghana, Malawi and Tanzania, giving her a broader understanding of the diverse issues affecting training in Sub-Saharan Africa. She has also pioneered distance learning initiatives and brought innovative teaching methods back to the UK, enriching surgical training in Yorkshire and Humber. Her work embodies humility, pragmatism, and the conviction that safe and effective surgery can — and must — be accessible everywhere.

This book is a testament to that vision. What makes it stand out is not only its authority, but also its readability. Global surgery can often seem daunting, layered with statistics, systems, and jargon. Yet in Lesley's hands, the subject becomes clear, compelling, and even personal.

This volume offers an authoritative yet accessible introduction to global surgery. It is written with clarity and economy, making a complex field comprehensible to students, practitioners, educators, and policymakers alike — and making a complex subject approachable without sacrificing rigour.

The chapters follow a logical progression, beginning with definitions and scope, and moving through barriers, solutions, and practical guidance for those seeking to engage in this work. Each section is concise, informative, and easy to read, while firmly grounded in evidence and practice.

The structure of the book reflects the breadth and depth of the field. The Introduction: A Call to Arms sets the stage, reminding us that billions still lack access to essential surgery. What is Global Surgery? defines the field and its core tenets — need, access, and quality — while Maternal Health and Surgical Capacity illustrates how maternal mortality serves as a mirror of broader inequities.

The chapters on Barriers and Delays and The Bare Necessities of Adequate Surgical Care explain, with vivid examples, why poverty, distance, and lack of infrastructure continue to cost lives, and what resources are truly essential. The World's Best Operations identifies the lifesaving procedures that bring the most value, while Major Initiatives in Global Surgery charts the rise of global collaborations and commissions that have pushed the agenda forward.

Quality and safety are at the heart of this book. In Quality Matters and Anaesthesia and Safety Culture, the reader is reminded that surgery is not just about access but also about outcomes and culture. Money, Money, Money underscores the financing challenges, while Task Shifting and Sharing provides pragmatic models for strengthening the workforce in constrained settings.

The book also highlights the importance of knowledge generation and creativity. Research in Global Surgery and Innovation in Global Surgery stress how data, evidence, and ingenuity shape progress. NSOAPs (National Surgical, Obstetric and Anaesthesia Plans) illustrate how governments can translate vision into national strategies, while Humanitarian Surgery reflects on lessons from disaster and conflict.

Later chapters move from policy into practice. Global Surgery Organisations introduces the networks that connect individuals and institutions worldwide. From Policy to Practice explores delivery models, while Motives, Skills and Readiness and Choosing Your First Program encourage reflection for those considering involvement. Finally, Self-Improvement, Practical Matters, and Poor Behaviour — Primum Non Nocere provide candid, practical advice on resilience, logistics, and ethics. The Afterword closes with a call to collective action.

Each of these chapters is concise, clear, and easy to read. Together they form an indispensable guide to a field that is growing in importance and urgency. They are evidence-based, accessible, and pragmatic — qualities that mirror the professional ethos of the author herself.

This book is both a guide and an invitation: an invitation to understand, to act, and to believe that surgery can be part of health for all. Lesley Hunt has shown us that it is possible to build capacity, transfer skills, and nurture systems that endure. This book equips us with the knowledge, perspective, and inspiration to continue that work.

Nobhojit Roy MS, MPH, PhD, FCS (ECSA)
Professor of Surgery and Chair, Center for Leadership in Global Health Equity, Butaro, Rwanda
Director, WHO Collaborating Centre for Emergency, Critical and Operative Care, Program for Global Surgery & Trauma, The George Institute of Global Health, New Delhi, India
Previously, Lead, Surgery & Anaesthesia, Clinical Services & Systems, WHO Headquarters, Geneva
Lancet Commissioner for NCD & Injuries in the poorest billion
Lancet Commissioner for Global Surgery

PREFACE

> *If ar bin no*
>
> *"If (only) I had known"*
>
> —SIERRA LEONE KRIO

My global surgery career began relatively late in life — a classic case of empty nest syndrome. By that stage, I'd been a surgical trainer, and running hands-on courses, for more than a decade. Yet, when I went to Sierra Leone, I was poorly prepared and consequently less useful than I should have been. Initially, the training we gave was generic and patchy.

My lack of preparation was not for want of trying. I searched the internet and the medical literature but found precious little advice. There was also a rather casual attitude prevailing at that time — "just go out and see what you can do...." It inevitably takes time and enduring relationships to make meaningful change, but a few pointers and insights at an early stage might well have shortened my learning curve.

So, this is the book that I wish had existed 15 years ago — a plain English introduction to global surgery and anaesthesia, leavened with some lived experience and pragmatic advice for early-years involvement. I hope it increases the chances that your efforts are productive and helps you avoid some common pitfalls. For some, it may even open a door onto a world they were unaware of — one of our readers commented that if he had read this book when newly qualified, he might have taken a different career path.

Despite being unprepared, I was warmly welcomed in Sierra Leone, and over time, a high-quality general surgery training programme was developed. This resulted in a cohort of excellent local surgeons, and burgeoning trainers, specifically prepared to manage the unique realities faced in their country. The pleasure I get from seeing their capability and patient outcomes is the ultimate professional reward.

In the book, you get to hear from some of them, and from high-income country colleagues. Those who have developed pragmatic solidarity with colleagues and communities in low-resource settings say this is the most professionally rewarding work they do. Take inspiration from their diverse contributions, and together we can make life a bit more equitable.

Lesley Hunt
Sheffield, UK
October 2025

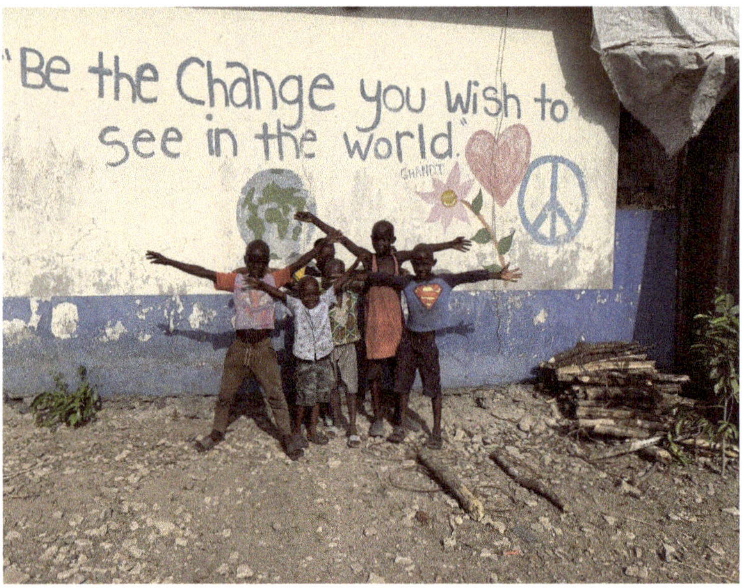
"Be the Change you wish to
see in the world."

Figure 1. Hatfield Archer Memorial Hospital, Rotifunk, Sierra Leone 2024.
Photo: author's own.

CONTRIBUTORS

Anita Eseenam Agbeko, Vascular Surgeon, Kwame Nkrumah University of Science and Technology; Deputy Director, NIHR GSU Ghana Hub, Ghana

Noel Aruparayil, Hepato-Pancreatic and Biliary Surgical Fellow, Glasgow Royal Infirmary, UK

Soham Bandyopadhyay, Academic Clinical Fellow, Oxford University, UK

Vijna Boodhoo, Clinical Innovation Fellow, University of Glasgow, UK; Vice-President, Global Anaesthesia, Surgery and Obstetrics Collaboration (GASOC), 2025

Mark Chapman, Consultant Colorectal Surgeon, University Hospitals Birmingham, UK

Samantha Conroy, Specialist Registrar in Urology, Sheffield Teaching Hospitals NHS Foundation Trust, UK

Jonathon Dean, Consultant Anaesthetist, East Suffolk and North Essex NHS Foundation Trust, UK

Donal Farrell, General Practitioner and volunteer with The Virtual Doctors, Sheffield, UK

Ibrahim Sorie Fofanah, Surgical Officer, Sierra Leone

Sandi Gangha, Surgical Officer, Sierra Leone

Qaiser Jalal, Consultant Surgeon, Sheffield Teaching Hospitals NHS Trust, UK

Anthony Abbot Kamara, Senior Surgical Officer, Sierra Leone

Sayoh Kanneh, Surgical Officer, Sierra Leone

Ishiaka Konneh, Surgical Officer, Sierra Leone

Sushil Maslekar, St James University Hospital, Leeds, UK

Peter Robert Mboma, Surgical Officer, Sierra Leone

Mwayi Darwin Nyirenda, Surgical Resident, Blantyre, Malawi

Raymond Nyirenda, Consultant Surgeon, Blantyre, Malawi

Ong Pei Jean, Specialty Registrar in Anaesthesia, Sheffield, UK; GASOC President, 2025

Helen Please, Surgical Registrar/Resident, Oxford Deanery, UK

Carolyn Ramwell, Pediatric Clinical Coordinator, Children's National Hospital, Washington, US

Ibrahim M. Sesay, Surgical Officer, Sierra Leone

Hassan Ahmad Sheriff, Surgical Officer, Sierra Leone

Marianne Stephen, Consultant, Obstetrics and Gynaecology, University Hospitals Plymouth NHS Trust, UK

Mark Szymankiewicz, Consultant Colorectal and General Surgeon, Salisbury NHS Foundation Trust, UK; Visiting Lecturer and Fellow, University of Winchester Centre for Global Health, UK; Founder and Trustee, Surgical teams Working in aFrica Together for Safer Surgery (SWIFTSS)

Dominik von Malsen, General and Abdominal Surgeon, Germany; International Medical Educator (IME), Physicians for Peace

Jen Watt, Surgeon and Post-CCT Fellow, London, UK

Jan Man Wong, Specialist Registrar in Anaesthesia, London; GASOC Anaesthetic Representative

With grateful thanks to Andy Dennis and Rob Atcheson for commenting on the manuscript.

CONTENTS

CHAPTER 1
INTRODUCTION: A CALL TO ARMS — SURGERY AND HEALTH FOR ALL

IN 1980, Dr Halfdan Mahler, then Director-General of the World Health Organization (WHO), addressed the World Congress of the International College of Surgeons in Mexico City. His speech, *Surgery and Health for All*, was a call to arms for the world's surgical community with an ambitious goal: train enough surgical teams so that everyone in the world could access lifesaving and essential surgery.

> *The vast majority of the world's population has no access, whatsoever, to skilled surgical care and little is being done to find a solution. Is the international surgical community ready to prepare training modules for essential surgery? Modules for training doctors, nurses, and auxiliary personnel in the first-line referral hospitals, both for work in operating theatres and for pre-operative and postoperative care. Finally, are the surgeons of the world ready to give top priority to training of this nature, both for undergraduate and postgraduate doctors, nurses, and other types of health worker involved, so that increasing numbers of people are proficient in providing essential surgery to all who need it.*[1]
>
> —DR HALFDAN MAHLER, 1980

Unfortunately, little happened after Dr Mahler's rallying cry. For the next thirty years, very few surgeons and public health professionals responded, and surgery remained firmly out of reach for five billion people, i.e. "the vast majority of the world's population."

Communicable diseases such as malaria, HIV, and tuberculosis continued to take precedence and universal access to surgery remained a low priority for major global public health initiatives. Surgery was perceived as just too complex to address and efforts to improve surgical care remained largely individual and small-scale.

THE SCALE OF NEGLECT

In 2025, the world's poorest continue to die from readily treatable conditions such as appendicitis and hernia. The progress achieved by international health organisations in controlling and treating communicable diseases puts the shortcomings of global surgical care into even starker relief.

Approximately one-third of global annual deaths are from conditions requiring surgical care — more than malaria, HIV/AIDS, and TB combined.

The statistics speak for themselves:[2,3,4]

- Five billion people lack access to safe emergency and essential surgery when they need it most.
- A third of the global burden of disease requires some form of surgery.
- Fifteen percent of all disability stems from untreated surgical conditions.
- Seventy-seven million disability-adjusted life-years (DALYs) are lost annually because of untreated surgical conditions.

WHAT IS CHANGING?

The plight of five billion people is no longer being completely ignored. In 2008, Paul Farmer, Professor of Global Health at Harvard, famously described surgery as "*the neglected stepchild of global public health*."[5] This maxim struck a chord and is repeated in hundreds of publications about the state of surgical care worldwide.

In many low-and middle-income countries (LMICs), the situation has changed little. Only a privileged minority can access essential and life-saving surgery. Nevertheless, the crisis is now widely acknowledged, measured, and investigated. The "neglected stepchild" may still not be receiving her fair share of attention, but at least people know she exists.

Improving access to surgery at the district hospital level has been identified as one of the thirty best mechanisms for advancing global welfare.[6] Timely access to safe, essential surgery is now accepted as both a cornerstone of functional healthcare systems and a highly cost-effective public health measure. With this recognition has come consensus among surgical teams: something must be done and done urgently.

> The World Bank classifies countries by gross national income (GNI) per capita (2023):
>
> **Low income:** ≤ US$1,145
>
> **Lower-middle income:** US$1,146–4,515
>
> **Upper-middle income:** US$4,516–14,005
>
> **High income:** > US$14,005

EXPLORE FURTHER

1. Meara, John G., Andrew J. M. Leather, Lars Hagander et al. "Global Surgery 2030: Evidence and Solutions for Achieving Health, Welfare, and Economic Development." *The Lancet* 386, no. 9993 (2015): 569–624. https://doi.org/10.1016/S0140-6736(15)60160-X.
2. Farmer, Paul E., and Jim Y. Kim. "Surgery and Global Health: A View from Beyond the OR." *World Journal of Surgery* 32, no. 4 (2008): 533–36. https://doi.org/10.1007/s00268-008-9525-9.

CHAPTER 2
WHAT IS GLOBAL SURGERY?

GLOBAL SURGERY IS a new field of expertise, study, and advocacy that endeavours to define the world's unmet need for surgery and seek mechanisms to address it. Its goal is universal access to safe, timely, and affordable emergency and essential surgery. Global surgery therefore focuses on underserved populations, found predominantly in LMICs, displaced populations and people in crisis because of disasters or conflict.

The term global surgery is a catch-all, encompassing not only the surgical specialties, obstetrics, and anaesthesia, but also epidemiologists, logisticians, economists, policymakers, and decision makers in funding organisations.

For years, public health monitoring systems ignored surgical disease and surgical care, but advocacy from global health organisations has resulted in huge efforts to measure the unmet need and accept that surgical care is a necessary part of healthcare.

Advocacy is a major element of global surgery. Lobby groups, like the Lancet Commission on Global Surgery, urge governments in LMICs to improve surgical services and pressure international partners and funding organisations to support this work.

The easiest way to define global surgery is to start with the desired end and work back. The aim is to make life saving and essential surgery available to all the world's population. This requires a diverse skill set, ranging from influential policymakers working in global institutions to individuals and small groups providing long-term training and supporting single institutions and colleagues in LMICs.

Three tenets underpin global surgery: **need**, **access**, and **quality**.

THE RISE AND RISE OF GLOBAL SURGERY

Social media, 24-hour news and the global consumer marketplace mean rich and poor nations are connected like never before. We can no longer overlook our global responsibilities, and there is growing discussion — and increasingly, action — from thousands of individuals and hundreds of professional associations.

In high-income countries (HICs), most surgical and anaesthesia societies and training institutions now have global surgery faculties or interest groups. Academic and educational meetings routinely include sessions on global surgery. We are still a long way from global surgery being seen as everybody's responsibility, however, a generation of surgical care providers are coming through who see involvement in global surgery as part of a conventional career.

Please note these acronyms as they are used consistently throughout this book:

LIC: Low-income-country

MIC: Middle-income-country

LMICs: Low-and-middle-income countries

HIC: High-income country

THE RISE AND RISE OF GLOBAL SURGERY INFORMATION

The two decades up to 2021 saw an exponential rise in research addressing global surgery themes, resulting in a body of literature exposing and quantifying unmet surgical need and the human suffering and economic implications of failing to meet it.

UNDERSTANDING UNMET SURGICAL NEED

Mapping processes in different countries have helped broadly define the extent of unmet surgical need worldwide. Assessment is complicated because surgery is not a disease entity, but a mode of treatment that crosses boundaries between specialities, forming part of the care of many diseases and reproductive health. But by using a variety of metrics, there has been some success in defining and estimating the extent of surgical disease.

Estimating unmet need is harder as many of those affected are not seen by healthcare professionals. Using data from countries where surgical needs are met and comparing the density of skilled healthcare workers in these countries with those in LMICs has been useful. If the surgical workforce in a country is very small, this suggests most of that country's surgical need is not being met. Similar comparisons can be made for infrastructure and systems, such as hospitals, clinics, and ambulance services. Systematic household (door-to-door) surveys have also proven useful, documenting unmet need in communities who do not present to health services.

Unmet Need: Headline Figures

5 billion people cannot access lifesaving and essential surgery

9 out 10 people in LICs cannot access lifesaving and essential surgery

At least 143 million essential and lifesaving operations are not done annually

17 million avoidable deaths annually

77 million lost DALYs annually

Figures published by the Lancet Commission on Global Surgery (LCoGS, 2015), indicate five billion people cannot access essential surgery when they need it (**Figure 2**).[1] Every year millions of essential operations simply do not happen, and people die or suffer real disability as a result. Annually, 17 million deaths occur which could have been prevented by safe, timely, affordable surgery. Seventy-seven million disability-adjusted life-years (DALYs) are lost because of untreated surgical conditions.

Unmet surgical need is defined as *those operations, essential to save life or prevent disability, that are not performed*. Unsurprisingly, LMICs carry the heaviest burden of unmet need, with 90% of people living in LICs unable to access lifesaving and essential surgery.

INEQUITY

Access to surgery is largely a privilege enjoyed by the wealthy. Rich nations average a hundred times as many surgeons and ten times as many operating theatres per capita than poor ones.

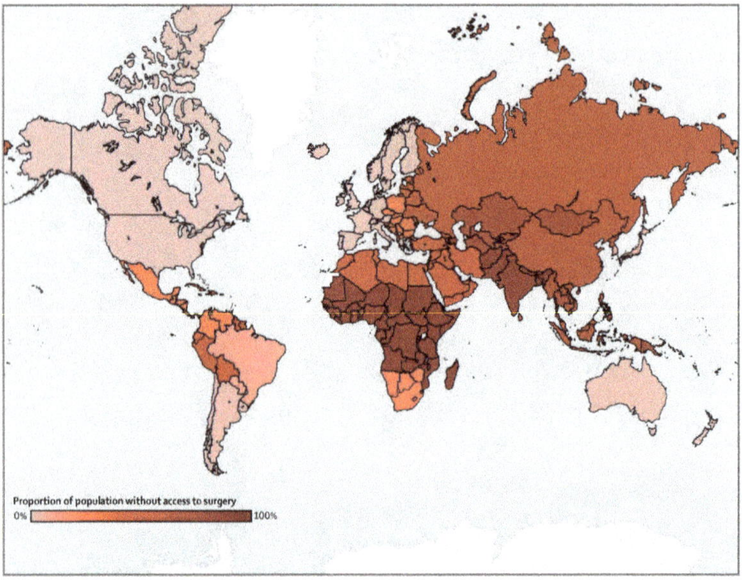

Figure 2. Proportion of the population without access to safe, affordable surgery and anaesthesia by region. From: Alkire BC, Raykar NP, Shrime MG, Weiser TG, Bickler SW, Rose JA, Nutt CT, Greenberg SL, Kotagal M, Riesel JN, Esquivel M, Uribe-Leitz T, Molina G, Roy N, Meara JG, Farmer PE. Global access to surgical care: a modelling study. *Lancet Glob Health*. 2015 Jun;3(6):e316-23. doi: 10.1016/S2214-109X(15)70115-4. Epub 2015 Apr 27. PMID: 25926087; PMCID: PMC4820251. Copyright © 2015 Alkire et al. Open Access article distributed under the terms of CC BY. Published by Elsevier Ltd. Reproduced under Creative Commons by licence.

In 2012, an estimated 313 million operations were performed across the world. Only 6% of these took place in the world's poorest countries, despite those countries being home to 37% of the world's population. The poorest third of the world's population undergo only 3.5% of the world's operations. Unmet need varies widely between countries and is close to zero in Western Europe. The figures presented here are already out-of-date, as the population is growing faster than surgical capacity in many LMICs (**Table 1**).

How were these figures calculated?

What is the benchmark?

Given the cross-cutting role surgery plays in treating disease, trauma and reproduction, calculating its minimal safe level is complex. The role of surgery therefore needs to be benchmarked for each disease,

Region	Essential Operations not Done (Gross, Annual)	Per 100,000 Population
Caribbean	131,050	301
Central Asia	919,432	1136
Central Europe	678,358	570
Central Sub-Saharan Africa	4,192,980	4343
East Asia	27,956,507	2000
East Sub-Saharan Africa	17,555,748	4935
North Africa and Middle East	2,115,011	474
Oceania	55,196	555
South Asia	57,791,550	3582
Southeast Asia	12,480,939	2045
Southern Sub-Saharan Africa	291,000	413
Western Sub-Saharan Africa	18,909,507	5625
Global Total	143,068,278	n/a

Table 1. Estimated unmet need for surgery by Global Burden of Disease epidemiological region. Abridged from: Meara JG, Leather AJ, Hagander L et al. "Global Surgery 2030: Evidence and Solutions for Achieving Health, Welfare, and Economic Development." *Lancet* 2015;386:569–624.

injury and reproductive function, which requires accurate documentation and coding.

New Zealand provides exemplary healthcare with universal access at a reasonable fraction of the country's Gross Domestic Product (GDP) and achieves excellent health outcomes, despite its rate of surgery being amongst the lowest in HICs. They are clearly good at providing what is really needed, while minimising unnecessary surgery. New Zealand combines this with robust data collection, allowing mathematical modellers to use their data as a baseline, giving us the expected frequency of surgery for given conditions, in a high-quality health service, at reasonable cost.

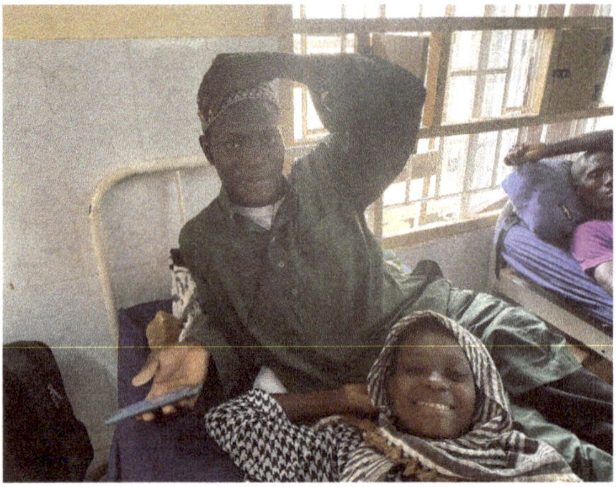

Figure 3. This patient required specialist reconstructive surgery after treatment for abdominal TB in Mauritania. Via word of mouth, she had heard there was "somebody doing the surgery in Sierra Leone," and in an amazing leap of faith, travelled with her husband more than 2000 km by public transport, enquiring at hospitals along the way until they found us. Photo: author's own.

Correlating the incidence of disease in New Zealand against that in other countries then allows calculation of surgical need in those countries. If data is available in that country on the number of operations currently being performed (the *met need*), the shortfall (the *unmet need*) can then be calculated. Using this method, the global annual requirement is estimated at 321 million operations, with a shortfall of about 143 million.[2] Even this figure probably underestimates true need, as diseases treated promptly in New Zealand are less likely to progress to the point where they require surgery.

The Three Tenets of Global Surgery

Need: operations, essential to save life or prevent disability, that are not performed.

Access: understanding the financial, logistic and cultural barriers that prevent people accessing surgery.

Quality: operations being performed, case mix and avoidance of key complications and post-operative mortality.

Using DALYs

Quality-adjusted life-years (QALYs) and DALYs are commonly used in healthcare measurement. DALYs, developed in the 1990s by the Global Burden of Diseases, Injuries, and Risk Factors (GBD) initiative, measure the burden imposed by conditions at the population level. [3] They describe years of life lost, and years lived with disability and facilitate comparisons of population health across geographical areas.

Estimates suggest at least 11% of global DALYs relate to surgical conditions. Surgery is needed for almost every disease, and poor access to medical care in LMICs increases the likelihood, for example, of untreated pulmonary infections progressing to empyema.

Using observational data

The greatest unmet need for surgery is in Sub-Saharan Africa and South and Southeast Asia — places where it is also hard to ascertain what surgery is currently being done. Measuring operative volume is time consuming and not straightforward, as LMICs often lack systematic, central reporting systems. Efforts to count the current volume of surgery therefore use multiple methodologies and proxy measures.

Data is gleaned from demographic surveillance systems, household surveys, verbal autopsies, facility-level data inquiries, and a mixture of modelling methods. A common method is field data collection, i.e. physically going to healthcare facilities to gather information. Facility-level enquiries may be as crude (or as gloriously simple) as medical students trawling through paper theatre registers and manually counting the number of operations performed.

The mixed methods Surgical Assessment Tool (SAT), developed by the Harvard Program in Global Surgery (PGSSC) and the World Health Organisation (WHO), and its forerunner the WHO Situational Analysis Tool, are validated for use in LMICs. Randomly selected primary care facilities, district hospitals and tertiary centres are visited, and key staff are interviewed about the infrastructure, services provided, how the surgery is paid for, what medical records are kept and the workforce. Operative logbooks and theatre records are interrogated, collecting data for the preceding 30 days. The SAT has provided a reasonable picture of the national surgical volume in countries such as Madagascar, Rwanda, Sierra Leone, Liberia, and Uganda.

A proxy measure

Proxy measures can also be used. For instance, the number of births by caesarean section, compared to the total number of live births, can be used as a surrogate marker of surgical provision. The WHO, the United Nations International Children's Emergency Fund (UNICEF), and

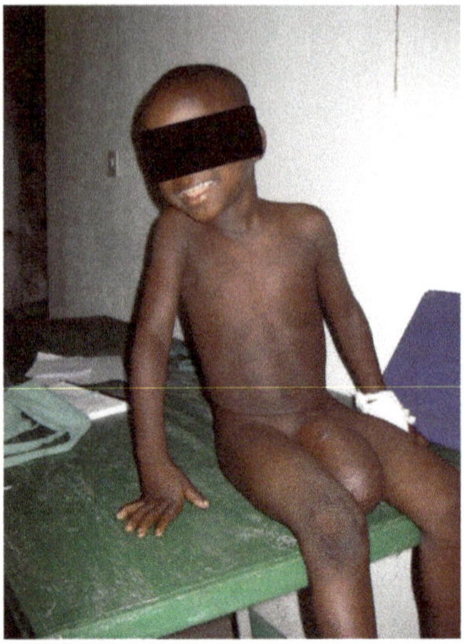

Figure 4. The human cost of unmet need: child with untreated congenital hernia. Photo: author's own.

United Nations Population Fund (UNFPA) recommend a caesarean rate of 5–15% is necessary, and 100% of obstetric complications should be treated, to limit maternal deaths.[4]

In 2002/2003, only 0.1–1% of births in Uganda, Kenya, South Sudan, and Rwanda were by caesarean section, and only 2–18% of expected obstetric complications were treated.[5] These figures obviously demonstrate unmet need in obstetric surgery, but low caesarean rates almost always also indicate unmet need across the breadth of surgery, allowing them to be used as a proxy marker for unmet need across all essential surgery.

Caesareans are also a useful marker for case mix and change over time can indicate a country's surgical development. Across Sub-Saharan Africa, caesareans make up 25–40% of all operations, rising to as much as 60% in the most deprived areas because not much else gets done.

Compare this with HICs, where caesareans account for only 2.6% of all operations. In countries like Rwanda, as surgical volume has increased, the absolute number of caesareans has also risen, but their proportion relative to other procedures has fallen. This change in proportion is a proxy indicator of growth in other surgical fields.

. . .

Using mathematical modelling

Using probability modelling and proxy measures where direct data were unavailable, the LCoGS estimated the likelihood of individuals being able to access surgery after serious injury. They looked at timeliness (availability of ambulances), surgical capacity (number of surgical procedures undertaken as a proportion of those needed), safety (presence of pulse oximetry), and affordability.

The modelling concluded that 5.3 billion people do not have access to safe, timely, and affordable surgery. At 2015 capacity levels, 94% of people in LICs and LMICs do not have access.

GLOBAL INDICATOR PROJECT

The LCoGS is discussed in more detail later in this book. However, it is useful to briefly discuss some of its indicators here.

Two indicators measure capacity: the proportion of the population living near a surgical hospital, and the density of key staff — surgeons, obstetricians, and anaesthetists.

Two indicators measure delivery: surgical volume, i.e. the annual number of surgical procedures per 100,000 population, and perioperative mortality.

The Global Indicator Data Collection Project measured performance against the LCoGS indicators in 2015 and 2017, across 215 countries. This was the first attempt to gather primary data on surgery to use with the modelled estimates. Data was obtained by direct contact with official bodies, systematic literature reviews and internet searches of grey literature.

The LCoGS target for surgical volume is 5000 operative procedures per 100,000 population per year. Some data was available on surgical volume from 184 countries, in which volume varied from 258 procedures per 100,000 in South Sudan to 30,091 per 100,000 in Monaco. No LMICs met the target.

Initially, only 16 countries provided data on in-hospital perioperative mortality, however this did include three MICs. Unsurprisingly, the project concluded that surgery remains an underrepresented part of the global healthcare agenda, as is borne out by just how few countries could even provide data.

WHY IS OPERATIVE VOLUME SO LOW?

Infrastructure, surgical equipment, and drugs are all necessary to provide high-quality care and support surgery. However, the principal determinant of operative volume is the number of surgical, obstetric and anaesthetic staff available. It seems that, wherever surgical teams are available, they will improvise to provide lifesaving surgery, despite the lack of seemingly essential items, such as running water, electricity and even a blade.

In simple terms, there are not enough surgeons, obstetricians, and anaesthetists in LMICs. Forty-eight percent of the world's population live in LMICs, yet these countries have only 19% of the world's surgeons and 15% of its anaesthetists. There are approximately two million surgeons in the world and, to reach the workforce numbers necessary to ensure essential surgery for everybody, we need another 1.27 million by 2030. Even then, this figure does not consider additional issues related to their level of training, postgraduate support and morale. Unsupported surgeons working in difficult conditions for low wages are likely to be less productive than those getting appropriate professional and financial reward.

Measuring and publishing average operative volume across a country is not necessarily a reflection of unmet need, as skilled workers tend to congregate in cities and affluent areas, and the rural poor struggle to travel. A more accurate reflection therefore requires collecting data across a country, and low levels of surgery in rural areas strongly suggest unmet need. In India, for example, the wealthy and geographically well-located enjoy some of the world's best healthcare, while in other parts of the country, and amongst other social groups, access to essential surgery is limited.

MICs that have undergone rapid development have also increased their surgical staffing and infrastructure. They have seen rapid growth in surgical volume and a reduction in unmet need. Although most development is positive, it can bring new problems, such as the rise in trauma from road and railway accidents in LMICs.

EXPLORE FURTHER

1. Kamali, Parisa, Issy Marks, Godfrey Sama, Dominique Vervoort, and Justine Davies. "Measuring Surgical Systems

Worldwide: An Update." *World Bank Blogs*, February 12, 2018. https://blogs.worldbank.org/en/opendata/measuring-surgical-systems-worldwide-update.

2. Bickler, Stephen, Doruk Ozgediz, Richard Gosselin et al. "Key Concepts for Estimating the Burden of Surgical Conditions and the Unmet Need for Surgical Care." *World Journal of Surgery* 34, no. 3 (2010): 2014. https://doi.org/10.1007/s00268-009-0261-6.
3. World Health Organization. *Emergency and Essential Surgical Care Situational Analysis Tool (SAT) Database.* https://www.who.int/surgery/publications/WHO_EESC_SituationAnalysisTool.pdf.
4. Blavatnik Institute Program in Global Surgery and Social Change: WHO-PGSSC Surgical Assessment Tool (SAT) https://www.pgssc.org/_files/ugd/d9a674_f2b179abea9e4b0a9a103fbe93ac6479.pdf .

CHAPTER 3
MATERNAL HEALTH AND SURGICAL CAPACITY IN LOW- AND MIDDLE-INCOME COUNTRIES

> *When women thrive, all of society benefits, and succeeding generations are given a better start in life.*
>
> —KOFI ANNAN (UN SECRETARY-GENERAL, 2003)

MATERNAL MORTALITY IS a key measure of human development that is morally important in its own right. As a clearly defined, measurable marker, it is also a valuable proxy for a country's health services, providing a reasonably accurate reflection of overall health and a benchmark for improvement.

Poor maternal health and death also contribute to infant and childhood mortality. Loss of the mother and the associated reduced household income bring hardship to families. When women die, their children lose out on food, healthcare, and education. Poor nutrition is a major contributor to one in three deaths under the age of five.

WHY DOES MATERNAL MORTALITY MATTER TO SURGEONS?

Maternal health data provides valuable information about the provision of safe surgery and disparities in access to surgical care. Obstetrics and the surgical specialities are distinct fields in rich countries, but surgical specialisation is a relative luxury. They are indivisible in many LICs and impoverished areas in MICs — dependent on the same infrastructure and often the same team. A single-handed surgeon is often responsible for the full gamut of surgery, from orthopaedics to obstetrics to oral surgery.

DEFINITIONS

The World Health Organization (WHO), United Nations Population Fund (UNFPA), United Nations Children's Fund (UNICEF), and the World Bank all record maternal mortality following the same metrics. Maternal mortality is defined as the death of a woman from any cause related to, or aggravated by, pregnancy or parturition or its management, occurring during pregnancy or within 42 days of the end of pregnancy.

Maternal mortality rate

Maternal deaths are commonly reported in two ways. The maternal mortality rate is the number of maternal deaths divided by the number of women of reproductive age. It is dependent on wide-ranging factors such as access to contraception, attitudes to female schooling, and female nutrition. It therefore reflects the value placed on women in society as well as the quality of their healthcare.

Maternal mortality ratio (MMR)

By contrast, the maternal mortality ratio (MMR) is the number of maternal deaths per 100,000 live births. As such, it is more specific to obstetric risk, and therefore a succinct and much studied indicator of surgical provision.

In 2023, the global MMR was 197 per 100,000 live births, with massive disparities between countries; the average MMR was just 11 in Europe, compared to 669 in West and Central Africa.[1]

In 2023, women in Western Europe had a 1 in 14,283 lifetime risk of dying because of pregnancy and childbirth. The rate in Chad and the Central African Republic was 1 in 24. Physical immaturity and possibly low social status result in the MMR being higher amongst teenagers, who represent a significant proportion of those giving birth in LMICs.

Safe surgery

Maternal mortality is a concise indicator of surgical provision generally. Maternal deaths indicate public health and inequality issues, and their reduction requires societal and general healthcare improvement, but access to safe surgery is also essential. About 15% of pregnant women require emergency obstetric care, including surgery, yet 951 million of them cannot get it. The World Bank's *Essential Surgery* (volume 1 of *Disease Control Priorities*, third edition) gives a comprehensive overview of the types of conditions and management seen by those caring for women in pregnancy in LMICs (see chapter 7, page 43).[2]

Three complications — haemorrhage, puerperal sepsis, and pre-eclampsia/eclampsia — cause three-quarters of all maternal deaths. Most of the remainder are due to complications of labour and delivery and unsafe abortion. Safe and timely surgery is an indispensable component in the management of all these conditions. For some conditions surgery is necessary only when medical treatment fails, but for others, like obstructed labour and ruptured ectopic pregnancy, only surgery can save the patient.

Simple surgery has the capacity to transform the obstetric end of maternal care. Caesarean section alone has the power to avert 40% of all maternal deaths, and reduce neonatal mortality by 30–70%.[3]

Ideal caesarean rates

The consensus is that caesarean rates of less than 10% of births are inadequate to meet the needs of the population.[4] Parts of Sub-Saharan Africa have rates of less than 5%, which is way too low. Rates higher than 20%, on the other hand, are not associated with improved maternal or foetal outcomes and increase the risk of some complications.

Some countries that have recently expanded surgical provision have seen caesarean rates rise to as high as 45% among richer women, who often perceive the procedure positively. There are providers willing to operate — perhaps motivated by financial gain.

SURGICAL WORKFORCE DENSITY AND MATERNAL MORTALITY

Low caesarean rates result in avoidable maternal deaths and indicate a failure of surgical provision generally. Getting the rates up to safe levels requires infrastructure and equipment. But most importantly, it requires surgeons, obstetricians and anaesthetists.

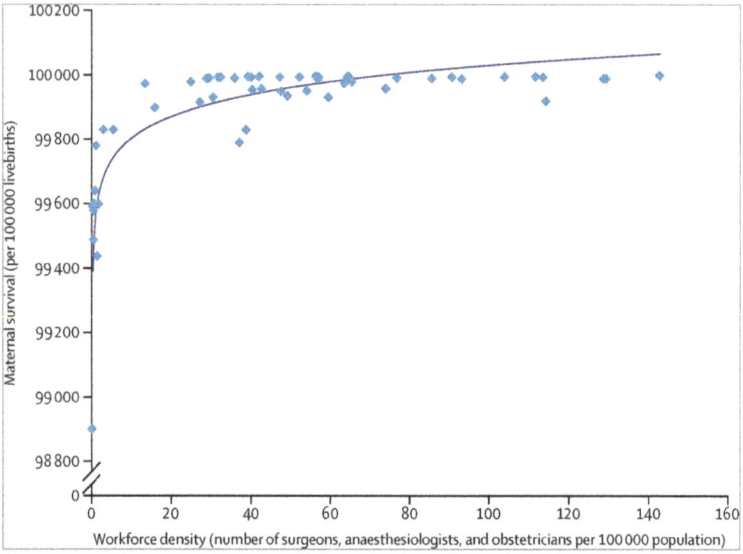

Figure 5. Specialist surgical workforce density and maternal survival. A density of under 20 per 100,000 specialist surgeons, anaesthetists, and obstetricians correlates with lower rates of maternal survival. Reprinted from Meara, JG, Leather, AJ, Hagander, L et al. "Global Surgery 2030: Evidence and Solutions for Achieving Health, Welfare, and Economic Development." *The Lancet* 386, no. 9993 (2015): 569–624. Lancet special credit: Reprinted from *The Lancet*, Meara, JG, Leather, AJ, Hagander, L et al. "Global Surgery 2030: Evidence and Solutions for Achieving Health, Welfare, and Economic Development." *The Lancet* 386, no. 9993 (2015): 569–624. With permission from Elsevier.

The term "SAO provider" is used to denote surgeons, anaesthetists and obstetricians regardless of cadre. Surgical workforce density is often defined as the number of SAO providers per 100,000 of population. As the number of specialist SAO providers increases from 0 to 20 providers per 100,000, caesarean section becomes available and rapid improvements in maternal survival are seen. Above this level, the line quickly flattens off, making 20 SAO providers per 100,000 something of a sweet spot in maternal care (**Figure 5**).[5,6]

> **To prevent women dying in childbirth, we need twenty SAO providers per 100,000 people in every region.**

The Lancet Commission on Global Surgery (chapter 7, page 56) therefore recommended targeting resources towards getting all countries up to 20 SAO providers per 100,000. Four years later, sampling suggested that the average SAO density was nearer 1 per 100,000 in LICs and 3 per 100,000

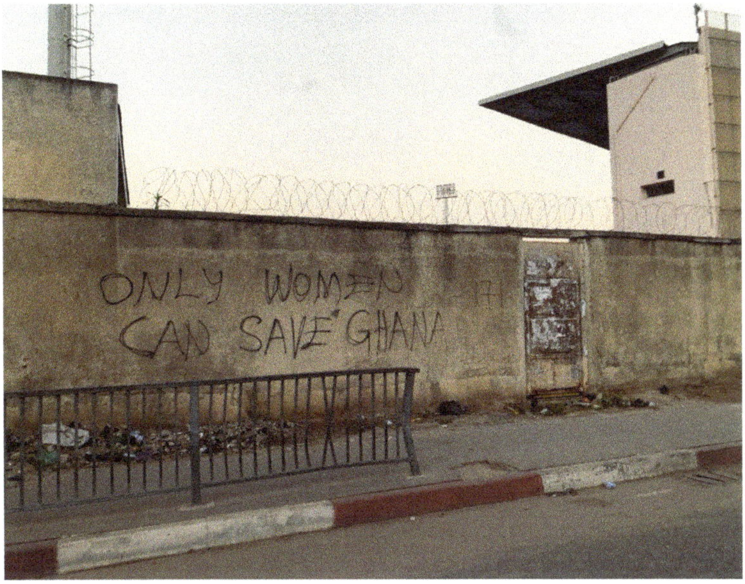

Figure 6. Accra, Ghana 2024.Photo: author's own.

in lower MICs, an increase on 2015 levels, but well below target.[7]

MILLENNIUM DEVELOPMENT GOAL NO. 5 (MDG 5)

In 2000, eight Millennium Development Goals were agreed by the UN (we will discuss these further in chapter 6).[8] Goal five was "to improve maternal health by 2015." More specifically, Target 5A stated: "Reduce by three-quarters, between 1990 and 2015, the maternal mortality ratio."[9]

Although this was not achieved, dramatic improvements were seen due to reduced fertility rates, improved per capita incomes and female educational attainment and increases in skilled birth attendants. Some countries invested in SAO training, and this may partially explain differences in mortality between countries within the same geographical region. In 2023, for example, the MMR in Liberia was 628, whereas it had fallen to 354 in neighbouring Sierra Leone.[10]

The anticipated improvements in some regions were undermined by the HIV epidemic, and spikes in MMR were seen internationally during the COVID-19 pandemic.[11] Despite these setbacks, worldwide maternal deaths fell by 40% and MMR fell from 328 to 197 per 100,000, between

2000 and 2023. Sub-Saharan Africa and Southeast Asia saw the greatest improvement. Nepal doubled health spending, concentrated funds on the poorest and cut the MMR from 480 to 142.

However, there is no room for complacency. More than a quarter of a million women still died of maternal causes in 2023. Nearly all deaths were in LICs and easily preventable with adequate resources.

OBSTETRIC FISTULA

Obstetric fistula usually results from prolonged obstructed labour in the absence of a skilled birth attendant. The foetus dies and may eventually lyse and pass, but the bladder and/or rectal walls are trapped between the pelvic ring and the foetal head, causing pressure necrosis and either vesicovaginal fistula (VVF) or rectovaginal fistula (RVF), or both. It occurs in about 1:1000 unattended labours, affecting 50,000 to 100,000 women worldwide each year. In 2002, there were 2 million women in Asia and Sub-Saharan Africa living with untreated obstetric fistula.[12]

Fistula has special significance in global surgery, as it is preventable with basic obstetric care and access to caesarean section. It is vanishingly rare in countries with functional health systems, and its continuing existence indicates poor surgical health systems, and the need to increase surgical provision. The United Nations Population Fund (UNFPA) launched the "Campaign to End Fistula" in 2003.

Fistula affects some of society's most marginalised individuals — young women, often teenagers, living in remote, impoverished communities. Corrective surgery is highly cost-effective and allows ostracised women to return to their communities. Surgery is usually carried out in referral hospitals, which build up expertise, sometimes supported by expatriate organisations and teams, including surgical camps.

The International Federation of Gynecology and Obstetrics (FIGO), the International Society of Obstetric Fistula Surgeons (ISOFS) and other partners have come together to develop competency-based training for fistula surgery. This is particularly significant in global surgery, where formal competency-based training and standard-setting remain largely absent.

With its seemingly impossible challenges, global surgery can feel daunting, but find inspiration in the story of Catherine and Reginald Hamlin, as told in *The Hospital by the River: A Story of Hope*. It describes the development of the world-renowned Addis Ababa Fistula Hospital, where tens of thousands of women have received transformative treatment and many LMIC surgeons have been trained in fistula repair. It is a humbling and inspiring account of what determined individuals can achieve.

EXPLORE FURTHER

1. World Health Organization, United Nations Children's Fund, United Nations Population Fund, World Bank Group, and United Nations Department of Economic and Social Affairs, Population Division. *Trends in Maternal Mortality: Estimates 2000 to 2023.* World Health Organization, 2025. https://www.unfpa.org/sites/default/files/pub-pdf/9789240108462-eng.pdf.
2. International Federation of Gynecology and Obstetrics (FIGO). *Competency-Based Fistula Surgery Training Manual.* FIGO, 2020. https://www.figo.org/sites/default/files/2020-05/FIGO_Global_Competency-Based_Fistula_Surgery_Training_Manual_0.pdf.
3. Hamlin, Catherine. *The Hospital by the River: A Story of Hope.* New edition. Monarch Books, 2004.

CHAPTER 4
BARRIERS AND DELAYS

BARRIERS TO ACCESSING surgery are multifactorial but mostly come down to money. Patients cannot afford to pay for the surgery or the costs involved in accessing it. Governments cannot afford to spend on hospitals, healthcare workers, or supplies. The education of new health workers is not adequately funded, and prospective trainees cannot afford the fees.

Poor countries tend to be poor across the board, and wider societal problems also stop people accessing surgery. Low levels of general education and literacy reduce healthcare-seeking behaviour. Roads connecting populations to hospitals are inadequate and impassable at certain times of year. Even where the roads are good, the cost of transport can be too much.

TOO FAR TO WALK: THE THREE DELAYS MODEL

The Three Delays Model (**Table 2**) describes critical delays seeking emergency maternity care, but the same issues apply to other surgical emergencies:[1]

1. Delay in **decision** to seek care
2. Delay in **reaching** care
3. Delay in **receiving** adequate care

Delay in Decision to Seek Care	Delay in Reaching Care	Delay in Receiving Adequate Care
Low status of women	Distance to facility	Poor facilities and lack of supplies, electricity or water
Poor understanding of pregnancy and when to seek help	Availability and cost of transport	Insufficient or inadequately trained or poorly motivated staff
Acceptance of maternal death	Poor roads	Inadequate referral pathways
Anticipated cost of care	Geography, e.g. rivers or estuaries without bridges	

Table 2. Thaddeus and Maine's Three Delays Model summarises the major obstacles women face when seeking, reaching, and receiving emergency maternity care. Source: Thaddeus, Sereen, and Deborah Maine. "Too Far to Walk: Maternal Mortality in Context." *Social Science & Medicine* 38, no. 8 (1994): 1091–1110. https://doi.org/10.1016/0277-9536(94)90226-7.

DELAY #1: THE DECISION TO SEEK MEDICAL CARE

Low levels of education and literacy delay the recognition of serious problems, and people are unsure when professional help is needed. Traditional healers and drug pedlars are often consulted first, with the hospital being the last resort. In LMICs, the decision to go to hospital is usually a big one, and the social and cultural barriers to seeking help

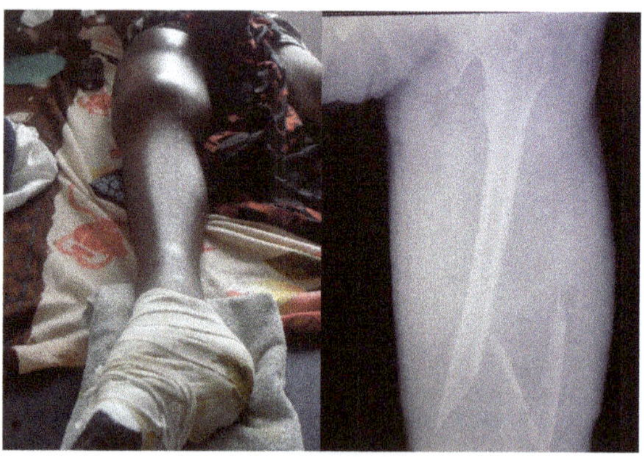

Figure 7. Left: Patient presenting with an ischaemic foot ulcer. Right: The X-ray of his swollen thigh is poor quality but reveals an old injury, undisclosed until this stage. Photos: author's own.

are influenced by the anticipated financial hardship it will bring. A senior member of the family is often called in to make the decision, and delay occurs while they make their assessment. Some family members might be considered less deserving of family money, with women and children often having a lower status than men.

Cultural suspicions of healthcare often have roots in poverty and tend to decrease, or even disappear, as education and financial circumstances improve. There is logic to the cultural distrust of hospitals and surgery in impoverished areas. Late presentation results in complications and mortality. For example, in regions where limb fractures are usually treated by local bone setters, those with simple fractures may do well. However, those with open and complicated fractures eventually get taken to hospital, sometimes days or weeks after injury. Amputation and death are therefore not rare, and the hospital is blamed.

When a decision is made to go to hospital, families frantically try to raise the money as their relative is dying of peritonitis. Money may be found by promise and debt. When late presentation means survival is far from guaranteed, families face very difficult dilemmas. Should they proceed with catastrophic expenditure in the face of a low likelihood of success, knowing that the loss of this money will seriously affect the life chances of the next generation?

In countries where life expectancy is low and infant and maternal mortality are high, acceptance of death is understandable. Suffering is normal and high birth rates are closely associated with high infant mortality.

"I worked in obstetrics in a rural hospital in India. A patient who remains with me to this day is a young woman, my age, who presented heavily pregnant. She had been experiencing heavy vaginal bleeding for several days, but her family had prevented her from seeking medical care, mainly due to patriarchal norms and cultural beliefs surrounding women's health.

By the time she reached us, the foetus had already died, and she was haemodynamically compromised. Unfortunately, despite our best efforts to resuscitate her, we were unable to save her. It was hard as we knew this could have been prevented. This episode stays with me still, as it made me realise a painful truth: no matter how skilled or well-prepared we are in the operating theatre, our efforts are meaningless if the patient does not arrive there in time."

—Vijna Boodhoo, Clinical Innovation Fellow (Glasgow, UK)

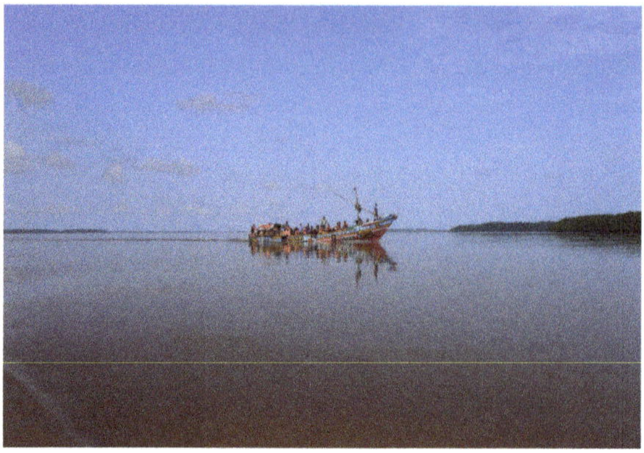

Figure 8. Sherbro Island ferry, Sierra Leone. The journey takes two hours, followed by several hours by road to reach the hospital. Photo: author's own.

DELAY #2: REACHING CARE

The next challenge is getting to hospital. Transport infrastructure is rarely distributed fairly, with poor people living in poor areas, with poor infrastructure. The term "hard to reach" has been coined to describe areas away from cities, often with unsealed roads. Hospitals, healthcare workers and aid agencies tend to cluster in urban and affluent areas, so the "local" hospital may be several hours away.

A boy acted as caretaker for his sick father, who died during treatment. Unable to afford his return home, the community abandoned him. Imagine a family losing a child because a 50 km journey is unaffordable....

Ambulances are rare in LICs, and private journeys are expensive and difficult. Imagine travelling three hours by motorbike with peritonitis, or while having a post-partum haemorrhage. Maternal complications are often particularly acute, and women and babies die before getting to hospital or arrive in a moribund condition.

In India, mortality from acute abdominal conditions correlates with distance to hospital. Living over 100 km from a well-resourced hospital is an independent predictor of poorer survival, even after adjusting for other socioeconomic factors.[2]

The cost of transport and of living away from home mean that, even if care is free at the point of delivery, the poorest may not be able to access it. In many LMICs, inpatient nursing care is limited to specific interventions. Feeding, washing, and moving patients is done by a caretaker or guardian staying alongside, so money must be found to transport and support two people living away from home.

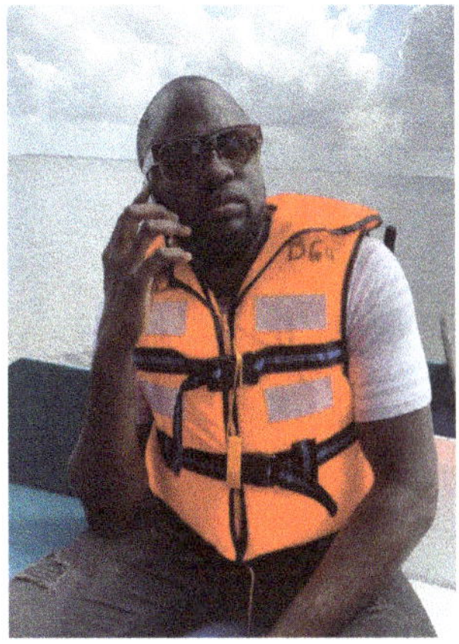

Figure 9. Emergency Surgical Officer Foday Daddy Mansaray travels 30 minutes by speedboat to Bonthe Government Hospital, Sierra Leone. The fuel costs alone would bankrupt most families. Before a resident surgeon was posted, islanders needing emergency surgery faced long, dangerous journeys, leading to deaths enroute or care foregone. Photo: author's own.

DELAY #3: RECEIVING ADEQUATE CARE

In some places, arrival at hospital does not equate with arrival at adequate surgical care. Necessities of are often lacking, even in ostensibly appropriate facilities. The hospital needs at least one surgeon, who needs to be available, and some essential equipment and drugs. This includes the ability to transfuse blood, if needed, and to provide oxygen. If things are missing, the surgery either goes ahead in the knowledge it is unsafe, or the patient needs to be transferred elsewhere, repeating the transport challenges.

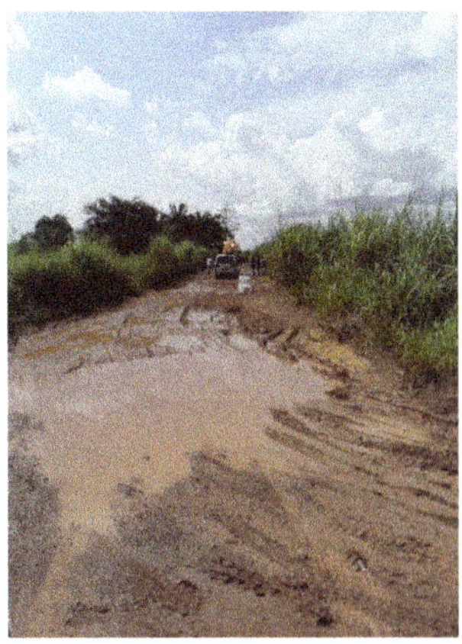

Figure 10. Typical West Africa: unsealed roads can be challenging in rainy season. Photo: author's own.

Resources may be available but first need to be located. The patient's relative or caretaker is often given a shopping list of consumables needed for the surgery, which cannot begin until they return with the cannula, anaesthetic drugs, IV fluids, antibiotics, sutures, and dressings. Even if everything is available, there can still be delays if staff are overrun with patients. In obstetrics, trauma, and emergency surgical practice, these additional delays can result in preventable deaths.

IN SUMMARY

The three delays — hesitation in seeking care, challenges reaching facilities, and obstacles to receiving timely and adequate treatment, all compound each other, increasing the risk of harm and death. Addressing these barriers means not only investing in health infrastructure and staff, but also improving education, wider infrastructure, and financial protection.

On top of the day-to-day barriers represented in the Three Delays Model, war, natural disasters, and displacement further disrupt care for millions of people.

"A 25-year-old man presented to a district hospital with a perforation and free air on X-ray. The diagnosis was made and resuscitation commenced, but they did not have the resources to operate there. He arrived at the central hospital late afternoon. The one operating theatre was in use into the night. We wanted to operate early morning but had to wait for the day-shift anaesthetist. From arriving with us, there was an additional delay of more than 16 hours. This increases mortality."

—Dominik von Malsen, surgeon and international medical educator (Blantyre, Malawi)

EXPLORE FURTHER

The Three Delays Model: Thaddeus, Sereen, and Deborah Maine. "Too Far to Walk: Maternal Mortality in Context." *Social Science & Medicine* 38, no. 8 (1994): 1091–110. https://doi.org/10.1016/0277-9536(94)90226-7.

CHAPTER 5
THE BARE NECESSITIES OF ADEQUATE SURGICAL CARE

VACCINATION PROGRAMS CAN BE CONDUCTED as standalone processes, with relatively simple infrastructure and rapidly trained staff. Surgery is more complex, requiring interconnected resources and at least one or two highly trained people. This may be why policymakers have shied away from surgery in the past. But is it really as complicated as we fear?

The Lancet Commission on Global Surgery's (LCoGS) report, Global Surgery *2030: Evidence and Solutions for Achieving Health, Welfare, and Economic Development*, outlines the necessities for safe surgical care as follows:[1]

> **Using the bevel tip on a hypodermic needle when there is no blade:**
>
> **"We used to improvise by using razor blades or an injectable (hypodermic) needle to go through the skin."**
>
> **—Ishiaka Konneh, surgical officer (Sierra Leone)**

- Trained surgical and anaesthesia providers
- Infrastructure, equipment, and supplies for safe general and regional anaesthesia, laparotomy, caesarean delivery, and open fracture treatment (e.g. electricity, water, PPE, basic labs, and HIV testing)
- Decontamination and sterilisation facilities
- Safe, affordable, screened, and cross-matched blood
- Essential drugs, including antibiotics, analgesics, and anaesthetics (per WHO Model List)

- Nursing care with appropriate physiological monitoring
- 24-hour surgical cover with capacity to monitor and manage deteriorating patients
- Quality-improvement systems, including perioperative mortality audits
- Risk assessment and operation planning for scheduled procedures

Due to the resourcefulness of surgical teams in LMICs, lifesaving surgery often goes ahead despite the absence of items on this list — things the rich regard as essential. Operations are completed by the light of mobile phones, using instruments boiled in a kettle, and with the knowledge that somebody in the team has the same blood group as the patient.

THE FIVE Ss

The US non-governmental organisation (NGO) Partners in Health (PIH) strengthens local health systems in LMICs. PIH popularised the Five Ss necessary for healthcare: Staff, Stuff, Space, Systems, Social Support. The LCoGS uses the approach for scaling up surgical provision.

STAFF

For safe surgery, a hospital needs at least one surgical, anaesthesia and obstetric (SAO) provider who is available, has received adequate training and has the necessary skill set (**Figure 11**).

Although the LCoGS states that surgeons and obstetricians cannot function in isolation, the reality is that, in rural areas, they often do. They may be the only person competent to resuscitate the patient, administer the spinal, perform the caesarean, and provide the postoperative maternal and neonatal care. This is far from ideal; a team of SAO providers, nurses, and laboratory technicians has a better chance of delivering high-quality, sustainable care. There also needs to be enough of them to meet demand. Teams that are completely overrun with patients do not have the time to deliver quality care.

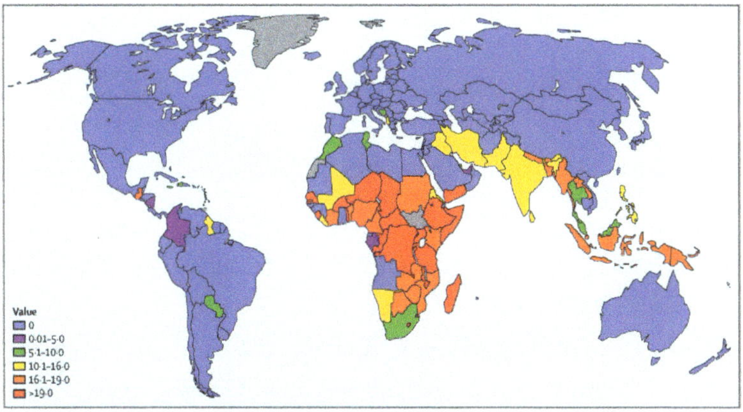

Figure 11. Change in surgical workforce density needed for specialist SAO-only model to meet 20 SAO providers per 100,000 population by 2030. Reprinted from Meara, JG, Leather, AJ, Hagander, L et al. "Global Surgery 2030: Evidence and Solutions for Achieving Health, Welfare, and Economic Development." *The Lancet* 386, no. 9993 (2015): 569–624. Lancet special credit: Reprinted from The Lancet, Meara, JG, Leather, AJ, Hagander, L et al. "Global Surgery 2030: Evidence and Solutions for Achieving Health, Welfare, and Economic Development." *The Lancet* 386, no. 9993 (2015): 569–624. With permission from Elsevier.

It is inevitable a single-handed SAO provider cannot always be available. The expectation of 24/7 cover leads to problems such as low morale and burnout, and these issues are exacerbated when staff are sometimes not paid for long periods. People struggle to cope and can be lured away into managerial roles or by organisations offering better salaries to administer projects and collect data.

"I enrolled in the surgical training program because I lost my elder brother to an incarcerated hernia due to the lack of quality surgical care in the country."

—Ibrahim M. Sesay, surgical officer (Sierra Leone)

Even if SAO providers are present and willing, they may not be adequately trained for the cases they face. Increasing access to surgery is only beneficial if it is done properly. Unfortunately, in countries with weak regulation, both local and foreign staff may "have a go" at surgery without proper training.

Safe, meaningful surgery in difficult circumstances requires training that matches or exceeds the quality of that provided in HICs. More high-quality training programs with competency assessment are badly needed. To make the most impact, the focus needs to be on providing workforce for rural and hard-to-reach areas and needs to be backed up with context-appropriate licensing and credentialing.

The term "SAO provider" encompasses everybody who does the job, both medically qualified and other cadres.

Experienced SAO trainers should take note: you can play important roles — whether by formally teaching new providers, upskilling existing ones, mentoring and offering ongoing support, or providing hands-on expertise to help establish new services.

Inequality between regions is a significant issue in some countries. Indian investigators mapped their country in terms of SAO providers.[2] Data for 2018/2019 shows the distribution of the workforce varied enormously, especially between urban and rural areas. The SAO provider density in India's most rural region was just 0.385 per 100,000 population. Surgical volume differed widely between demographic, socioeconomic, and geographic groups, as did perioperative mortality rates. The authors concluded India fell short of achieving its targets and called out an evidence gap in India's surgical care planning.

STUFF

Extreme frugality is the norm in low-resource settings, but all surgery requires equipment and consumables. The LCoGS recommends all district hospitals carry the equipment for caesarean section, laparotomy and open fracture management.

Sutures, for example, are often in desperately short supply, and compromises are made daily. A single suture may be used for the uterus, sheath, and skin, whereas six or seven would be used in wealthy countries. Certain drugs are also essential. Analgesia is often limited, and expectation and tolerance of postoperative pain is the norm in some settings.

"After graduating, I was honoured to be selected as a national trainer. This role allowed me to help shape and deliver both theoretical and practical surgical training for students, graduates, and doctors — a vital step in addressing Sierra Leone's growing surgical needs. It was more than a role; it was a calling. I enjoyed learning alongside international experts, growing professionally, and, most importantly, passing on knowledge that could save lives. I believed in the mission."

—Hassan Sherriff, emergency surgical officer and trainer (Sierra Leone)

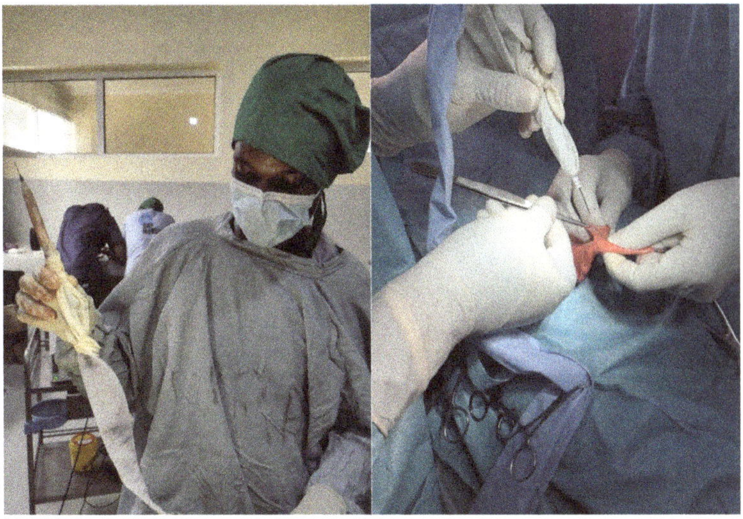

Figure 12. This innovative waterproof gown and glove cover allows reuse of a disposable diathermy pencil, with sterilisation of the tip only. The author was taught this in Tanzania (left) and showed the photograph to a colleague in Sierra Leone. The next day it was in use there (right). Photos: author's own.

Many of the surgical instruments used in LMICs are donated from rich countries. Despite efforts to "green" operating theatres, we are profligate and some of our discards find their way to other countries. There can be a tendency for HICs to donate malfunctioning and less-often used instruments, which remain malfunctioning and less-used after travelling abroad.

When operations are done using inadequate materials, quality can be compromised. Across Sub-Saharan Africa there is a paucity of surgical mesh. Groin hernia repair, one of the commonest operations in Africa, is often done by suture — a method virtually obsolete in rich countries because of its high recurrence rate. This means African surgeons are knowingly performing substandard surgery, for want of the correct materials. Similarly, although it is possible to give an anaesthetic without pulse oximetry, it is infinitely safer when it is used. Yet in 2010, oximetry was missing from 55% of operating theatres in Sub-Saharan Africa.[3]

Dependence on donated materials is unsatisfactory. Stuff needs supply chains, and supply chains need transport infrastructure and honest brokers along the way. Commercial vendors sometimes have more reliable supply chains than governments in LMICs, so essential resources may be available in-country but not stocked in hospitals. Patients or their relatives must obtain them, if they can afford to do so.

SPACE

Other than the most minor procedures, surgery requires hospitals and to be effective, emergency surgery requires hospitals *close to the population*. There is a tendency for surgical teams and facilities to cluster in cities and centres of political importance, significantly reducing their impact. The district hospital is recommended as the core site for surgical and anaesthetic delivery. It is large enough to house all the necessary elements of care, yet close enough to the population to allow meaningful emergency care.

> "On some days, soap is cut into slivers to stretch across shifts. On others, it runs out entirely. Still, the team carries on — adapting, innovating, and caring for patients with dignity. What stands out is not the lack of infrastructure, but the strength of the people within it. Nurses who improvise dressings, anaesthetists who monitor vitals with unreliable equipment, and surgeons who teach and train despite a crushing clinical load — they are not waiting for change. They are already doing the work, often without recognition."
>
> —Soham Bandyopadhyay, academic clinical fellow (Oxford), on working in Tanzania

The Copenhagen Consensus, a 2008 project identifying the smartest investments for advancing all aspects of global welfare, ranked improving access to surgery at district hospitals among the world's top thirty priorities.[4] This is not only because of the benefits of the operations themselves, but also because the infrastructure necessary to deliver safe surgery enables care for a wide range of other conditions.

Raising the quality of district hospitals begins with running water and sanitation and moves on to provision of electricity and oxygen. They then need laboratory space, blood banking, and functioning operating theatre suites, replete with lighting and sterilisation facilities.

SYSTEMS

Some hospitals in LMICs have adequate staff and stuff, and yet the system is so grinding that lives are still lost unnecessarily. Management

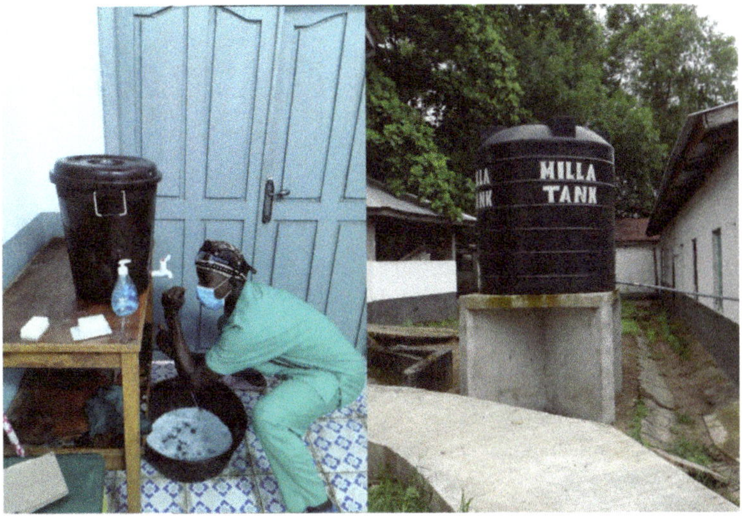

Figure 13. Sierra Leonean surgical officer Ibrahim Fofanah scrubbing up without running water (left). Provision of simple tanks can provide running water for operating theatres (right). Photos: author's own.

and decision making may not be focused on patients, and resources are not prioritised for those with time-sensitive conditions. Good local leadership, governance, and financial practice are essential to change this. In many places, supply chains are embryonic, and some healthcare systems have an entrenched culture of dependency on donations, which reduces the impetus to develop sustainable logistics.

System improvements focusing on clinical policies, protocols, and a culture that ensures escalation, referral, and timely review are needed, with key clinical decision makers involved in the care of urgent cases. Some institutions have adequate staff, but the distribution of workload is skewed and does not meet patient need.

The LCoGS recommends national planning of the number and distribution of emergency surgical facilities, integrating governmental, NGO, and private providers; establishing a central framework for ordering and purchasing equipment; implementing a national blood plan; improving connectivity and referral systems; and paying close attention to referral logistics.[5] In reality, manpower planning has not always ensured the correct staff are in the correct facilities. For example, some countries have high-quality district hospital buildings, with excellent theatre facilities, lying largely unused. The system has failed to staff them with SAO providers, or posted single-handed surgical officers there, while surgeons in the cities compete for theatre space.

Emergency patients therefore must travel to central hospitals. Even if ambulances are present, there may not be enough fuel for everybody. Services are often reserved for maternity cases, so if you present with peritonitis and are referred on, the ambulance cannot take you until it is also carrying a pregnant woman.

When patients finally arrive at the hospital where the surgeons are, they find emergencies are not prioritised, and they wait for their laparotomy, despite being critically ill. The staff are there, the space is there, the stuff is just enough — but without effective health system leadership and strategic planning, patients needlessly suffer and die.

A telling example of where clinical systems fall short is the limited adoption of the WHO Safe Surgery Checklist,[6] even though teams are aware that its use substantially reduces surgical mortality in LMICs. Non-Technical Skills for Surgeons (NOTSS) training may be done, but without governance structures and leadership, it is rendered useless.

Effective clinical governance processes, quality outcome monitoring, and quality-improvement programs are all essential for safe surgery but are in their infancy in many LMICs. A telling insight into this is how surgical residents in a large teaching hospital categorised deaths

"TB took the use of the teenager's legs. I held little hope of his pressure sore healing, without specialist dressings, expert wound care and plastic surgery. Would these be available in the capital, 3.5 hours away?

'He just needs to get the few hundred metres here.... we have more than enough', said the clinic nurse. She knew the San Bushmen and demonstrated what was needed was in abundance:

- Patient-centred care: listening to context, recognising his concerns
- Communication: explaining, demonstrating, empowering his informal carers to relieve pressure areas
- Nutritional support: simple foodstuffs ensuring calories, protein, vitamins and minerals to promote healing
- Judicious use of resources: saline or sterile water to clean and wet-to-wet gauze dressings
- Holistic care: psychosocial well-being, with the patient's drawings bringing a smile, a laugh, improved self-confidence, and a growing social circle

The wound was tamed, and I learned what effective care and leadership looks like."

—Donal Farrell, doctor, N/a'an ku sê Lifeline Clinic (Namibia, 2018)

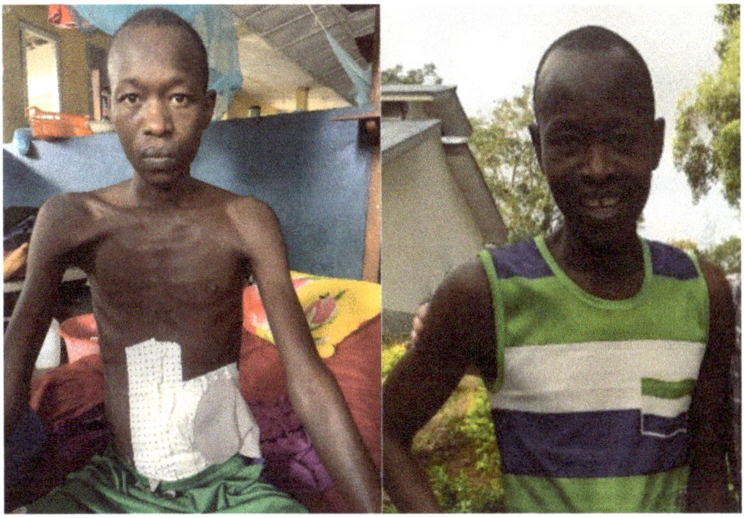

Figure 14. (Left) Patient who developed serious complications after elective surgery. His money ran out and he was left without food. (Right): Same patient after four months of preoperative nutritional support and stoma reversal. Photos: author's own.

during their morbidity and mortality (M&M) meetings. Instead of categorising them as "preventable" and "unpreventable," deaths were designated as "expected" and "unexpected." As nobody stopped to ask if the death was preventable, nothing was done to stop it happening again.

SOCIAL SUPPORT

The best health systems in the world cannot deliver benefit without community engagement and buy-in. Social support is essential for patient care, recovery, and maintaining good health. For surgical care to be fully effective, it must go hand-in-hand with food, housing, transportation, and financial support for patients and their families. Even when care is free at the point of delivery, the costs associated with accessing it are prohibitive for many.

EXPLORE FURTHER

1. Meara, John G., Andrew J. M. Leather, Lars Hagander et al. "Global Surgery 2030: Evidence and Solutions for Achieving Health, Welfare, and Economic Development." *The Lancet* 386,

no. 9993 (2015): 569–624. https://doi.org/10.1016/S0140-6736(15)60160-X.

2. Partners In Health. "Our Approach: Staff, Stuff, Space and Systems." https://www.pih.org/our-approach.
3. World Health Organization. "The WHO Model Lists of Essential Medicines." Updated biennially. https://www.who.int/groups/expert-committee-on-selection-and-use-of-essential-medicines/essential-medicines-lists.

CHAPTER 6
THE WORLD'S BEST OPERATIONS — DEFINING ESSENTIAL SURGERY

WHAT IS LIFESAVING SURGERY? What is essential surgery?

Lifesaving surgery might seem easy to define, but the concept is more complex than it first appears. For example, an inguinal hernia in a young man left untreated for twenty years eventually strangulates and he dies. Would an elective procedure two decades earlier have been regarded as "lifesaving"?

Essential care is also challenging to define. Are procedures for club foot essential? The condition does not kill people, but it blights lives and can lead to poverty and social exclusion, both of which are causes of untimely death.

"Essential Surgical Care" has been defined as "basic surgical procedures that save lives and prevent permanent disability or life-threatening complications."[1] The aim of global surgery is for everyone to get access to these procedures.

In a world where five billion people lack access to surgical care, expediency also matters. Every day, people die for lack of simple surgery. Which operations represent the best value when rapidly increasing surgical capacity? We need procedures that are relatively easy to learn and deliver the most benefit to the most people — the "low hanging fruit" of surgical practice.

In LICs and rural, impoverished regions of MICs, surgeons are generalists to a greater or lesser extent. Procedures must be feasible in resource-constrained environments, easy to implement, and within the repertoire of surgeons expected to cover a broad scope of practice.

THE BEST OPERATIONS IN THE WORLD

In 2004 and 2005, the World Health Organization (WHO) launched two overlapping and complementary initiatives. The Emergency and Essential Surgical Care (EESC) programme develops and implements training materials to improve surgical care in LMICs, including the textbook *Surgical Care at the District Hospital.*[2]

The Global Initiative for Emergency and Essential Surgical Care (GIEESC) is an international forum of global surgical bodies and policymakers. It advises on policy and aims to stimulate collaboration, and has been crucial in defining essential surgical procedures.[3]

Since then, several expert groups have described different versions of an "Essential Surgical Package." Details vary, but all agree on a core set of truly essential operations. These are surgery's "Best Buys" — delivering them should result in maximum gain for the maximum number of people within a reasonable time frame.

ESSENTIAL SURGERY DISEASE CONTROL PRIORITIES

Disease Control Priorities (*DCP*) are a series of publications produced by the World Bank that review the cost-effectiveness of health interventions to allow rational use of resources and improve care in low-resource settings. The third edition (2015) is a nine-volume textbook that, for the first time, included a separate volume on essential surgery; *DCP3: Essential Surgery.*[4]

This volume identifies an Essential Surgery Package of 44 surgical procedures that address significant need, are cost-effective, and are feasible to implement in LMICs. Estimates suggest that universal access to surgical care would avert 4.7 million deaths annually. Worldwide provision of just these 44 procedures could avert 1.5 million deaths. This is 6–7% of all avertable deaths in LMICs.

Among the 44 are 23 emergency procedures (shown in red in **Table 3**) that can be delivered at district hospitals, if infrastructure, systems and personnel are sufficiently upgraded.

Type of Procedure	Community or Primary Care Facility	First-Level (District) Hospital	Second- and Third-Level Hospital
Dental	Extraction		
	Drainage of dental abscess		
	Treatment of caries		
Obstetrics, Gynaecology and Family Planning	Normal delivery	Caesarean birth	Repair obstetric fistula
		Vacuum extraction/forceps delivery	
		Ectopic pregnancy	
		Manual vacuum aspiration and dilation and curettage	
		Tubal ligation	
		Vasectomy	
		Hysterectomy for uterine rupture or intractable postpartum haemorrhage	
		Visual inspection with acetic acid and cryotherapy for precancerous cervical lesions	
General Surgery	Drainage of superficial abscess	Repair of perforations: for example, perforated peptic ulcer, typhoid ileal perforation	
	Male circumcision	Appendicectomy	

Table 3. The Essential Surgery Package: procedures and platforms. From: Debas, H. T., P. Donkor, A. Gawande, D. T. Jamison, M. E. Kruk, and C. N. Mock, editors. 2015. *Essential Surgery. Disease Control Priorities*, third edition, volume 1. World Bank. doi:10.1596/978-1-4648-0346-8. License: Creative Commons Attribution CC BY 3.0 IGO.

Type of Procedure	Community or Primary Care Facility	First-Level (District) Hospital	Second- and Third-Level Hospital
General Surgery *(cont.)*		Bowel obstruction	
		Colostomy	
		Gallbladder disease, including emergency surgery	
		Hernia, including incarceration	
		Hydrocelectomy	
		Relief of urinary obstruction: catheterisation or suprapubic cystostomy	
Injury	Resuscitation with basic life support measures	Resuscitation with advanced life support measures, including surgical airway	
	Suturing laceration	Tube thoracostomy (chest drain)	
	Management of non-displaced fractures	Trauma laparotomy	
		Fracture reduction	
		Irrigation and debridement of open fractures	
		Placement of external fixator; use of traction	
		Escharotomy/ fasciotomy	
		Trauma-related amputations	

Table 3. (cont.)

Type of Procedure	Community or Primary Care Facility	First-Level (District) Hospital	Second- and Third-Level Hospital
Injury *(cont.)*		Skin grafting	
		Burr hole	
Congenital			Repair of cleft lip and palate
			Repair of club foot
			Shunt for hydrocephalus
			Repair of anorectal malformations and Hirschsprung's Disease
Visual Impairment			Cataract extraction and insertion of intraocular lens
			Eyelid surgery for trachoma
Non-Traumatic Orthopaedic		Drainage of septic arthritis	
		Debridement of osteomyelitis	

Table 3. (cont.)

TRAUMA

Trauma is a crucial part of the Essential Surgery Package. It causes two-thirds of the disability that could be averted by increasing access to essential surgery (**Figure 15**). Road accidents account for the largest percentage, followed by fire, heat and hot substances. Burns, it should be noted, are frequently a disease of poverty.

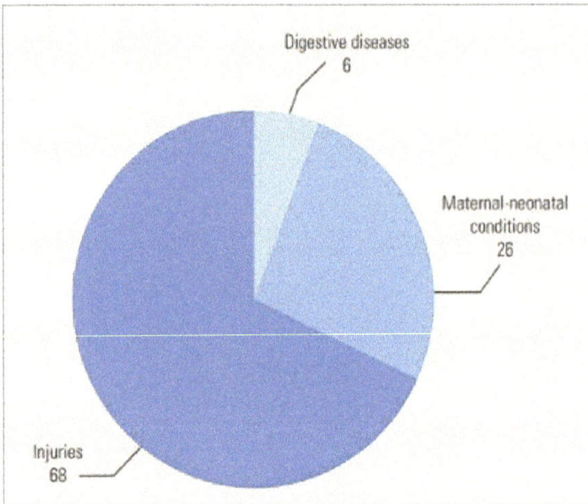

Figure 15. Percentage distribution of disability burden avertable by scaling up basic surgical care deliverable at first-level hospitals in LMICs. Note: Percentages based on a package treating gastrointestinal diseases, maternal-neonatal conditions, and injuries managed by simple interventions. From: Debas, H. T., P. Donkor, A. Gawande, D. T. Jamison, M. E. Kruk, and C. N. Mock, editors. 2015. *Essential Surgery. Disease Control Priorities*, third edition, volume 1. World Bank. doi:10.1596/978-1-4648-0346-8. License: Creative Commons Attribution CC BY 3.0 IGO.

Much essential trauma care is simple. The Essential Surgery Package includes:[5]

- **Airway**: manage appropriately
- **Breathing**: support until independent
- **Pneumothorax/haemothorax**: diagnose and treat promptly
- **Bleeding**: stop, whether internal or external
- **Shock**: recognise and treat; provide intravenous fluids
- **Brain injuries**: decompress space-occupying lesions as early as possible
- **Abdominal injuries**: identify and treat promptly
- **Extremity and spinal injuries**: immobilise and manage properly
- **Rehabilitation services**: provide to minimise long-term impairment
- **Medications**: supply for treatment and pain control

Readers from rich countries may be surprised by the simplicity of this list and assume all these things are available. They are not, or at least not quick enough for millions of people in LICs and the poorer parts of MICs. To die for lack of a chest drain when teams in rich countries squander plastic tubing every day is an outrage.

THE AMSTERDAM DECLARATION

In 2014, a consortium of surgical organisations and NGOs supporting global surgical aims met in Amsterdam. They represented diverse and authoritative organisations such as the College of Surgeons of East, Central and Southern Africa (COSECSA), the International Committee of the Red Cross (ICRC), the World Federation of Societies of Anaesthesiologists (WFSA), and the Association of Surgeons of Great Britain and Ireland (ASGBI).

In 2015, they issued the *Amsterdam Declaration on Essential Surgical Care*, listing 15 essential surgical conditions and the procedures necessary to address them (**Table 4**).[6] They solicited support from governments, the UN, WHO, World Bank, major donors, NGOs, and professional bodies to scale up surgery and deliver these procedures.

As you can see, this is not high-end stuff. These relatively simple, inexpensive operations are the ones that are the most powerful. It is within the gift of surgical teams in HICs to pass these skills on to emergency teams in countries where they are most needed.

USING BELLWETHER PROCEDURES

A bellwether is a tame, castrated ram that carries a bell around its neck and leads the flock. The term is also used metaphorically to mean "a reliable indicator of trends." The Bellwether Procedures in global surgery are caesarean section, emergency laparotomy and the treatment of open fracture.[7]

The Bellwether Procedures:

1. Caesarean section
2. Emergency laparotomy
3. Procedures for open fracture

Condition	Intervention
Obstructed labour	Caesarean section, symphysiotomy, assisted or manipulative delivery, repair of uterine perforation
Severe uterine bleeding	Evacuation of retained products of conception, B-Lynch suture, repair of uterine perforation
Surgical infections	Incision and drainage of abscess, fasciotomy, dental extraction, tympanotomy, bone drilling, arthrotomy
Severe wounds, including burns	Debridement, haemostasis, suturing, escharotomy, skin grafting
Severe head injury	Management of head injury, cranial burr holes, elevation of depressed skull fracture
Airway obstruction	Management of compromised airway, tracheostomy, cricothyroidotomy, removal of foreign body
Chest injury and infections	Intercostal drainage, thoracostomy
The acute abdomen	Emergency laparotomy including appendicectomy
Fractures and dislocations	Reduction of fractures and dislocations, casting and splinting, external fixation
Severe limb ischaemia, sepsis and injury	Amputations
Urinary outflow obstruction	Suprapubic catheterisation
Hernia	Hernia repair
Cataract	Cataract extraction and intraocular lens insertion
Club foot	Casting and splinting, tenotomy
Simple cleft lip	Cleft lip repair

Table 4. Amsterdam Declaration list of fifteen proposed surgical procedures. From: Botman et al., *World J. Surg.* 39 (2015): 1335–1340.

All are straightforward, acute, and high value in terms of reducing morbidity and mortality in LMICs. They are also a useful proxy marker, i.e. a bellwether of a facility's more general capability. Hospitals providing them are considered capable of delivering the full range of emergency procedures in the Essential Surgery Package. The systems in place to deliver these means those facilities are usually also able to manage a wide range of non-surgical conditions. Blood transfusion, for example, is necessary to provide safe surgery but also benefits medical patients. The Bellwether Procedures are therefore a marker of adequately functioning healthcare systems.

BELLWETHER MAPPING

The Lancet Commission on Global Surgery's access target is: "A minimum of 80% coverage of essential surgical and anaesthesia services per country by 2030." Progress is measured by "the proportion of the population who are within two hours of a facility providing the Bellwether Procedures."

A handful of countries have published data on this. In 2016, for example, 30% of Ghana's population could not reach a Bellwether-competent hospital within two hours.[8] This type of data is useful for strategic planning. The time to get to hospital depends not just on distance, but also on the affordability of transport. The two-hour target is a cost/distance analysis, and solutions range from building new hospitals to providing an ambulance service.

The Ghanaians used the information to identify five first-level (district) hospitals performing fewer than twelve of each Bellwether Procedure per year. They reasoned that strengthening these facilities would have the greatest effect on population-level spatial access to essential surgery within two hours.

Distance is not the only barrier; physical geography can also work against people. The Milne Bay Province of Papua New Guinea is an archipelago of islands with only one Bellwether-competent hospital. Staff there found that only 28% of patients who made it to hospital reached them within two hours.[9]

A 2021 study in Malaysia found the country had 49 Bellwether-competent hospitals and that 94% of the population lived within two hours of one. However, 1.8 million people in East Malaysia did not have timely access. Malaysia's Ministry of Health used this data to guide national surgical planning.[10]

However, countries with data are exceptions; most have not measured or reported two-hour spatial access to surgical care. In 2021, only 31 countries provided two-hour access data to World Bank researchers.[11] Millions of impoverished people still measure travel time to surgical hospitals in days, not hours.

EXPLORE FURTHER

1. World Health Organization. *Global Initiative for Emergency and Essential Surgical Care*. Accessed August 2025. https://www.who.int/initiatives/who-global-initiative-for-emergency-and-essential-surgical-care
2. World Health Organization. *Surgical Care at the District Hospital: The WHO Manual*. WHO, 2013. https://www.who.int/publications/i/item/9241545755
3. Debas, H. T., P. Donkor, A. Gawande, D. T. Jamison, M. E. Kruk, and C. N. Mock, editors. 2015. *Essential Surgery. Disease Control Priorities*, third edition, volume 1. World Bank. doi:10.1596/978-1-4648-0346-8. License: Creative Commons Attribution CC BY 3.0 IGO.

CHAPTER 7
MAJOR INITIATIVES IN GLOBAL SURGERY

FOR THE LAST FIFTY YEARS, people have been talking and writing about the plight of those without access to essential surgery. Yet despite Dr Halfdan Mahler's appeal to the global surgical community in 1980, his aspiration to train sufficient surgical teams gained little traction.

In 2005, the WHO Global Initiative for Emergency and Essential Surgical Care (GIEESC) brought together global surgical bodies, healthcare professionals, policymakers, and public health experts to improve collaboration, knowledge sharing, and explore solutions to unmet surgical need. However, activity remained small-scale, even individual, and sometimes inappropriate. Over the last decade, things have started to change, with a consensus building that something must be done and done *now*.

2015: THE YEAR GLOBAL SURGERY BECAME A THING

2015 marked a seismic shift in activity and awareness. Initiative followed initiative and surgical institutions and professional bodies in HICs began to debate and contribute. Global surgery had finally become a thing.

THE WORLD BANK'S *DCP3: ESSENTIAL SURGERY*

In 1993, the World Bank published *Disease Control Priorities in Developing Countries* (*DCP1*). *DCP1* systematically assessed the cost-effectiveness of disease interventions for LMICs to inform World Development Reports.[1]

The second edition of *Disease Control Priorities* (*DCP2*) appeared in 2006 and promoted interconnected platforms and packages, rather than standalone interventions. It highlighted surgery's role, estimating that 11% of the global disease burden was surgical.[2]

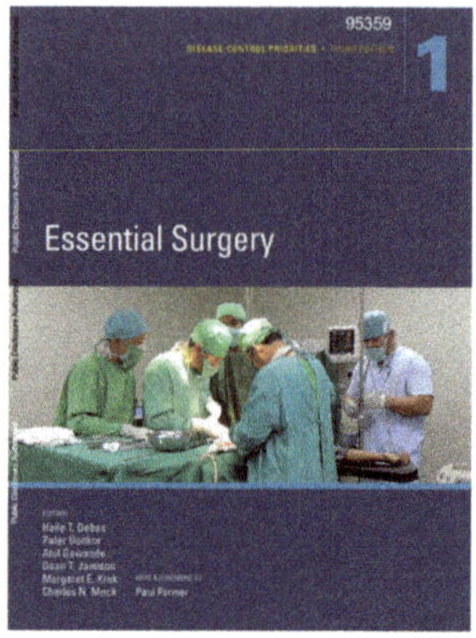

Figure 16. Cover of *Essential Surgery* (*Disease Control Priorities*, third edition).

Four key areas were defined:

1. Competent, immediate care of injury victims to reduce death and long-term disability.
2. Management of obstetric complications such as obstructed labour and haemorrhage.
3. Timely surgical management of various emergency and life-threatening conditions.
4. Elective care of easily treatable conditions such as hernia, clubfoot, and cataract.

In March 2015, the third edition of *Disease Control Priorities* (*DCP3*) introduced a separate volume on surgical conditions.

Essential Surgery defined the health burden of surgical disease, identified cost-effective and cost-beneficial procedures, and described policies and platforms for delivery. It explored financial protection against catastrophic out-of-pocket (OOP) spending and analysed access to surgery across income groups.

The book covers the whole range of surgical conditions and pathologies. It describes the fundamental importance of surgical care; the burden surgical conditions impose, and the cost-effective and cost-beneficial nature of surgical care.

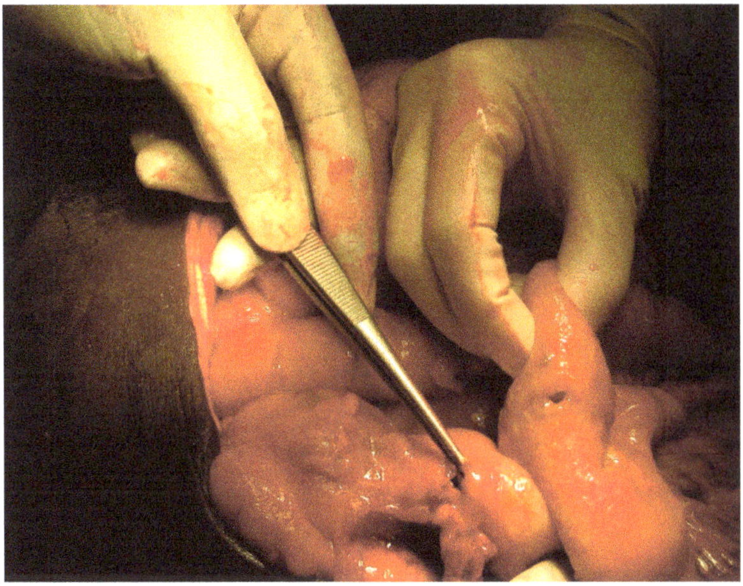

Figure 17. Terminal ileal perforations secondary to *S. Typhi* infection. Photo: author's own.

Essential Surgery challenges the myth that surgery is not feasible in impoverished communities. It cites successful programs in difficult settings, identifies key surgical conditions that cause a heavy health burden, and cost-effective, feasible procedures to manage them in LMICs (**Table 5**). The text's Essential Surgery Package lists 44 essential procedures that meet those criteria (chapter 6, page 52). Universal health coverage (UHC) that includes these procedures could prevent 1.5 million deaths per year — 6–7% of all preventable deaths in LMICs.[3]

Surgical conditions result in 401 million lost disability-adjusted life-years (DALYs) annually in LMICs, 116 million of which are avertable with the Essential Surgery Package.[4] This compares well with HIV/AIDS, TB and malaria, which together cause 214 million lost DALYs annually.

Twenty-eight of the procedures in the Essential Surgery Package can be delivered at district hospitals, and 23 are time-sensitive emergencies, which makes the surgically competent district hospital the key site for delivery of essential surgery. Caesarean section can be provided in hospitals with basic surgical facilities and 50–200 beds, serving 50,000 to 200,000 people.

Condition	Deaths (1000s)	DALYs (1000s)
Category 1. Communicable, maternal, perinatal, nutritional		
Maternal conditions	280	19,000
Birth asphyxia and birth trauma	780	78,000
Category 2. Noncommunicable diseases		
Cataracts	<1	7000
Peptic ulcer disease	230	7000
Appendicitis	38	2000
Skin diseases	90	16,000
Cleft lip and palate	5	<1,000
Oral conditions	<1	13,000
Category 3. Injuries		
Road traffic crash	1160	72,000
Other unintentional injuries	1550	96,000
Intentional injuries	540	34,000
Totals		
Burden from these conditions	470	340,000
Total burden from all causes	45,000	2,400,000
Share of burden due to those conditions addressable by essential surgery	10.4%	14.2%

Table 5. Total burden of conditions addressed by Essential Surgery in LMICs in 2011. Source: Debas, H. T., P. Donkor, A. Gawande, D. T. Jamison, M. E. Kruk, and C. N. Mock, editors. 2015. *Essential Surgery. Disease Control Priorities,* third edition, volume 1. World Bank. doi:10.1596/978-1-4648-0346-8. License: Creative Commons Attribution CC BY 3.0 IGO.

DCP3: Essential Surgery notes that task sharing (see chapter 11, page 111) has been widely demonstrated to be safe, and saves lives while countries make long-term investments in their surgical, anaesthetic, and obstetric (SAO) workforce.

Essential Surgery drills down into specific diseases and proposes

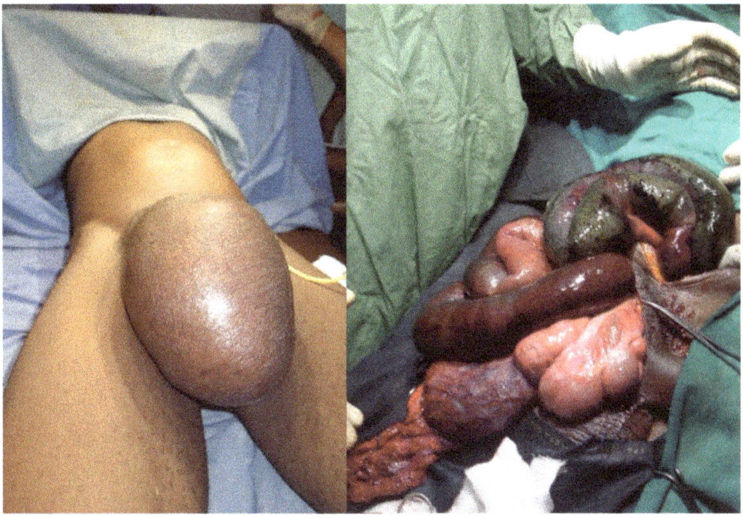

Figure 18. *DCP3: Essential Surgery* points out both the necessity of teaching bowel resection and anastomosis to save young men's lives in LMICs, and that this is not a complicated procedure for adequately trained surgeons. To be effective, the surgery needs to be provided close to the population. Photos: author's own.

management in low-resource settings for conditions ranging from congenital abnormalities to blindness and dentistry.

A clear understanding of what is killing people is needed, but defining surgical disease is not straightforward. Is a child dying of an ileal typhoid perforation the victim of a surgical or infectious disease?

Specific clinical direction is given. For example, limited access to surgery means hernias in LICs tend to be large, symptomatic, and frequently present with incarceration and strangulation, leading to high morbidity and a global mortality of 44,000 each year. For this reason, "wait and watch" is considered unsafe in LICs, and inguinal hernia repair is recognised as one of the most cost-effective of all health interventions.

APRIL 2015: THE AMSTERDAM DECLARATION

The Amsterdam Declaration on Essential Surgical Care, proposing a list of 15 essential surgical conditions and the procedures needed to treat them, was issued in April 2015 (chapter 6, page 47).[5]

APRIL 2015: THE LANCET COMMISSION ON GLOBAL SURGERY

At the initiation of surgeons, the Lancet Commission on Global Surgery (LCoGS) was launched in January 2014 and published Global Surgery *2030: Evidence and Solutions for Achieving Health, Welfare, and Economic Development* a year later.

The Commission systematically collected and reviewed published materials on the state of world surgery. Professors John G Meara (Harvard Medical School), Andy Leather (King's College, London), and Lars Hagander (Lund University) chaired the process. They worked with collaborators in 110 countries, including 22 commissioners representing professional societies, government agencies, NGOs, and academic institutions.

Experts in surgery, anaesthesia, obstetrics, oncology, healthcare policy, finance, economics, and research formed four working groups:

1. Healthcare delivery and management
2. Education and training
3. Economics
4. Information management

Structured expert opinion evaluated disease incidence data and estimated that 28–32% of the global burden of disease is surgical. Previous estimates had suggested that two billion people lacked access to surgery, but mathematical modelling revised this figure to 4.5–5.3 billion.

The Commission exposed profound inequalities; for example, 93% of the population in Sub-Saharan Africa and 97% in South Asia do not have access to safe, timely surgery. In contrast, only 3.6% in HICs lack access. Each year, 33 million people face catastrophic expenditure paying for surgery, and 48 million more incur catastrophic costs through non-medical expenses associated with accessing it.

Framework for action

Global Surgery 2030 evidences the key clinical, educational, financial, managerial, and political challenges, and the needs of global surgical delivery. It also proposed a framework for achieving universal access by developing National Surgical, Obstetric and Anaesthesia Plans (NSOAPs). NSOAPs are country-specific strategic plans that define infrastructure, workforce, service delivery, finance, and data collection priorities (see chapter 14, page 135).

Global Surgery: 2030 makes the moral and economic case for scaling up surgery. At the North American launch in Boston in May 2015, panels of experts met to discuss the way forward and produce a roadmap for HIC actors. Published in 2016, this called for the rich to abandon colonial narratives and instead work in partnership with teams in LMICs.[6]

LCoGS INDICATORS AND TARGETS

The Commission set ambitious 15-year targets for expanding and financing essential surgery. Six progress indicators were defined and targets set against them (**Table 6**). Ministries of Health are responsible for delivering the targets related to preparedness; Ministries of Health and hospitals are responsible for the delivery targets; the World Health Organization (WHO), World Bank, and USAID are responsible for the financial targets.

The Commission recommends seven basic surgical care packages, giving highest priority to the emergency package delivered at district hospitals (**Table 7**).

Global Surgery 2030: Key Messages

- 5 billion people cannot access safe surgical care.
- 313 million operations are done annually, but only 6% occur in the poorest countries, where one in three of the world's population lives.
- To prevent premature death and disability, 143 million more operations are required annually.
- 33 million people face catastrophic expenditure paying for surgery and anaesthesia each year.
- Investment in surgical and anaesthesia services is affordable, saves lives, and promotes economic growth.
- To be effective, district hospitals are the principal sites of delivery of essential surgery.
- Surgery is an indivisible, indispensable part of healthcare.

The publication of *Global Surgery: 2030* generated enormous publicity and interest amongst surgical teams and health economists internationally. Its key messages, illustrations and tables have been cited and

Indicator	Definition	Target
Preparedness for Surgical and Anaesthetic Care		
Access to Timely Essential Surgery	Proportion of the population that can access, within 2 h, a facility that can do the the Bellwether Procedures: caesarean delivery, laparotomy, and treatment of open fracture	A minimum of 80% coverage of essential surgical and anaesthesia services per country by 2030
Specialist Surgical Workforce Density	Number of specialist surgical, anaesthetic, and obstetric physicians working per 100,000 population	100% of countries with at least 20 surgical, anaesthetic, and obstetric physicians per 100,000 population by 2030
Delivery Of Surgical and Anaesthetic Care		
Surgical Volume	Procedures done in operating theatre per 100,000 population per year	80% of countries by 2020 and 100% of countries by 2030 tracking surgical volume; a minimum of 5000 procedures per 100,000 population by 2030
Perioperative Mortality	All-cause death rate before discharge patients who have undergone a procedure in an operating theatre, divided by the total number of procedures, presented as a percentage	80% of countries by 2020 and 100% of countries by 2030 tracking perioperative mortality; in 2020, assess global data and set national targets for 2030

Table 6. The LCoGS targets and indicators. OOP, out-of-pocket. *[Table continues on next page.]*

reproduced in thousands of publications and presentations. It also stimulated debate and a proliferation in global surgery research and documentation and helped clarify issues around missions from HICs.

Indicator	Definition	Target
Affordability Of Surgical and Anaesthesia Care		
Protection Against Impoverishing Expenditure	Proportion of households protected against impoverishment from direct OOP payments for surgical and anaesthesia care	100% protection against impoverishment from OOP payments for surgical and anaesthesia care by 2030
Protection Against Catastrophic Expenditure	Proportion of households protected against catastrophic expenditure from direct OOP payments for surgical and anaesthesia care	100% protection against catastrophic expenditure from OOP payments for surgical and anaesthesia care by 2030

Table 6. (cont.)

NSOAPs can provide both a framework for practical action and a jumping-off point for international agreements.

So, what's happened since 2015?

None of the LCoGS targets will be met by 2030. We are already ten years into the fifteen-year plan, and very few countries even measure the key indicators. However, there has been a change in attitude, with widespread recognition amongst policymakers and surgical professional bodies that the status quo is not acceptable.

It is also now well recognised that some approaches from previous decades, such as short-term missions, were not only unproductive — by failing to strengthen health systems — but at times even counterproductive. Arising from this, there is consensus that actors from HICs must work in equal partnership with teams in LMICs, placing surgical care within a broader strengthening of healthcare systems.

Most surgeons and anaesthetists in HICs are now aware of global surgery and professional bodies are beginning to develop collective responsibility for the problems, with some developing bilateral relationships to help solve them. Amongst surgical providers in HICs, there is a shift from the "glory" of high-volume, short-term trips to long-term commitment and enduring relationships with colleagues abroad.

Package Type	Package Name	Included Procedures
Emergency	Basic Trauma Surgery	Open and closed fracture care, chest tube placement, amputation, trauma laparotomy, burr hole, wound care, and debridement
	Basic Emergency Obstetric	Caesarean section, hysterectomy, salpingectomy, dilation and curettage (evacuation of retained products)
	Basic Emergency General Surgical	Laparotomy, appendicectomy, hernia repair (+ bowel resection), incision and drainage of soft tissue infection
Planned (Elective)	General Surgery	Hernia repair, hydrocoelectomy, cholecystectomy, ureteric or kidney stone removal, prostatectomy, thyroidectomy (in goitre endemic regions), excisional biopsy, lumpectomy or mastectomy, resection of early-stage oral tumours, and bowel resection
	Obstetric and Gynaecological	Treatment of cervical precancer and hysterectomy for cervical cancer
	Specialist Surgical	Cataract surgery, trachoma surgery (where endemic), cleft palate and lip repair, clubfoot correction, surgical repair of congenital heart anomalies, and obstetric fistula repair
	Palliative Care Surgical	Mastectomy, diversion colostomy, and appropriate analgesia

Table 7. The LCoGS seven basic care packages.

THE NEXT DECADE MUST BE DIFFERENT

Surgical Health Policy 2025-35: Strengthening Essential Services for Tomorrow's Needs has just been published.[7] It assesses progress towards the LCoGS aims, reviewing publications from the past decade, including new, as yet unpublished, information. It finds persistent, fundamental gaps in surgical workforce, volume and financial protection, with most countries off track to meet all of the LCoGS targets.

Unmet surgical need is estimated to have risen to 160 million procedures per year, as provision has not kept pace with population change. Care quality is also lacking, with an estimated 3.5 million post-operative deaths per year, exceeding those from HIV, malaria, and TB combined.

As economic instability and armed conflicts risk pushing global surgery down the international agenda, this review updates and reinforces the economic argument for embedding surgery in health systems and reframing surgery as essential to save lives and improve economic productivity. It emphasises the importance of reliable data and accountability, and preserving nascent data infrastructure in the face of uncertain global health funding.

MAY 2015: THE WORLD HEALTH ASSEMBLY RESOLUTION WHA 68.15 — "STRENGTHENING EMERGENCY AND ESSENTIAL SURGICAL CARE AND ANAESTHESIA AS A COMPONENT OF UNIVERSAL HEALTH COVERAGE"

The World Health Assembly (WHA) is the highest decision-making body of WHO, comprising the ministers of health of UN member states. It meets annually to approve WHO's budget, adopt resolutions on health priorities, and set policies for WHO's work. WHA resolutions are not binding on member states but exert influence over governments and donors and give WHO a mandate for directing resources to specific health problems.

> Surgical care must receive funding commensurate with the burden. Policy changes and financing are required, starting with recognition that surgical care is affordable, promotes economic success, and is a fundamental part of universal healthcare.

In May 2015, the WHA adopted resolution WHA68.15, "Strengthening emergency and essential surgical care and anaesthesia as a component of universal health coverage." This was the first time governments recognised surgery and anaesthesia as key components of UHC. High-level political commitments were made to address the public health gaps arising from lack of safe, affordable, accessible surgical and anaesthetic services.[8]

Professor Emmanuel Makasa, an orthopaedic surgeon and health attaché for Zambia, convinced his government to propose the resolution. Many countries, including the United Kingdom, then co-sponsored the resolution.

WHA 68.15 Resolution Recognises:

- Surgery and anaesthesia are neglected.
- Surgical conditions account for 11% of global disease burden, mostly affecting LMICs.
- Maternal and child mortality gaps and the Millennium Development Goals (MDGs) cannot be addressed without surgical expansion and inclusion of essential surgery in UHC and improving humanitarian response and preparedness.

It Encourages Governments to:

- Scale up surgery near populations.
- Identify and prioritise a core set of emergency and essential surgery and anaesthesia services (EESC) at local level.
- Ensure ministries of health lead EESC promotion.
- Implement reliable supply chains for essential drugs, equipment, supplies, and infrastructure.
- Enforce antibiotic stewardship and strengthen infection prevention and control for safe surgery.

It Agrees:

- Scaling up surgery is cost-effective.
- Financing is needed for access and affordability.
- Task sharing is one solution for workforce shortages.

It Stresses:

- Policy, professional standards, and core competencies.
- Strategies for surgical team training, and ongoing education.
- Policy and workforce standards.
- Mandatory monitoring and evaluation of capacity, volume, and safety data.

WHO committed to supporting these efforts through global partnership and collaboration. It aimed to raise awareness of the cost-effectiveness of upscaling surgery, and disseminate expertise to support measurement, benchmarking, data collection and reporting.

With the help of partners, governments would analyse current national surgical care and use the findings to develop NSOAPs integrated into national health policy. The aim was to strengthen essential surgical care as part of UHC by member states working with international partners to mobilise adequate resources. All surgical providers were expected to actively participate.

In 2015, 194 member states adopted the resolution. In 2017, the WHO and Harvard Medical School published *Surgical Care Systems Strengthening*, supporting the NSOAP process (see chapter 14, page 136).[9]

In 2023, WHA 76.2, "Integrated emergency, critical and operative care for universal health coverage (UHC) and protection from health emergencies," reinforced the objectives of WHA 68.15 and stated that "emergency, critical and operative care services are an integral part of a comprehensive primary healthcare approach."[10]

The Dakar Declaration further reaffirms the ambitions of the 28 signatory African countries to up-scaling surgery.[11]

SEPTEMBER 2015: 2030 SUSTAINABLE DEVELOPMENT GOALS

The 17 Sustainable Development Goals (SDGs) of the 2030 Agenda for Sustainable Development were adopted in September 2015 at the UN Summit.[12] The goals came into force on 1 January 2016.

UN development goals encourage collective action to address global challenges such as poverty, inequality, climate change and environmental degradation. All UN member states are expected to work towards the shared goals, which are designed to promote cooperation and partnership.

To understand the SDGs, we first need to go back to 2000 and review their predecessors, the eight MDGs.[i]

---

i Millenium Development Goals: https://www.un.org/millenniumgoals/

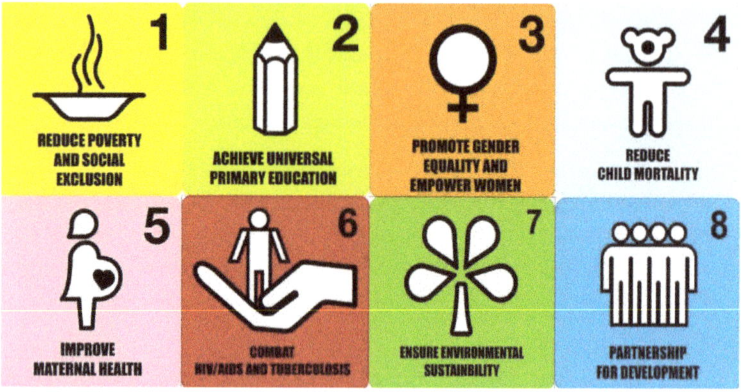
1
REDUCE POVERTY AND SOCIAL EXCLUSION
2
ACHIEVE UNIVERSAL PRIMARY EDUCATION
3
PROMOTE GENDER EQUALITY AND EMPOWER WOMEN
4
REDUCE CHILD MORTALITY
5
IMPROVE MATERNAL HEALTH
6
COMBAT HIV/AIDS AND TUBERCULOSIS
7
ENSURE ENVIRONMENTAL SUSTAINBILITY
8
PARTNERSHIP FOR DEVELOPMENT

Figure 19. The Millennium Development Goals.

The UN Millennium Development Goals (MDGs)

MDG 4, "Reduce child mortality," and MDG 5, "Improve maternal health," were directly relevant to surgery. Other goals, such as the fight against extreme poverty, had a huge bearing on the ability of people to access safe surgery.

Specifically, the goals were to reduce the under-five mortality rate by two-thirds, the maternal mortality ratio (MMR) by 75%, and achieve universal access to reproductive health by 2015 (**Figure 19**).

If the MDGs had been met in 2015, universal access to essential surgery would have been implemented and this little book would be unnecessary. However, they were not met and were also criticised in several aspects.

Some goals lacked legitimacy because the countries they were designed to assist were not properly represented when they were drafted. Measurement processes were lacking, and definitions and baselines unclear. It was also suggested that the wording of some documents made progress appear better than it was, and goals did not focus sufficiently on economic and development disparities within countries. In 2010, new plans were adopted, keeping the 2015 target, but with fresh initiatives and commitments on maternal and child health.

Despite the criticisms, the MDGs had positive effects. They acknowledged and focused attention on major issues and stimulated efforts to help the world's poorest people.[13] There was progress, in the provision of safe water and the fight against HIV/AIDS. Extreme poverty was halved. Many wealthy nations fulfilled their pledge to contribute 0.7% of GDP, although some later reneged on their promise.

Between 1990 and 2013, the world's under-five mortality fell 49%, to 46 deaths per 1000 live births. In 2013, 6.3 million children still died before their fifth birthday, but this was significant progress compared to 12.7 million in 1990.

Over the same period, maternal deaths fell from 523,000 to 289,000 worldwide.[14] Progress was patchy, with some countries such as Benin failing to meet any of the targets. Nevertheless, the overall trend was positive and showed what can be achieved when the will and funding is present.

By 2017, UN estimates indicated that under-five mortality had fallen further to 43 per 1,000 live births. Globally, MMR reached 211 per 100,000; an average annual reduction of 2.9% since 2000. Despite this, maternal mortality remained the leading cause of death for girls aged 15 to 19.[15]

Death from noncommunicable diseases fell marginally, however this group contains major non-surgical disease groups, so the impact of surgery is difficult to assess. Road traffic deaths remain three times higher in LMICs than HICs, despite there being less vehicles per capita. Wealthier countries reduced traffic deaths by introducing regulation and improving infrastructure and surgical care.[16]

The UN 2030 Agenda for Sustainable Development

In September 2015, 193 UN member states adopted the *2030 Agenda for Sustainable Development*, aiming to end extreme poverty and ensure wellbeing for all.[17] This renewed global strategy set out 17 SDGs to be achieved by 2030, building on the partial success of the MDGs. World leaders promised to secure the rights and wellbeing of everyone on a healthy, thriving planet.

The SDGs are wider ranging than the earlier MDGs and include climate and environmental issues, as well as more specific targets and measurements, enabling much clearer tracking of global progress. The strategy is also different, focusing on systems and partnerships to strengthen health systems by building local capacity.

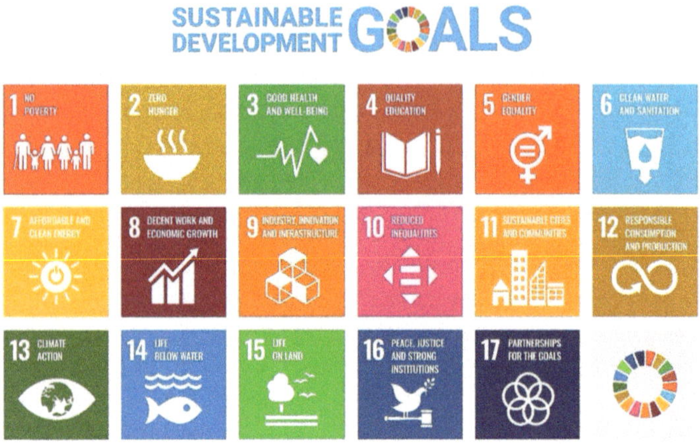
SUSTAINABLE DEVELOPMENT GOALS
1 NO POVERTY
2 ZERO HUNGER
3 GOOD HEALTH AND WELL-BEING
4 QUALITY EDUCATION
5 GENDER EQUALITY
6 CLEAN WATER AND SANITATION
8 DECENT WORK AND ECONOMIC GROWTH
9 INDUSTRY, INNOVATION AND INFRASTRUCTURE
10 REDUCED INEQUALITIES
12 RESPONSIBLE CONSUMPTION AND PRODUCTION
13 CLIMATE ACTION
14 LIFE BELOW WATER
15 LIFE ON LAND
16 PEACE, JUSTICE AND STRONG INSTITUTIONS
17 PARTNERSHIPS FOR THE GOALS

Figure 20. The 17 UN Sustainable Development Goals.

SDG 3: Ensure healthy lives and promote well-being for all at all ages

SDG 3 has sweeping aims with 13 health targets and 28 progress indicators, nine of which are outcome targets (**Figure 20**).

Key surgery-related targets are:

- Reduce MMR to ≤ 70 per 100,000
- End preventable deaths in children under five and reduce under-five mortality ≤ 25 per 1,000 live births
- Lower mortality from noncommunicable diseases
- Halve global deaths from road traffic accidents
- Achieve UHC, including financial protection for essential care

There are also targets focused on the "means to achieving," which include increasing health financing and supporting workforce development.

WHERE ARE WE NOW?

The UN SDGs Report 2024 makes depressing reading.[18] The world is "severely off track" to realise the 2030 targets. Of targets for which we have sufficient data, 17% are on track to be achieved, 48% are moderately or severely off the trajectory, 18% show stagnation, and 17% have regressed below the 2015 levels.

The report also comments on how the COVID-19 pandemic reversed a decade of improvements in life expectancy. Most health indicators are now improving again, but slowly. We are a long way from achieving UHC — minimal progress was achieved between 2015 and the pandemic, leaving 4.5 billion people without coverage in 2021, but financial hardship from OOP health spending has worsened since 2015. Without ensuring UHC, there can be no universal access to essential surgery.

Globally, between 2000 and 2017, the number of women dying from reproductive complications fell by 38%, with Sub-Saharan Africa and Southeast Asia seeing the greatest improvement. The rapid gains in MMR running up to 2017 have largely stalled, falling from 227 per 100,000 live births in 2015 to 223 in 2020, three times the 2030 target. Conflict is to blame in some countries with the MMR in fragile states twice the global average. Under-5 deaths reached an historic low in 2022, but progress here has also slowed.

EXPLORE FURTHER

1. Debas, H. T., P. Donkor, A. Gawande, D. T. Jamison, M. E. Kruk, and C. N. Mock, editors. 2015. *Essential Surgery. Disease Control Priorities*, third edition, volume 1. World Bank. doi:10.1596/978-1-4648-0346-8. License: Creative Commons Attribution CC BY 3.0 IGO.
2. Meara, John G., Andrew J. M. Leather, Lars Hagander et al. "Global Surgery 2030: Evidence and Solutions for Achieving Health, Welfare, and Economic Development." *The Lancet* 386, no. 9993 (2015): 569–624. https://doi.org/10.1016/S0140-6736(15)60160-X.
3. Ng-Kamstra, Joshua S., Sarah L. M. Greenberg, Fizan Abdullah et al. "Global Surgery 2030: A Roadmap for High-Income Country Actors." *BMJ Global Health* 1, no. 1 (2016): e000011. https://doi.org/10.1136/bmjgh-2015-000011.
4. United Nations Development Programme. Sustainable Development Goals. Accessed August 21, 2025. https://www.undp.org/sustainable-development-goals.

5. United Nations General Assembly. Resolution 70/1, "Transforming Our World: The 2030 Agenda for Sustainable Development." Adopted September 25, 2015. A/RES/70/1. https://sdgs.un.org/2030agenda.

CHAPTER 8
QUALITY MATTERS

INCREASING access to surgery in LMICs will only save lives and be cost-effective if the procedures are done competently.

LANCET COMMISSION QUALITY INDICATORS

The Lancet Commission on Global Surgery (LCoGS) recommends tracking perioperative mortality, and two of its other indicators are also interesting to consider in relation to quality.

ACCESS TO TIMELY ESSENTIAL SURGERY

This is considered a preparedness indicator, although all surgical teams know it is also a key quality indicator. Few governments worldwide have reliable data on access. Many surgical teams and NGOs prefer to work in cities, whereas to be effective, emergency surgery needs to be delivered in the districts close to the population. Countries that have positively targeted poor communities, such as Nepal, have seen huge strides in maternal mortality rate (MMR) and other quality indicators.

SURGICAL VOLUME

Increasing surgical volume is automatically considered evidence of improvement, however, this is only true when surgical care is *competently* delivered. In some countries, people are permitted to operate and give anaesthesia if they have MBChB, even if they have never had a single day's surgical or anaesthetic training. This illustrates the disconnect between HIC perspectives and realities on the ground.

Perioperative mortality

The LCoGS's quality measure is perioperative mortality, specifically the: "all-cause death rate before discharge after a procedure in an operating theatre, divided by the total number of procedures, presented as a percentage."[1] The target was for 80% of countries to track this by 2020 and 100% by 2030, and for the 2020 results to allow targets to be set for 2030.

Little is known about the indications for, and the quality, safety and outcomes of, surgical care in LMICs. What about the situation closer to home? Do we know mortality rates in HICs?

The difficulty in assessing this is basic: what is the denominator? In Britain, this varies from 1.5 to 7.9 million procedures per year, depending on what is counted. Similarly, deaths around the time of surgery can be extracted, but it is not easy to say whether these were procedure-related or simply temporally related. Does somebody dying within three months of an ascitic tap for malignancy represent a post-procedural death?

Using the British United Provident Association (BUPA) classification,[i] 2.8 million intermediate and 1.8 million major procedures were performed annually in Great Britain in the five years up to 2014.[2] The mean 30-, 60-, and 90-day post-procedure mortality was 1.1%, 1.8% and 2.3%, respectively. Even with the sophisticated data monitoring systems used in the UK, understanding postoperative mortality is not easy, so it is unsurprising that LMICs struggle.

The UK National Emergency Laparotomy Audit (NELA) forced better data collection.[3] Risk-adjusted 30-day mortality is high, with variation between the poorest and best performing quintiles (11.4% vs. 6.6%), despite equivalent predicted mortality. Projects like NELA show the value of monitoring for quality improvement, as they allow resources to be directed to the areas most needed.

Where LICs and lower MICs have been able to report mortality, this has been much higher than in HICs. Compared to Sweden, for example, death after caesarean section is two to four times higher in Latin America, six to ten times higher in South Asia, and a hundred times higher in Sub-Saharan Africa.[4] Similarly, mortality after appendicectomy and inguinal hernia repair are forty times higher in Sub-Saharan Africa.

---

i "Code search," BUPA, https://codes.bupa.co.uk/home (accessed September 29, 2025).

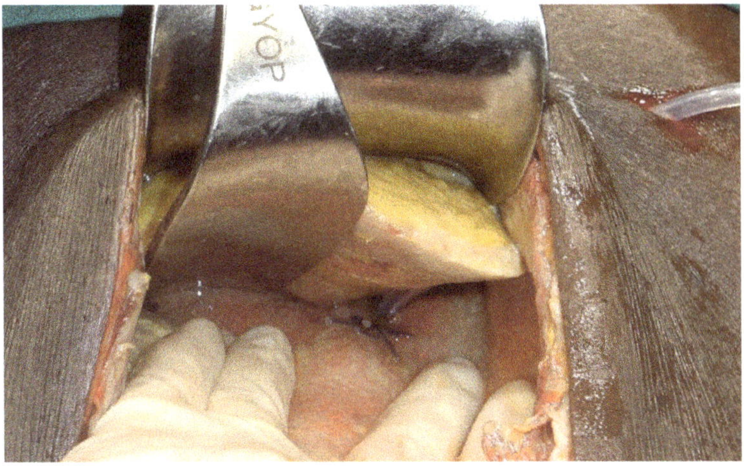

Figure 21. Poor healing may occur in acutely malnourished patients presenting days after perforation of a peptic ulcer. Here, the omental patch repair failed, necessitating a controlled fistula and distal enteral feeding. Photo: author's own.

Understanding risk

High mortality may reflect poor care or inadequate resources. But case mix will also make a substantial difference. The rate of surgery was recently reported as twenty-eight times higher in the UK than Sierra Leone. In 2014, the surgical volume in the UK was estimated at 10,487 procedures per 100,000 people, compared with 372 per 100,000 in Sierra Leone in 2017.[5,6] The more surgery you do, the more will be elective. When a country's surgical volume is extremely low, a significant proportion of the cases will be life-threatening emergencies.

The mitigating factors for mortality vary across different health economies. In HICs, risk is very dependent on age, co-morbidity and ASA grade,[ii] whereas teams in LICs predominantly operate on young patients without co-morbidity but often presenting late against a background of poverty and malnutrition.

African authors report mortality from ileal typhoid perforation according to the number of days between the perforation and the operation, with mortality far higher among those presenting late.[7] Deaths

[ii] The American Society of Anesthesiologists (ASA) Physical Status Classification system assesses a patient's preoperative health, ranging from ASA 1 (healthy patient) to ASA 5 (moribund patient not expected to survive without the operation). Emergency cases are denoted with "E" (e.g. ASA 3E).

depend on what is happening outside the hospital as well as the quality of care within it.

These factors mean surgical teams may be unfairly criticised. It can also lead to a systemic acceptance of death and failure of learning, such as when deaths are categorised as "expected," even though they could have been prevented with different management.

In HICs, risk scoring systems such as the NELA score and the Portsmouth Physiological and Operative Severity Score for the enUmeration of Mortality and Morbidity (P-POSSUM) are commonly used for high-risk surgical interventions. Both have also been used in LMICs. However, while they tend to overestimate risk in the UK, Egyptian investigators found they u*nderestimated* risk among their patients. Scores were designed and validated in HICs, addressing the risks prevalent in those environments.

Key factors influencing perioperative mortality:

HIC	LIC
Age	Late presentation
ASA grade	Poverty / malnutrition
Co-morbidity	Lack of monitoring
	Delays in care

We need risk scores tailored to the distinct challenges in LMICs, enabling teams to accurately assess and compare their performance with peers facing similar constraints.

ANAESTHESIA

Safe anaesthesia is discussed in chapter 9 (see page 87).

WHO PATIENT SAFETY PROGRAM

Perioperative safety and avoidance of needless complications and death is a major global public health issue.[8] In 2012, 313 million operations were performed worldwide, following which one million people died and seven million developed significant complications. HICs report 0.4–0.8% perioperative mortality and major complications occurring after 3–22% of inpatient operations. Half of all adverse events in HICs are preventable.

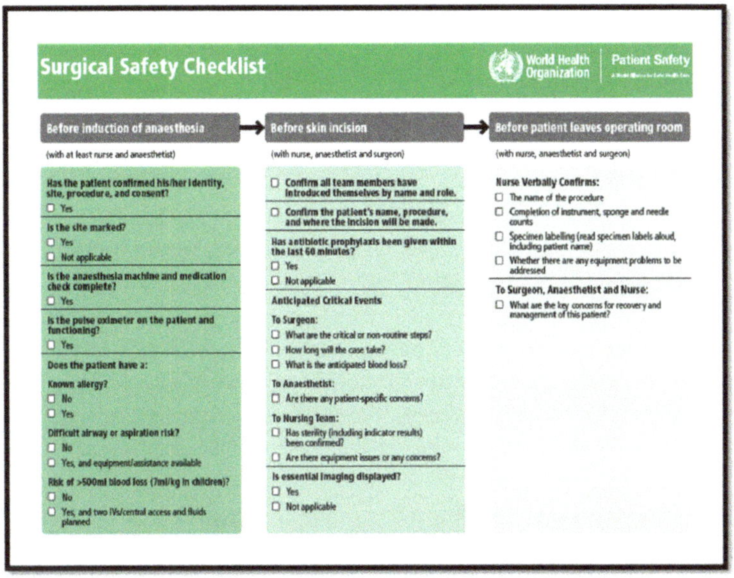
Surgical Safety Checklist

World Health Organization | Patient Safety

Before induction of anaesthesia
(with at least nurse and anaesthetist)

Has the patient confirmed his/her identity, site, procedure, and consent?
☐ Yes

Is the site marked?
☐ Yes
☐ Not applicable

Is the anaesthesia machine and medication check complete?
☐ Yes

Is the pulse oximeter on the patient and functioning?
☐ Yes

Does the patient have a:

Known allergy?
☐ No
☐ Yes

Difficult airway or aspiration risk?
☐ No
☐ Yes, and equipment/assistance available

Risk of >500ml blood loss (7ml/kg in children)?
☐ No
☐ Yes, and two IVs/central access and fluids planned

Before skin incision
(with nurse, anaesthetist and surgeon)

☐ Confirm all team members have introduced themselves by name and role.

☐ Confirm the patient's name, procedure, and where the incision will be made.

Has antibiotic prophylaxis been given within the last 60 minutes?
☐ Yes
☐ Not applicable

Anticipated Critical Events

To Surgeon:
☐ What are the critical or non-routine steps?
☐ How long will the case take?
☐ What is the anticipated blood loss?

To Anaesthetist:
☐ Are there any patient-specific concerns?

To Nursing Team:
☐ Has sterility (including indicator results) been confirmed?
☐ Are there equipment issues or any concerns?

Is essential imaging displayed?
☐ Yes
☐ Not applicable

Before patient leaves operating room
(with nurse, anaesthetist and surgeon)

Nurse Verbally Confirms:
☐ The name of the procedure
☐ Completion of instrument, sponge and needle counts
☐ Specimen labelling (read specimen labels aloud, including patient name)
☐ Whether there are any equipment problems to be addressed

To Surgeon, Anaesthetist and Nurse:
☐ What are the key concerns for recovery and management of this patient?

Figure 22. WHO Safe Surgery Checklist. Available from: https://www.who.int/teams/integrated-health-services/patient-safety/research/safe-surgery/tool-and-resources.

The limited data available on perioperative safety suggests things are worse in LMICs.

A few critical safety checks minimise common and avoidable risks during surgery and anaesthesia. The WHO Safe Surgery Checklist (**Figure 22**) is used routinely in HICs. Randomised controlled trials show it is simple, ultra-low-cost, and associated with a reduction in major complications from 11% to 7% and a reduction in mortality after major surgery from 1.5% to 0.8%.[9]

Checklist use not only prevents complications from the "misses" the checklist identifies but, when implemented with full engagement, also fosters a safety culture that encourages consistent general procedural compliance. This improves theatre safety, teamwork, and communication, all of which positively impact patient outcomes.

CHALLENGES

WHO identifies four key safety challenges:[10]

1. **Acknowledging the issue:** Measures to improve the safety and reliability of existing surgical provision have not received much attention.
2. **Lack of basic data**: International surveillance systems in obstetrics are in place, but most surgical disciplines lack robust outcomes monitoring.
3. **Safety practice failures:** Widespread failure to use existing safety practices most effectively (e.g. perioperative antibiotics are used liberally, but administration is not always timed for the skin incision).
4. **Failure of operating department teams to fully use their knowledge and abilities on behalf of the patient:** Surgery and perioperative care present multiple opportunities for error and omission. For example, checking of swabs is careless or not done at all in some LMIC hospitals. Effective teamwork can avert a considerable proportion of life-threatening complications, necessitating culture change rather than increased resources.

FAILURE TO ENGAGE WITH SAFE SURGERY IN LMICS

LICs have more to gain from implementing the WHO Safe Surgery Checklist than HICs, in terms of greater reductions in complication rates and perioperative mortality. Yet, despite the evidence, many facilities in LMICs have not engaged with the program, even though it is an easy win requiring minimal resources.[11]

BARRIERS TO IMPLEMENTING SAFE SURGERY

Widespread awareness of the value of the checklist and Non-Technical Skills for Surgeons (NOTSS) makes them popular for international teams to teach. Some countries, such as Mozambique, have embraced Safe Surgery and managed to sustain good practice.[iii] However, in other places, as soon as visiting teams depart, these straightforward ways to save lives are dropped, or performed in such a tokenistic way as to be useless or even detrimental.

Understanding why efforts pay off in some places and not in others can

[iii] By "Safe Surgery," we mean adoption of the WHO Surgical Safety Checklist, its associated safety standards and equipment requirements.

provide insight on how to improve implementation. Qualitative studies have suggested that the most important barrier to implementation is often a single dominant, negative individual. Hierarchical relationships are a major barrier to implementation in all settings, and these are typically more pronounced in LICs, where entrenched hierarchies are quite common and can make workplace relationships more difficult. It is just not considered appropriate to check whether a more senior person has done their job correctly.

During introduction of the WHO Checklist in the UK, a few people felt it was a waste of their valuable time. However, in the UK, no matter how important individual clinicians think they are, they rarely have the power to *totally* block evidence-based change. In some LMIC institutions, on the other hand, "the boss is the boss" and can block change no matter how strong the case for improvement.

Quality governance structures may be absent, or draconian punishment for human error may be a problem. Qualitative studies indicate that health workers in LMICs have great concerns about reporting errors and near misses. If governance systems and powerful individuals do not accept that human error is normal, then openness and safety practices do not afford protection.

People fear speaking out, or are simply ignored, so that those lower down the hierarchy cannot implement change even when they have the evidence behind them. Workers report that they feel it might be better to make misleading records than admit mistakes. Meaningful introduction of the WHO Checklist requires governance structures and good leadership and struggles to succeed where either are lacking.[12]

District hospitals and practice variation

As part of the FALCON trial (reducing surgical site infections [SSIs] in LMICs) and the ChEETAh trial (glove and instrument changes before abdominal wall closure), a report on 15,000 patients in 80 hospitals across six countries examined compliance with the WHO Checklist.[13]

> In countries with immature surgical systems, failure to adhere to the WHO Safe Surgery Checklist means easily avoidable errors can, will and do happen.

Unsurprisingly, they found that district hospitals had fewer full-time surgeons and medically trained anaesthetists and higher rates of emergency surgery than referral centres. But, district hospitals demonstrated significantly higher use of the WHO Checklist than referral hospitals and showed no difference in mortality or SSIs despite their higher rates of emergency surgery. This may be because people treated each other better in the smaller hospitals, enabling them to implement safety change more readily than institutions dominated by powerful individuals.[14]

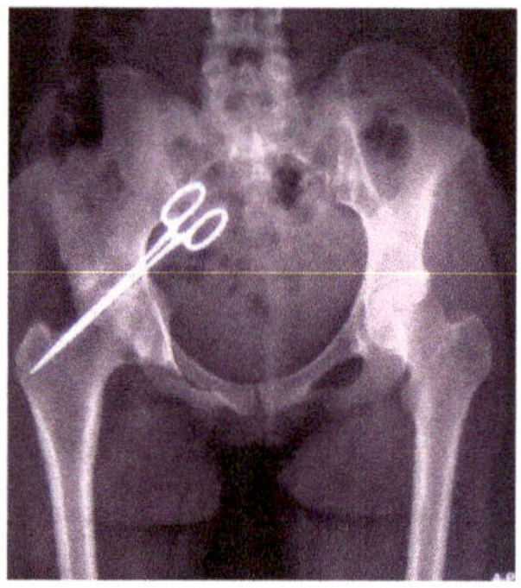

Figure 23. This patient presented with abdominal pain and an unhealed abscess on her thigh. The tip of a retained artery forceps had pierced the obturator foramen. Photo: author's own.

Equipment shortages

Shortage of materials can also be a barrier to improving perioperative safety. Attempts to ensure global use of the WHO Checklist threw light on the widespread lack of safety equipment and helped focus resources and donations to correct this. Anaesthetic teams in much of Sub-Saharan Africa simply could not comply with Safe Surgery as they had no pulse oximeters.

This led to the Patient Safety Pulse Oximetry project. WHO Patient Safety worked with the Harvard School of Public Health, the World Federation of Societies of Anaesthesiologists (WFSA), the Association of Anaesthetists of Great Britain and Ireland[iv] and other partners to develop high-quality, low-cost devices. Donations of these to the sites most in need were paired with a training bundle that included a toolkit for managing hypoxaemia.[15]

This demonstrates where the value of the WHO Checklist exceeds simply "checking things off a list." The list helped teams appreciate the critical importance of vigilance, which in turn focused attention on the essential role of oximeters in operating theatres, setting in motion a virtuous circle where improvements in monitoring led to further adoption of safety practices and ongoing quality gains.

The fact that this project included small bits of kit may have helped its uptake. In some settings the very simplicity of the WHO Checklist can work against its adoption. To some, it appears too simple to work and people may prefer higher tech solutions to their problems. For this reason,

[iv] Now known as the Association of Anaesthetists

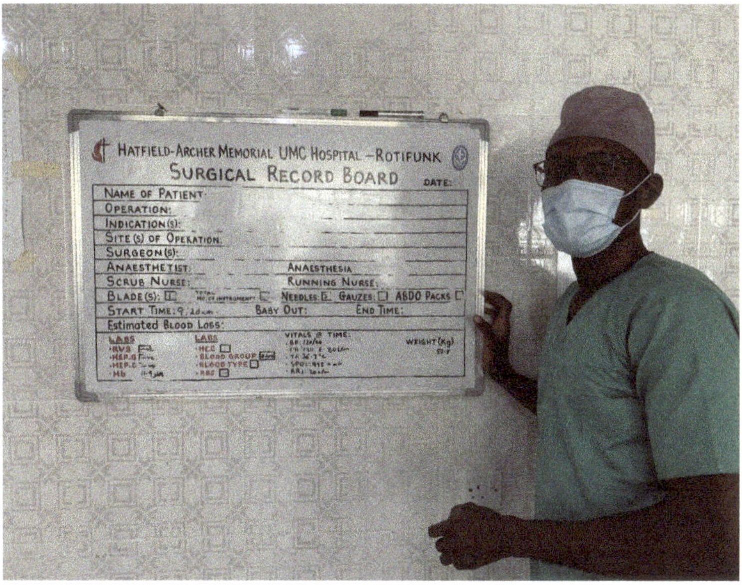

Figure 24. Several years ago, Surgical Officer Mohamed Mousa Tommy introduced the WHO Safe Surgery Checklist and counting of all operative materials at his small rural hospital in Sierra Leone. Many large Sierra Leonean hospitals still do not comply. Photo: author's own.

visiting teams bringing physical resources may be better received than those solely bringing education.

QUALITY IMPROVEMENT

Quality-Improvement (QI) initiatives in HICs include morbidity and mortality (M&M) conferences, surveillance of complications, and policies for the investigation of errors and near misses. Hospitals in LMICs do have QI activity, but their effectiveness is variable and sometimes they even reinforce suboptimal practice.

The status of the person voicing their opinion can carry more weight than scientific evidence. Visitors from HICs can be afforded unearned respect and should therefore be particularly careful of their comments, which can be misunderstood, applied inappropriately and even become local "lore." A case in point: because of something once said by an international visitor, a surgical team in a large African hospital believed it was unsafe to anastomose the terminal ileum, leading to this essential bit of gut being routinely sacrificed in countless operations.

Isolation means teams can also get stuck in a time warp. Twenty-five years ago, when the threshold for Bogota bag application was briefly lowered in HICs, [v] visitors passed on this technique to African teams. The negative effect of the practice was quickly appreciated in HICs and emphasis returned to getting the abdomen closed. However, isolated teams in low-resource settings may not be updated, and risk continuing with practices long since abandoned elsewhere.

Where the audit measures and corrective action loops recommended in *DCP 3: Essential Surgery* are not yet present, M&M meetings may pass obsolete practice to new residents, reinforcing rather than correcting the problem. Sharing updates is one reason enduring relationships and partnerships are so essential to lasting change.

The WHO has a "multimodal toolkit" approach for trauma QI involving M&M reviews, preventable death panel reviews, audits, and surveillance.[16] Uptake of activities like these can be limited when the culture of QI is not yet established, awareness is low, or teams are simply overwhelmed with work.

> "In the UK, a serious incident would trigger a cascade of structured responses: root cause analyses, multidisciplinary reviews, and systematic learning. But in a country where underlying issues such as drug shortages or lack of training remain unresolved, would such reviews still be meaningful if the findings can't be acted on?
>
> These are the uncomfortable questions you ask yourself, and often others, in the corridors of the hospital. The answers are rarely simple. While improvements can be made, there are few quick fixes. Real change requires investment in long-term, respectful partnerships, not transient interventions."
>
> —Jonathan Dean, consultant anaesthetist (UK)

THE GLOBAL INDICATOR DATA COLLECTION PROJECT

The Global Indicator Data Collection Project requested information on the annual number of people who die after surgery (either in-hospital or 30-day mortality) and the total number of surgical procedures done. Only 25 countries were able to provide this, and in only 16 was the data robust enough to be used. Data came from ten HICs, four upper MICs

[v] A Bogota bag is a temporary plastic covering to an open abdomen.

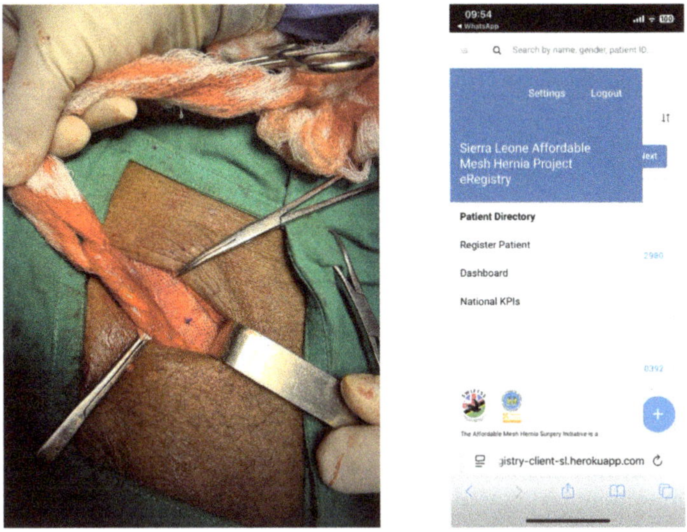

Figure 25. The Surgical teams Working in aFrica Together for Safer Surgery (SWIFTSS) Affordable Mesh Hernia Project provides training and free mesh to African hospitals. Because of the concerns around mesh complications, data is collected prospectively on all cases. Photos: author's own.

and two lower MICs. No LICs and no countries in Sub-Saharan African provided data, but then neither did the USA or the UK.[17]

The median postoperative mortality was 0.46% (range 0.062% to 1.7%). For countries reporting both inpatient and 30-day mortality rates, substantial differences were seen. Kosovo, for example, found a 6.4-fold difference. Latvia showed a 27% increase in reported deaths when counting total patients rather than unique procedures.

Countries providing post-operative mortality data:

Australia, New Zealand The Solomon Islands, Taiwan, Tonga, Tuvalu, Andorra, Belgium, Cyprus, Finland, Kosovo, Latvia, Monaco, Spain, Belize, and Brazil.

What this really demonstrates is the difficulty in collecting, understanding and responding to what would appear to be the simplest and crudest quality measure: did the patient survive the operation? But the surprising reality is that few countries, including most HICs, can provide this information. Oceania leads the world in being able to provide this data, with Australia able to show trends over time.

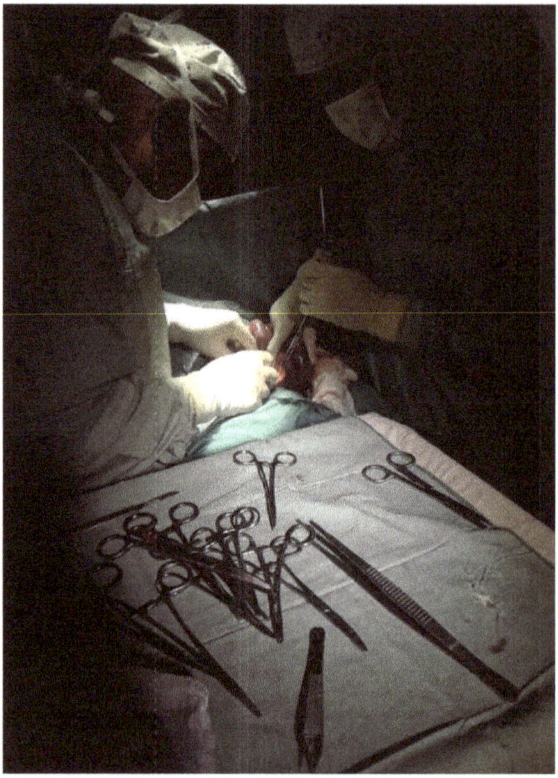

Figure 26. Operating with inadequate light. Photo: author's own.

POOR QUALITY INFRASTRUCTURE AND LACK OF STUFF

Poor quality buildings, lack of running water and power cuts are the daily challenges faced by teams trying to deliver quality surgery and anaesthesia in LMICs. Oxygen comes from concentrators (£180 second-hand on eBay), and more than one child may be on the same machine.

Equipment taken for granted in HICs is often absent. Functional overhead theatre lights are often absent or cast-offs from rich countries. Operations are regularly done using headtorches, and when these are broken or out of batteries, by the light of a mobile phone.

Diathermy is a luxury, scissors are blunt, and extreme suture economy slows down surgery. Inevitable compromises, such as closing laparotomies with rapidly absorbable suture, are made. Skilful local surgeons are fighting adversities unknown to those in rich countries.

Can surgeons do their best work in these conditions?

WORKFORCE QUALITY

The output of training in medical schools and allied-health worker training institutions in LMICs varies. In Malawi, visiting teams often comment that the knowledge of medical school graduates is higher than in their own countries. However, in other regions, not all schools are properly regulated, and corruption can occur. Some training can be of very low quality, for example, a lecturer reading from a textbook for an hour and then leaving. Occasionally, one meets doctors in LICs whose knowledge and clinical understanding are breathtakingly poor.

Licensing, regulation and continuous professional development may also be lacking in some countries, allowing doctors to operate without any surgical training. The concept of direct supervision and competency assessment can be absent, so that it is down to the individual doctor as to whether they have the insight to be safe. In contrast, efforts have been made to report the results of surgery performed by Associate Clinicians and Health Officers (see chapter 11, page 113).

The quality of expatriate surgeons working in LMICs, particularly in Sub-Saharan Africa, is largely unregulated. Some of the most highly committed and skilful professionals in the world work in unglamorous positions for low salaries in poor countries. However, others do not meet the standards expected in their own countries. Unearned privilege and respect are often afforded to expatriates, especially those with white skin, and this may be combined with self-belief and entitlement. Lack of regulation and governance allow these people to work in roles they are unfit for in their home countries, and hospitals in parts of Sub-Saharan Africa can find themselves the employers of last resort for people who have failed elsewhere.

Trainees from HICs may also work beyond their level, either because they feel pressured, mistakenly perceive there is no-one else around, or lack respect for locally trained providers.

QUALITY OF SURGICAL, ANAESTHETIC, AND OBSTETRIC (SAO) TRAINING

In some LMICs, absence of regulation extends to the quality of training provided within SAO training programs. Many countries have established postgraduate training colleges over the past 20–30 years, to develop curricula, examinations and residency programs.

The Royal College of Surgeons of Edinburgh was founded in 1505. Compare this to the West African College of Surgeons (WACS) and College of Surgeons of East Central and South Africa (COSECSA), which have been in existence since 1960 and 1999, respectively. Progress can be impressive. The Ghana College of Physicians and Surgeons was established in 2003 and quickly began an in-country credentialing process that graduated 284 specialist surgeons and obstetrician-gynaecologists by 2014. These emerging colleges are battling big problems: immature systems, financial constraints and difficulty establishing new regulatory bodies.

However, in many LICs, the concept of regulating trainers and training is still in its infancy. Focus may be placed on passing exams and the exams themselves may be poor or unvalidated. Insufficient attention may be paid to developing competent providers and things HIC trainees take for granted, such as supervised procedure training, formative assessments and competency-based progression are unusual.

The quality of training provided by expatriates is even *less* regulated. The Essential Surgery Package should provide clear guidance and aims for such training, yet it is possible to deliver training without any regard to local need or concern for trainer competency. Some training missions lack defined aims aligned with the Package or ignore it altogether. Instead, they may organise training more around the skills and knowledge of their staff and volunteers than the needs of the host country.

Training missions tend to measure what is easy, not what matters. Reports typically provide trainee numbers, trainee satisfaction, and short-term knowledge, but not the quality of the alumni, change in practice or clinical outcomes.

Some involved in global surgery even put forward the concept of "over-training." No, this doesn't mean exercising too much but reflects a neo-colonial attitude that the Essential Surgery Package is "too much" for

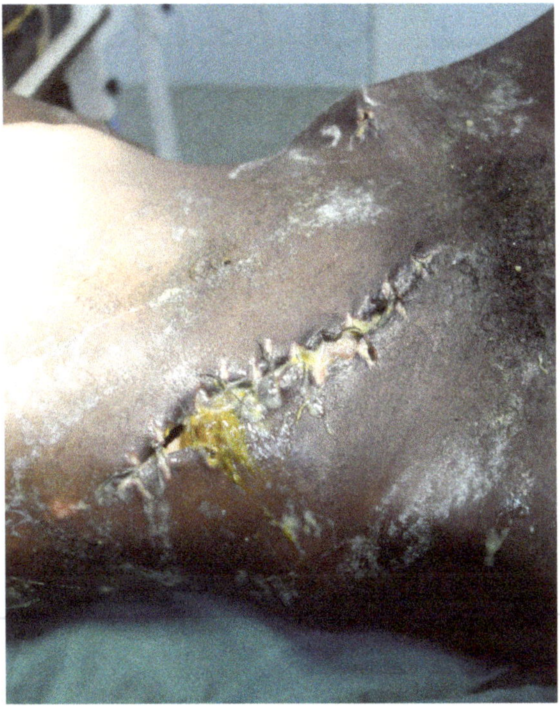

Figure 27. Faeces leaking from a teenager's wound after an appendicectomy performed by an untrained provider. Photo: author's own.

local personnel and systems, who are not (currently) considered capable. As a result, they suggest that key emergency skills should be withheld, thereby maintaining dependence. The fact that dumbing-down an already straightforward list of procedures even gets voiced is indicative of the lack of quality control and governance in expatriate training.

The absence of quality controls in training and competency assessment is a major concern. Five billion people do not have access to safe surgical care, and if HIC actors are to help train the way out of this, poor quality training must be addressed. It is simply not acceptable that anybody can rock up and teach what they fancy. Training quality must match or exceed that carried out in HICs.

Focusing on sound technical skills and safe practice is paramount in settings where lack of resources means there's nowhere to hide. The people being trained as part of the upscaling process are the seed corn, who will set the standard of surgery in their countries for the next 20 years.

Robust assessment is necessary for this. In *Surgical Training in Low-Resource Settings*, Klein and Park sum it up nicely "standardized curricula and consequential, validated examinations must be part of training,"[18] to which we would add "regardless of cadre."

MEASURING THE QUALITY OF SHORT-TERM MEDICAL MISSIONS

In 2008, 6,000 short-term medical missions (aka camps) originated from the US alone, mostly focused on elective surgery.[19] Some camps provide valuable care in LMICs but risk giving temporary relief while undermining the efforts of local teams. Chapter 17 (see page 183) discusses how camps work and the ethical questions they raise. Chapter 10 (see page 106) covers their financial implications.

How do camps assure the quality of their clinical results? Despite the size of this industry, there is no organisation policing short-term missions. Although some measure their impact, they are under no obligation to do so, and they often lack clinical governance and QI mechanisms. Only 20% of US mission personnel reported they felt post-operative follow-up was adequate to assess the impact of their work.

There is no standardised method to assess clinical outcomes. However, a consensus has emerged over the last decade that missions should report measurable goals, cost, efficiency, impact, preparedness for the local context, educational outcomes, and sustainability. Other positive indicators include long-term data collection and volunteer qualifications.[20]

In both the UK and USA, groups providing short-term missions operate outside specific legislation. The UK Medical Council requires UK doctors working abroad to uphold the same standards as at home. This obligation not only covers our own behaviour, but also the need to report sub-standard practice observed within the mission.

In 2008, 60% of reporting missions provided training and education,[21] but the quality and relevance of the educational content is rarely scrutinised. Education may be recorded as "delivered," not whether this translated into improved outcomes.

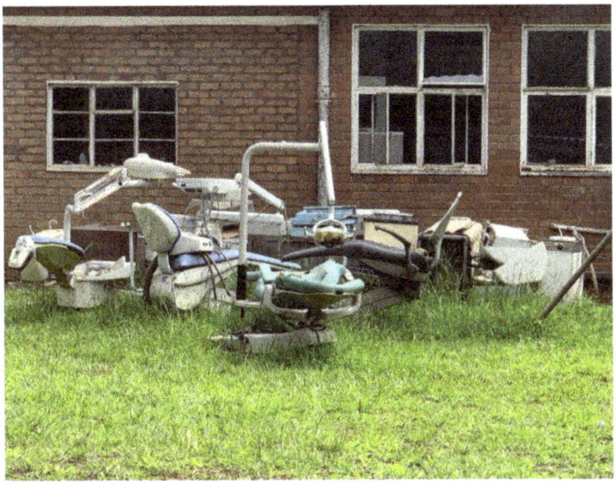

Figure 28. Hospital in Southern Africa — where dental chairs go to die. Photo: author's own.

The USA is taking a leading role in encouraging short-term missions to adopt best practice and quality assurance, while working sustainably in partnership with local healthcare teams.[vi]

QUALITY OF DONATIONS

Equipment is frequently donated by those seeking to improve access to surgery. Some donations are valuable, well-received and put to good use. HIC teams in long-term relationships with LMIC partners are adept at learning what is most needed.

However, at the risk of sounding like a broken record, this sector is unregulated and, in some countries, up to 75% of donated equipment is scrapped.[22] Donated items are often inappropriate, poorly functioning, or just plain broken. Well-intentioned donors may be unfamiliar with local needs or fail to appreciate the lack of trained biomedical engineers in LMICs. The US term "Junk for Jesus" has been co-opted to describe the burden that useless equipment places on LMICs.

Guidelines and best practice policies emphasise the importance of meeting recipient needs, complying with local regulations, and planning for long-term maintenance. However, there is little evidence that these frameworks are followed.[23]

---

vi Americares.org

Donating consumables is not ideal as it can disrupt efforts to develop sustainable supply chains. However, this is a counsel of perfection and in many LICs, surgery relies heavily on donated consumables, particularly sutures. For more on donating equipment, see chapter 21, page 264.

EXPLORE FURTHER

1. World Health Organization. "WHO Safe Surgery Checklist: Data and Implementation Tools." https://www.who.int/teams/integrated-health-services/patient-safety/research/safe-surgery/tool-and-resources.
2. Park, Adrian, and Raymond Price, eds. *Global Surgery: The Essentials*. Springer, 2017. https://doi.org/10.1007/978-3-319-49482-1.
3. Americares. https://www.americares.org.
4. World Health Organization. "Information and Policy Standards for Donations." https://www.who.int/teams/health-product-and-policy-standards/medicines-selection-ip-and-affordability/donations.

CHAPTER 9
ANAESTHESIA AND SAFETY CULTURE

ANAESTHESIA HAS BEEN EVEN MORE OVERLOOKED in global health than surgery. "If global surgery was a neglected stepchild, then anaesthesia was its invisible friend."[1] Yet, surgical and obstetric care rely entirely on safe anaesthesia. The Lancet Commission on Global Surgery's (LCoGS) report *Global Surgery: 2030* references anaesthesia 267 times, most often in the phrase: "surgical and anaesthesia care."[2]

Access to safe anaesthesia and patient safety systems is lacking in countries with the lowest Human Development Index (HDI), with unmet need being greatest in Southeast Asia and Sub-Saharan Africa. Universal access to essential surgery will save millions of lives, but only if supported by safe anaesthesia — without it, preventable death and disability will continue.

ANAESTHESIA-RELATED MORTALITY

Deaths due to anaesthesia are 100 to 1000 times higher in LMICs than in the Global North, and the difference is especially marked in obstetric and paediatric practice.[3] For 50 years, anaesthetic teams in HICs have embraced safety and vigilance, resulting in avoidable anaesthetic death being all but eliminated.

At the end of the 1980s, the risk of dying as a direct result of anaesthesia was estimated to be 1 in 185,000 in the UK, but in 2005 in Togo, it was still 1 in 133.[4] Most of these deaths occurred in fit, young people, with half occurring in obstetric practice. Forty-seven percent of the avoidable deaths were due to circulatory problems, including lack of blood for transfusion, and 30% were respiratory, i.e. airway problems.

> **Risk of dying from anaesthesia:**
>
> **1990 UK: 1 in 185,000**
>
> **2005 Togo: 1: 133**

Similar small studies in other countries have found the same pattern as in Togo — deaths of young adults and children from undetected hypoxia or hypovolaemia, with concerns about lack of training, supervision, and monitoring.[5]

SHORTAGE OF "STUFF"

Critical equipment can be absent from operating theatres and recovery areas in LICs and parts of MICs. Without effective monitoring, staff are not alerted to situations requiring urgent attention. Most critical is pulse oximetry. Rapidly adopted in HICs, it is now unthinkable to conduct anaesthesia without it, and unethical to conduct research into its value in LMICs.

Anaesthetists face many infrastructure challenges. Piped gas and cylinders may not be available. The World Health Organisation (WHO) Situational Analysis Tool (SAT) database survey of 800 LIC facilities found 24% did not have oxygen and 31% did not have reliable electricity, which is essential to make oxygen via concentrators.[6]

The LCoGS details the lack of basic equipment. In 2010, 55% of district hospitals across eight African countries had no anaesthetic machine.[7] Seventy percent of operating rooms in parts of Sub-Saharan Africa lacked a pulse oximeter, and 35% of Zambian district hospitals did not have a laryngoscope.[8,9] In 2012, Nigeria reported only 42% of district and 24% of regional hospitals had equipment to maintain a paediatric airway.[10] Essential medications, consumables and personal protective equipment were all in short supply.

Drugs for anaesthesia and pain control on the **WHO Model List of Essential Medicines** (see text box) are cheap, cost-effective and agreed by experts, but are not always available. Older agents like halothane are often used in LMICs and can cause myocardial depression, especially in patients with haemodynamic instability. Rescue drugs such as adrenaline may not be available. Although these problems can sometimes be mitigated by skilled anaesthesia, they are compounded when those providing the anaesthesia have limited training.

Effective analgesia such as opioids, are also often in short supply. Although cheap, LMICs sometimes struggle to manage opiates and secure supplies.

PRAGMATISM IN LOW-RESOURCE SETTINGS

In impoverished areas, protecting the airway is challenging, and using neuromuscular blocking agents can lead to airway loss and death if not skilfully managed. Hospitals also lack dedicated theatre recovery areas and trained recovery staff. Given such constrained circumstances, general anaesthesia is often provided with intravenous ketamine, allowing the patient to maintain their own airway. This approach is usually safer in places lacking the skills, equipment, or infrastructure required for anaesthesia using inhaled gases and airway maintenance. Local and regional anaesthesia are also widely used. Even so, concerns remain regarding aseptic technique, dosing, and the lack of rescue medicines.

The key anaesthesia skills needed in LMICs are:

1. Intravenous cannulation.
2. The ability to maintain an open airway and provide breathing and oxygenation, via bag and mask ventilation, or tracheal intubation.
3. Initiation of spinal or peripheral nerve block anaesthesia.

WHO Model List of Anaesthesia Essential Medicines List (2023)

- Inhalational agents: halothane, isoflurane, nitrous oxide, sevoflurane
- Injectable anaesthetics: ketamine, propofol (alternative: thiopental)
- Local anaesthetics: bupivacaine, lidocaine, lidocaine with adrenaline (dental cartridge)
- Preoperative/sedation: atropine, midazolam, morphine
- Medical gases: oxygen
- Muscle relaxants and cholinesterase inhibitors: atracurium, neostigmine, suxamethonium, vecuronium
- Pain management: acetylsalicylic acid, ibuprofen, paracetamol, codeine, fentanyl patch, morphine (alternative: oxycodone)
- IV fluids: glucose 5%, 10%, 50%; glucose with sodium chloride (dextrose saline); potassium chloride (ampoule); sodium chloride (normal saline); sodium bicarbonate; compound sodium lactate
- Allergy/anaphylaxis: dexamethasone, adrenaline, hydrocortisone, loratadine (alternatives: cetirizine, fexofenadine), prednisolone
- Palliative care/symptom control: ondansetron, diazepam, amitriptyline
- Rescue medications: atropine, naloxone, adrenaline

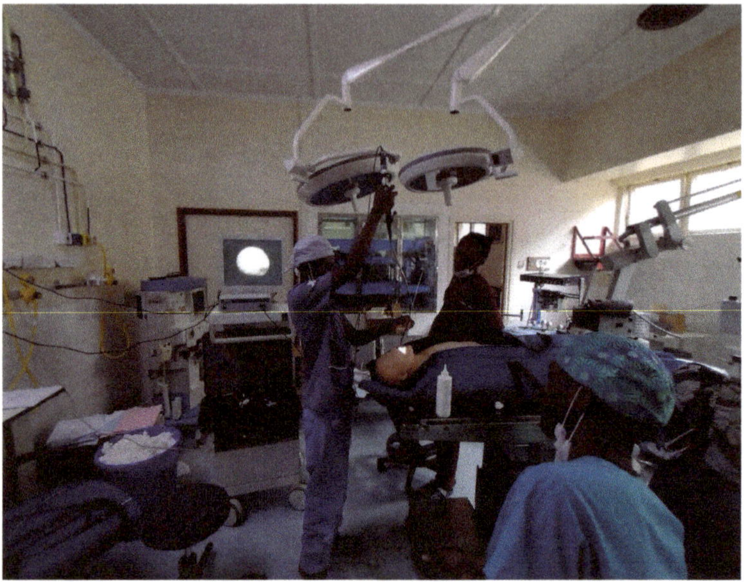

Figure 29. Learning awake fibreoptic intubation using a gastroscope in Malawi. Photo: Jonathon Dean.

Alongside these skills, staff need a working knowledge of basic physiology, an attitude of continuous vigilance, and the knowledge and skills to rescue things if key complications such as hypoxia or hypotension occur. The absence of providers with these skills for children is a particular concern.

Key Anaesthesia Skills in LMICs

1. Intravenous cannulation.
2. The ability to maintain an open airway, provide breathing and oxygenation via bag and mask ventilation, or tracheal intubation.
3. Initiation of spinal or peripheral nerve block anaesthesia.

Where equipment like pulse oximetry is not available, the vigilance which goes along with continuous monitoring is often also absent. It is difficult to maintain a safety culture in the face of inadequate equipment and staff training. Failure to adopt the WHO Safe Surgery Checklist — despite its proven benefit and almost zero cost — is telling.

TASK SHIFTING/SHARING

Task shifting for anaesthesia in LMICs is common. Nurses, health officers, and technicians form the backbone of delivery in many areas. Africa and Southeast Asia lack doctors but not talent and many in these cadres would have trained as doctors if they lived in HICs. With appropriate education and oversight, non-physician anaesthetic providers deliver high-quality care. While not universally accepted, task shifting generates less debate in anaesthesia than in surgery commensurate with practice in many HICs, where non-physician providers often deliver routine anaesthesia.

However, in the poorest places, even formally trained cadres may be absent. Hospitals fill the void as best they can, and people who have no specific qualifications or training provide anaesthesia. In Uganda in 2008, for example, 17% of those delivering anaesthesia reported no formal training and learnt on the job.[11]

TRAINING AND CREDENTIALING

Many countries are developing and implementing national anaesthesia training programs, often supported by NGOs and institutions from HICs. They frequently offer two tier training, with basic anaesthesia officers training for 6 to 24 months, ready to provide most of the care in district hospitals, where the bulk of essential surgery will be performed. Others undertake higher-level training for two to four years and go on to provide more complex anaesthesia, supervise staff, and train others.

There is an urgent need not only for structured education, but also for credentialing with minimum qualifications, and for systematic tracking of who is doing what. Increasingly, national societies are developing and implementing the necessary

> "Take tomorrow's caesarean section list as an example. Will there be spinal needles available, or will I need to improvise with a cannula for a neuraxial block? Will there be bupivacaine? If so, will it be in date — and will it even work? Frequently, it doesn't work fully. As a result, spinal anaesthetics are often repeated, increasing the risk of complications such as high spinals. And when one occurs, who comes running to help manage this emergency? Possibly no one. The resuscitation equipment, if present, may be incomplete or unreliable."
>
> —Jonathon Dean, consultant anaesthetist (UK), talking about Malawi

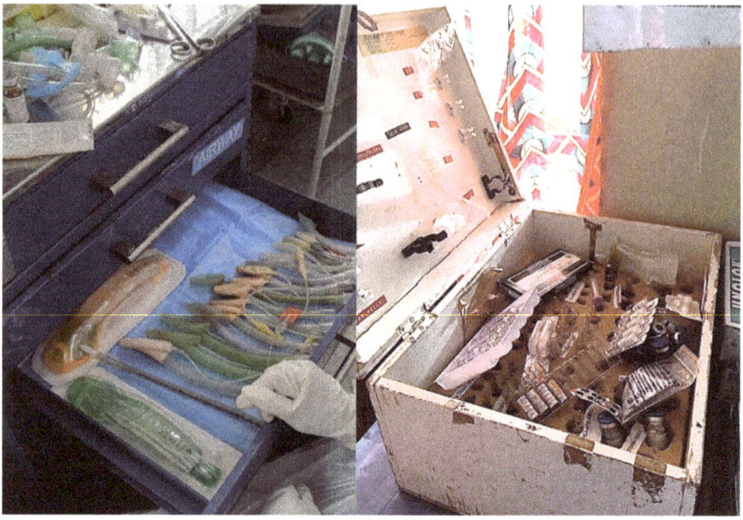

Figure 30. (Left) An attempt to instil order. Donated equipment is often underused because poor organisation makes it inaccessible when it is needed. Vital items may be hidden in boxes. Photo: Jonathon Dean. (Right) Emergency drug box in Zambian theatre. Photo: Pei Jean Ong.

oversight processes. The need for standard-setting and monitoring across all cadres is accepted by the anaesthetic community internationally, yet at present, some countries have scant knowledge or control over who is providing anaesthesia. A culture of constant vigilance, without distraction and time lapses, is absent in some places. One hears terrible stories, such as a night where five consecutive patients died before a hospital brought in training.

The low priority given to anaesthesia can mean training is technically available but unaffordable. In Uganda, doctors pursuing the three-year Master of Medicine in Anaesthesia pay fees, but do not receive a salary. Scholarships are more readily available for other careers, making anaesthetic training financially inaccessible. Partnerships with the Association of Anaesthetists (formerly AAGBI) and other UK and US groups fund allowances for trainees, and clinical attachments in North America and the UK. In-country Association of Anaesthetists volunteers support local trainers and local trainee research projects.

The World Federation of Societies of Anaesthesiologists (WFSA) also funds education. It provides fellowships in LMICs, supports and develops potential clinical leaders, strengthens institutions and establishes clinical networks. Standalone charitable organisations also fund scholarships in LMICs.

SAFER ANAESTHESIA FROM EDUCATION (SAFE)®

Developed by the AAGBI and WFSA, the SAFE project has been training anaesthetic providers and trainers in LMICs since 2011.[i] The AAGBI SAFE Steering Group oversees the process: it facilitates course updates, translations, and funding; monitors implementation; and evaluates both impact and strategy.[ii]

SAFE courses are delivered in small groups over two to three days. They have been developed by individuals knowledgeable in health education training and combine lectures, low-tech simulation, discussions and role-play. Participants receive a detailed course manual, handbook and logbook to continue to use. There are specialist courses in paediatric, obstetric and head and neck anaesthesia, and additional online training.

SAFE has delivered more than 230 courses in 50 countries, mainly in Sub-Saharan Africa and Southeast Asia, training over 8,000 providers and 1,350 trainers. Mercy Ships, Smile Train, some national societies, and other international organisations also run courses. SAFE peer-reviewed publications demonstrate both long-term retention of knowledge and skills and sustained improvements in clinical practice by course participants. As such, SAFE courses provide an exemplar of how to conduct short courses in low-resource settings.

MONITORING

The true test of effective training and instigation of safety culture will be a reduction in anaesthesia-related mortality. Tracking death within 24 hours of surgery is suggested as an indicator of avoidable anaesthesia deaths. Although this metric is affected by other factors, such as patient condition at presentation, the ease with which the data can be collected and parallels with existing mandatory MMR reporting could make it a crude but pragmatic first step towards quality monitoring.

---

i https://wfsahq.org/our-work/education-training/safe-training/

ii Safer Anaesthesia From Education®. https://safe-anaesthesia.org.

LIFEBOX®

A Cochrane meta-analysis confirmed that routine use of pulse oximetry reduces hypoxaemia in operating theatres and recovery.[12] Subjectively, one in five anaesthetists reported that an early warning from oximetry led to the avoidance of a potential complication. Studies do not show significant mortality reduction, which is not surprising given 22,000 patients were studied in a country where avoidable anaesthetic deaths would be expected to be nearer 1:200,000. However, in LMICs with high anaesthesia-related mortality, the gains from routine oximetry are likely to be considerable, particularly as hypoxia is harder to spot in darker skin.

"I thoroughly enjoyed coordinating projects with my resource-constrained colleagues — from curating a learning needs assessment, to the logistics of delivering educational content, to finally meeting in person. I really enjoyed walking hand-in-hand with anaesthetists from all over the world. It is humbling when they later call upon us to help fundraise and champion in times of need — a testament to the depth of authentic friendship and network."

—Jan Man Wong, specialist registrar in anaesthesia (UK)

Lifebox® have donated 35,000 robustly constructed, rechargeable battery-powered oximeters for use in low-resource settings, in conjunction with an educational package.[iii] In Malawi, they were able to show a reduction in desaturation episodes from 17.2% to 6.5%, occurring over the first 100 cases following the intervention.[13] The authors concluded that when anaesthetists could routinely measure oxygen saturation, their practice improved, with earlier detection of problems and more rapid responses, reflecting increased vigilance and good clinical practice. Furthermore, follow-up showed that the oximeters remained in use and could be located.

HOLISTIC PERIOPERATIVE CARE

There is robust evidence supporting many aspects of perioperative care, but almost all studies come from HICs. The Enhanced Recovery After Surgery (ERAS) Society published comprehensive guidelines for elective abdominal and gynaecological procedures at primary and secondary hospitals in LMICs. A team from the ERAS Society collabo-

iii https://www.lifebox.org/

rated with representatives from MICs (The Philippines and South Africa), to develop the document, which they see as a starting point to address sub-optimal perioperative care.[14] Pilot studies in LMICs are envisaged as the next step.

The ERAS team highlighted concerns about "Failure to Rescue," defined as "the death of a patient following one or more complications." This fits with lived experience in LICs. It is unnerving to institute early postoperative feeding when patients are on wards where there are no members of staff awake at night. (Maybe because staff are working two jobs to make ends meet....)

Advocates of safe anaesthesia in LMICs recommend:

- Prioritising patient safety
- Education, training, and credentialing for existing and future anaesthesia providers
- Creating a culture of vigilance and providing safety monitoring
- Ensuring oxygen and rescue medicines are available
- Collect 24-hour post-operative mortality rates (POMR)
- Universal reporting of POMRs, by the WHO

OBTAINING ANAESTHETIC EQUIPMENT FOR LMICS

Supply chain systems that prioritise anaesthesia items are urgently needed in many LICs and lower MICs. In the meantime, anaesthetic teams travelling from HICs often take equipment with them. They should make friends with their local resuscitation officer before their trip. The stock on resuscitation trolleys is rarely used and despite being made from durable materials, is routinely discarded and updated, making these trolleys a valuable source of anaesthesia consumables.

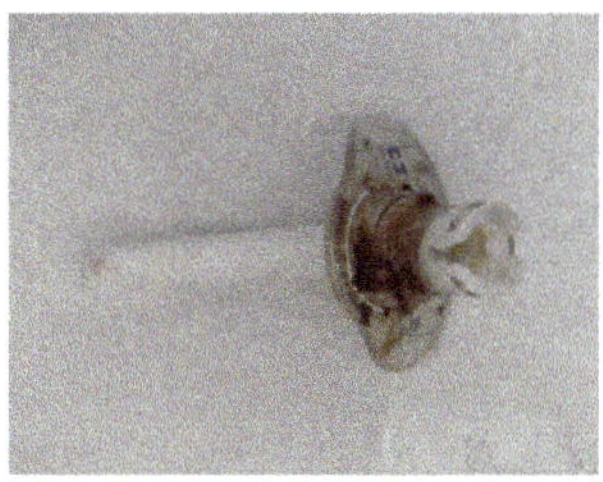

Figure 31. This tracheostomy tube was removed from a patient who had received intensive care for burns but was lacking tracheostomy care. Photo: Jonathon Dean.

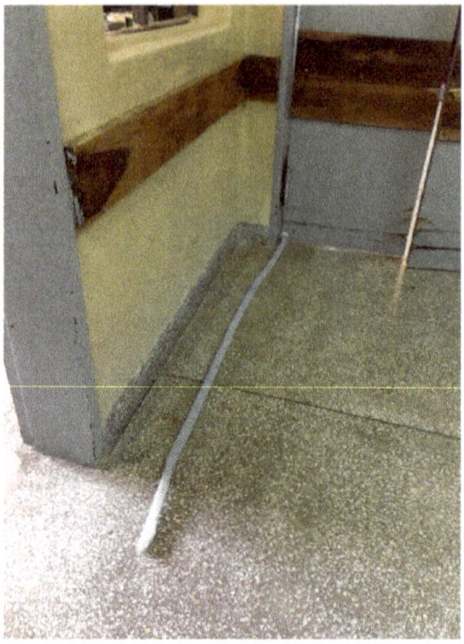

Figure 32. Scavenging pipe from anaesthetic machine leading out of theatre (through dedicated hole in the door) into the staff room, Zambia Photo: Pei Jean Ong.

EXPLORE FURTHER

1. Citron, Isabelle, and John G. Meara. "A Global Surgery, Obstetrics and Anaesthesia Metamorphosis: The SAFE-T Summit 2018 Reports." *Update in Anesthesia 33* (2019):39–44. https://resources.wfsahq.org/wp-content/uploads/uia33-Safe-anaesthesia-for-everybody-%E2%80%93-today%E2%80%99s-initiative-the-anaesthesia-patient-safety-perspective.pdf.
2. Safer Anaesthesia from Education®. https://safe-anaesthesia.org.
3. Association of Anaesthetists. *Anaesthesia Emergencies Quick Reference Handbook.* https://anaesthetists.org/Home/Resources-publications/Safety-alerts/Anaesthesia-emergencies/Quick-Reference-Handbook. — *An invaluable resource.*
4. Munasinghe, Baththirange Malaka, Jayasuriya N. J. A. Sahan Sachitra, and Martin F. Mayall. "Global Synergy in Anaesthesia Training: The Crucial Role of International Collaborations for Trainees from Low-Resource Countries." *British Journal of Anaesthesia* 135, no. 1 (2025): 220–22. https://doi.org/10.1016/j.bja.2025.03.020. — *This article explores international collaboration in anaesthesia training. It is behind a paywall but free for RCoA members.*

5. Craven, Rachael, Hilary Edgcombe, and Ben Gupta, eds. *Global Anaesthesia*. Oxford Specialist Handbooks in Anaesthesia. Oxford: Oxford University Press, 2020.
6. Dobson, Mike. *The Right Stuff: Anaesthetic Equipment and Techniques That Work Best in Low-Resource Countries.* Morrisville, NC: Lulu.com, 2017.

CHAPTER 10
MONEY, MONEY, MONEY

> *Surgery is an indivisible, indispensable part of healthcare ... these conditions are financially devastating for individuals and their families, economically damaging for countries, and disproportionately threaten the welfare of the poorest and most vulnerable people in our societies.*[1]
>
> —JIM YONG KIM, PRESIDENT, WORLD BANK, AT THE LAUNCH OF THE LANCET COMMISSION ON GLOBAL SURGERY, BOSTON, JANUARY 17, 2014

ECONOMISTS FEEL NOT enough attention is being given to financing in global surgery, perhaps because global health teams are dominated by health workers, who do not recognise the wider picture. **Figure 33** shows key factors that prevent people in LMICs from accessing surgery. People are often affected by more than one factor, but what the diagram highlights is the disproportionate impact of affordability.

In systems where care is free at the point of delivery, the idea of having to sell everything for an appendicectomy is hard to grasp. The concept is perhaps easier to understand in countries where healthcare is insurance-based, but even then, most HICs provide a safety net of basic care for life-threatening emergencies.

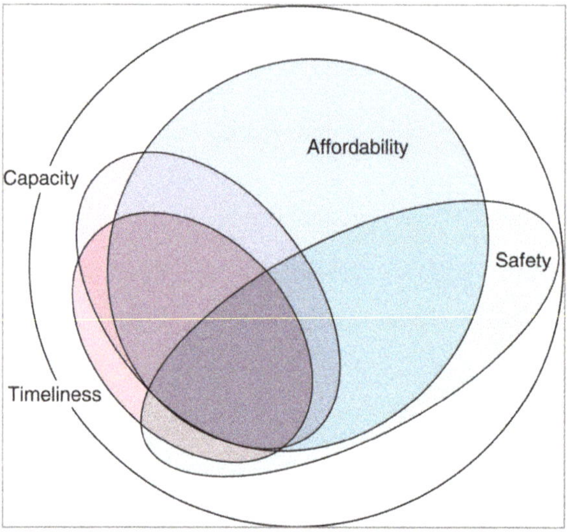

Figure 33. Area-proportional Euler diagram illustrating lack of access to surgery. The large circle shows global population; the ellipses show those without surgical care. Source: Niclas Rudolfson, Mark G Shrime, Blake C Alkire, Modelling why 70 per cent of the world's population lack access to surgery, *BJS*, Volume 110, Issue 4, April 2023, Pages 500–501, https://doi.org/10.1093/bjs/znad005 Reproduced under Creative Commons CC by Licence.

PATIENT-LEVEL FINANCIALS

Catastrophic expenditure

"Catastrophic expenditure" is defined as direct out-of-pocket (OOP) payments for surgery that are greater than 10% of total income or 40% of income after paying for food and shelter. For the world's poorest, the cost of an operation will not only consume the individual's entire income, but also that of their relatives. Families may never recover from the financial hit.

Currently, 3.7 billion people, mostly in Sub-Saharan Africa and South-east Asia, are at risk of catastrophic expenditure if they develop a surgical condition.[2] That's 81 million people per year, 33 million of whom face catastrophic expenditure paying for the surgery itself, and 48 million more when paying for the non-medical costs of accessing care. A quarter are bankrupted by surgery.

Many more are impoverished by surgery. Impoverishment is defined as being pushed into poverty, or being pushed further into poverty, by OOP for surgery.

> "They would often come to the government hospital, but for many, the financial burden of surgery was insurmountable. I did my best to help by performing surgeries for free whenever possible, but I often faced limitations. Once, the hospital management even asked me, "Are you trying to turn this government hospital into a charity hospital?"
>
> —Ibrahim M. Sesay, surgical officer (Sierra Leone)

The reality is probably much worse than this, as these figures do not include those who did not present at all. Data appears to suggest that the proportion of people facing catastrophic expenditure is higher in lower MICs than in LICs. This only makes sense once we realise that those at the very bottom do not even attempt to access surgery and are therefore not counted in the data. People will not seek care if they already know it is unaffordable or if they are unaware of it because it is not available in their area.

PROTECTION AGAINST OUT-OF-POCKET EXPENDITURE FOR SURGERY

Financial protection against catastrophic expenditure is essential if universal access to essential surgery is to be achieved. The WHO, the World Bank, and global health organisations all advocate protection against OOP costs.

Safeguarding people means moving from models where the user pays at the time of need to indirect systems that pool risk, funded by general taxation or insurance schemes that cover essential surgery. This allows healthcare development utilising both public and private services, while minimising user fees at the point of delivery. This pro-poor approach to funding requires both domestic and international health funding.

The Lancet Commission on Global Surgery (LCoGS) presented two affordability indicators:[3]

1. 100% of households to be protected from impoverishment from OOP payments for surgery by 2030.
2. 100% of households to be protected against catastrophic expenditure from OOP payments for surgery by 2030.

Both targets will be missed widely. Many LMICs do not factor surgical expenditure into their national health-care budgets, meaning there is no realistic financing or budget allocated for surgery.

Surgical interventions are highly cost-effective in LICs:

- Caesarean section for obstructed labour: 1–3× per capita GDP per DALY averted
- Groin hernia repair: <1× per capita GDP per DALY averted

[Source: ghcearegistry.org]

The Global Indicator Data Collection Project measured progress towards the LCoGS financial indicators in 2015 and 2017.[4] One-hundred and eighty-six countries provided information about the cost of surgery across representative geographical areas of their countries. They found that living in a HIC affords either complete, or near complete, protection from catastrophic expenditure. At the other end of the spectrum, 99% of Burundi's population were exposed to catastrophic expenditure should they need surgery.[5] Previously, some progress was being made to address affordability, but then the 2008 world financial crisis deflected attention, and many donor countries are now actively cutting development aid.

THE COST OF UPSCALING SURGERY

Increasing the availability of surgery is crucial if unmet need is to be addressed. The minimum number of procedures required annually is 5,000 per 100,000 population.[6] Scaling up to this level would allow Universal Coverage of the Essential Surgery Package (UCES), which is estimated to reduce mortality by 3.2%, lost DALYs by 3.5% annually, and reduce the maternal mortality ratio (MMR) to ≤100 per 100,000.[7]

Average annual growth in surgical procedures in LMICs has been 5.1%, but some countries have done particularly well. Desirable surgical volumes would be achieved if all countries followed the practice of the best performing ones. Mongolia, for example, achieved 8.9% growth and Mexico 22.5% growth in a year.[8] If Mexico's achievements had been replicated everywhere, the necessary upscaling would be on target for 2030. If the average country had done as well as Mongolia, two-thirds of countries would be on target.

Analysis by the LCoGS shows that scaling up essential surgery in LICs, lower MICs, and upper MICs requires significant but manageable

Category	LICs	Lower MICs	Upper MICs
Unit cost for surgical procedures	179	219	332
Surgical theatre construction cost	319,002	412,488	1,906,064
Historical rates of increase (5.1% per year)			
Cost of surgical procedures	14	115	86
Cost of operating rooms	6	37	40
Total cost	20	152	126
Annual cost (% of total annual health expenditures)	1 billion (4%)	8 billion (4%)	7 billion (1%)
Mongolian rates of increase (8.9% per year)			
Cost of surgical procedures	31	197	91
Cost of operating rooms	13	50	40
Total cost	44	247	31
Annual cost (% of total annual health expenditures)	2 billion (8%)	14 billion (6%)	7 billion (1%)
Mexican rates of increase (22.5% per year)			
Cost of surgical procedures	76	274	95
Cost of operating rooms	17	50	40
Total cost	93	324	135
Annual cost (% of total annual health expenditures)	5 billion (17%)	18 billion (8%)	8 billion (1%)

Table 8. Total and annual costs of scaling up basic surgical services (per billion 2012 US$), using historical, Mongolian, and Mexican rates for 33 low-, 33 lower-middle-, and 22 upper-middle-income countries. Source: Meara JG, Leather AJ, Hagander L et al. Global Surgery 2030. *Lancet* 2015;386:569–624.

investment. Total costs to expand surgical services between 2012 and 2030 for the 88 LMICs were estimated at US$300 billion (i.e. US$16 billion annually) moving at the average rate of expansion, and to achieve Mexican growth rates, US$550 billion (US$31 billion annually).[9]

Table 8 shows the cost of constructing, equipping and running the necessary operating theatres. While the costs of upscaling surgery are substantial, they are highly affordable, if there is the will amongst the international community to do it. Even at Mexican rates of expansion, in global economic terms the costs are not prohibitive and represent a small fraction of total healthcare spending. However, cuts in overseas development aid by HICs have the potential to derail progress for many years.

THE COST OF *NOT* UPSCALING SURGERY

Reducing early death and lost DALYs promotes economic growth. Failure to invest in surgical capacity ultimately costs more than the investment required to scale up surgical services, as countries continue to bear the economic burden of untreated surgical disease.

Five conditions — neoplasia, trauma, maternity care, neonatal conditions, and digestive disorders — were projected to cause a cumulative loss of US$21 trillion to the global economy between 2015 and 2030, about 1.3% of projected economic output, with more than half of these losses occurring in LMICs. In MICs, surgical disease will cost up to 2% of annual GDP growth by 2030, and the proportion is even greater in LICs.

Globally, neoplasia and trauma account for 95% of losses, but in LICs, maternal, digestive and neonatal problems make up 26% of losses. A multi-billion-dollar investment is needed to offset multitrillion-dollar losses.

Providing essential surgery at district hospitals in LMICs is highly cost-effective.[10,11] Economically, surgery compares well to programs such as vaccination, HIV care, malaria prevention, and basic public health campaigns. For instance, the cost-effectiveness of hernia repair in LMICs is better than breastfeeding promotion and oral rehydration therapy.

Investment in health results in economic returns by preventing early death and improving national income, and surgery is no exception. Countries that have invested in surgery have seen reductions in both maternal and under-five mortality. All countries wishing to bring themselves out of poverty need to improve surgical services as part of their development package.

COST-EFFECTIVE CARE

Trauma causes a million preventable deaths each year and leaves 20–50 million people permanently disabled.[12] Trauma care is highly cost-effective, at US$87 per DALY averted and managing obstructed labour costs US$82 per DALY.[13] However, for care to be cost-effective, it must also be clinically effective, which means it needs to be high quality and available close to the population.

Skilled birth attendants deliver excellent value. In 2000, for example, adding a trained birth attendant to antenatal care cost US$22 in Sub-Saharan Africa and US$37 in South and Southeast Asia.[14] This works out as US$67 million and US$96 million, respectively, for those entire regions — less than the transfer value of some English Premier League footballers.

The delivery of safe surgery brings other benefits, as hospitals providing the "five Ss" for surgery (see chapter 5, page 32) are also capable of dealing with a broad range of health problems.

Benefit–Cost Analysis (BCA) is an economic evaluation method that assigns monetary values to all costs and benefits, including intangible factors. BCA can quantify the economic benefit when an incapacitated person returns to the workforce after intervention, and balance these gains against the cost of treatment, allowing governments to compare health spending with other services, such as education or road building.

Caesarean section for obstructed labour has been assessed using BCA. One might argue this is unnecessary, as there is a moral imperative to provide it to save life and prevent fistula, but economic arguments can be more powerful. Thankfully, BCA demonstrates that investment in caesarean section is not only cost-effective but also brings positive net economic returns: "Death or morbidity in childbirth is a preventable tragedy. As societies develop and improve maternal health, all levels of society benefit."[15]

SURGERY IN LICs IS CHEAP

Direct costs per operation in LICs and LMICs vary, but all look cheap. For example, the cost of caesarean section in Africa ranges from US$40–200, and mesh hernia repair is about US$100, even with commercial mesh.[16]

In macro-economic terms, surgical expansion is also cheap. For example, at historical rates of increase of 5.1% per year, total annual costs are US$1 billion for LICs or 4% of health expenditure (**Table 8**, page 103). If countries can match Mongolian or Mexican rates, costs would increase to US$2–5 billion, but this would still represent only a small proportion of health budgets.[17]

Implementing UCES would be exceptionally cost-effective. In 2015, the estimated annual cost was around US$3 billion, with a predicted benefit-to-cost ratio better than 10:1. Prehospital trauma care is also highly cost-effective. Training first responders costs less than US$7 and basic ambulance services range between US$94–284 per life year saved. Trauma care is generally highly cost-effective, as injuries account for around one million preventable deaths each year, three-quarters of all surgically preventable deaths, and leave 20–50 million people permanently disabled.[18]

There is little data comparing the cost-effectiveness of different delivery platforms in LMICs. Missions and nongovernmental facilities may understate the cost of ongoing care and government hospitals may be better or worse value than the charitable sector. Mission hospitals appear expensive but, if they operate efficiently with high throughput, they may be good value.

However, all these estimates assume that procedures are both properly indicated and competently performed. Data on quality is essential to be able to understand the economic impact. Nobody gains from poorly conducted or inappropriate operations, except perhaps the operators, but let's not go there just yet.

COSTING SHORT-TERM MISSIONS

Short-term missions have variable attitudes to both money and sustainability. Some strengthen local services in partnership with local providers, improve infrastructure and meet local needs. Others focus on maximising the number of procedures performed and leave little or no legacy.

Self-assessment shows that surgical camps are expensive. The generosity of donors means this is not necessarily a limiting factor, but missions that provide no sustainable benefit represent opportunity cost; those resources could be used for interventions with greater long-term value elsewhere. For example, cleft lip and palate repair may cost between US$52 and US$1,827 per DALY averted, depending on who does it and how costs are counted.

In 1996, blindness cost US$168 billion in lost productivity. Cataract surgery is therefore one of the most cost-effective operations in LMICs, at approximately US$5 per DALY averted. Cataract camps appear cheap, at US$50 per case, but innovative systems such as Aravind Eye Care (see chapter 13, page 128) may be even better.

Most camps provide free surgery, and affordability is key for many patients. But is it good value to transport foreigners to do hernia operations? Why not just give the money to local teams to do free surgery?[19] Economic analyses tend to compare surgery versus no surgery, when what we should compare is surgery by the travelling team versus surgery by local teams. Surgical camps are usually only cost-effective when no other options exist. *DCP3: Essential Surgery* counsels caution interpreting the economic outcomes of short-term missions as some clinical outcomes have been unsatisfactory, and projected financial gains depend on operations being done well.

Local capacity can be increased if there is the will to do so. In settings where local delivery of routine surgery is available (i.e. most places), camps are unlikely to be either the clinically or financially the best method of delivery. Recognition of this has led teams to rethink their modus operandi, incorporating features to empower local teams. If you are considering volunteering, study the financial reports of prospective organisations to ensure resources are used effectively and support sustainable local capacity (see chapter 19, page 218).

Something not captured in economic analysis is the real-life truth that camps offer an accessible entry point for those new to global surgery, and some participants go on to make valuable sustainable contributions.

WHO-CHOICE

WHO's Choosing Interventions that are Cost-Effective (WHO-CHOICE) is a standardised tool to help assess the cost-benefit of sending surgical teams abroad.[20] However, since its introduction in 1998, most surgical missions have not made use of it, which is surprising, as one would think donors would insist on rigorous financial reporting.[21]

SELF-CONTAINED PLATFORMS

The record of camps in proving complex surgery is not encouraging (see chapter 8, page 84). However, self-contained mobile surgical facilities may provide an economically and morally appropriate alternative, until local healthcare provision reaches a level where complex surgery can be performed safely. Mercy Ships, for example, provide specialised surgical care in West Africa, via their "American hospital on a ship." This type of surgery is, by its nature, expensive. Complex maxillofacial surgery on the ship cost US$2,242 per DALY averted in 2018, but these patients currently have no viable alternative.[22]

EXPLORE FURTHER

1. Alkire, Blake C., Jeffrey R. Vincent, and John G. Meara. "Benefit–Cost Analysis for Selected Surgical Interventions in Low- and Middle-Income Countries." In *Essential Surgery*, edited by Haile T. Debas, Peter Donkor, Atul Gawande, Dean T. Jamison, Margaret E. Kruk, and Charles N. Mock. Vol. 1 of *Disease Control Priorities*, 3rd ed. World Bank, 2015. https://doi.org/10.1596/978-1-4648-0346-8.
2. World Health Organization. "New Cost-Effectiveness Updates from WHO-Choice." https://www.who.int/news-room/feature-stories/detail/new-cost-effectiveness-updates-from-who-choice.

CHAPTER 11
TASK SHIFTING AND TASK SHARING

TASK SHIFTING and task sharing are the reassignment of clinical tasks, including surgery and anaesthesia, from one cadre to another. Usually, this is moving tasks traditionally done by medically qualified providers to those without a medical degree.

The WHO defines task shifting as "the rational redistribution of tasks among health workforce teams ... from highly qualified workers to health workers with shorter training and fewer qualifications."[1] It implies the complete reassignment of certain responsibilities i.e. the substitution of a different cadre for a doctor. Task sharing is slightly different, with tasks completed collaboratively by providers with different levels of training who share responsibility. In practice, the line between the terms is blurred. Here we use the term "task shifting" as it is the most common scenario; however, most narratives use "task sharing."

> Initiatives aiming for task sharing may end up as task shifting, with health officers providing care in areas where doctors are scarce. Supervision may be nominal — perhaps by someone hours away or without procedure related training.

Numerous cadres exist. Here we use the term "health officer" as a generic term for cadres such as clinical officers, medical assistants, and other non-physician providers who may perform surgical procedures. But names and roles vary from country to country, and the role may be different from that implied by the name. These cadres are the backbone of surgical and anaesthesia care in many countries, particularly in rural areas. For instance, health officers perform 90% of major obstetric surgery in rural areas of Tanzania and Mozambique.[2]

WHY DO TASK SHIFTING?

Sub-Saharan Africa has 11% of the world's population, 24% of the global burden of disease and only 3% of its health workers. The region has three times the population of the United States, but less than 1% of the number of surgeons. To provide universal access to essential surgery, we need to double the number of surgeons worldwide.

National Surgical Obstetric and Anaesthesia Plans (NSOAPs) repeatedly find critical shortages of surgical, anaesthesia, and obstetric (SAO) providers the biggest barrier to increasing surgery (see chapter 13).

Where will these new SAO providers to come from? Sierra Leone has 2.4–4 doctors per 100,000 population, so dependence on those with a medical degree will fail to deliver. Significant increases in SAO providers would first require a massive increase in medical schools, requiring faculty and infrastructure, which is potentially decades away. Therefore, the only way to up-scale surgery rapidly is to train other cadres, maximising available human resources.[i]

COLONIAL MISCONCEPTIONS

Task shifting is not universally accepted, particularly by those unfamiliar with LICs. Such critics have concerns that the complexity of decision making necessitates a medical degree. The HIC perspective risks assuming that delegating tasks to non-medical cadres implies assigning them to individuals who lacked the intellect to enter medical school. The implicit inference is that Africa has too few doctors because it simply doesn't have enough 'clever' people.

In HICs, if someone wants to become a doctor and has the intellect and determination, then they can usually become a doctor. In LICs, however, individuals with the intellect and determination are busy working as health officers because they lacked the cash to pay for medical school. Africa is short of doctors, not short of talent. Many health officers would be doctors if they lived in other countries. You

---

i World Population Review. "Doctors per Capita by Country 2025." Accessed October 23, 2025. https://worldpopulationreview.com/country-rankings/doctors-per-capita-by-country.

don't have to be long in Africa to see how many go to medical school as soon as they get the money to do so. The individual is the same, the job title is different.

Sadly, the converse can also occasionally apply. There are LMIC doctors who graduated medical school through patronage rather than ability. Some may not be committed to healthcare but felt it would be a financially worthwhile profession. Having a qualification does not always guarantee intellectual ability or a genuine wish to serve patients.

Another relatively common colonial misconception is that health officer SAO providers should be trained to a lower level, as doctors will be doing the difficult cases. Yet, the raison d'être for training health officer SAO providers is because doctors are not there, and referral and transport problems preclude safe movement of emergency patients. Therefore, anyone being trained must be able to safely handle the situation they are assigned to. Their repertoire of procedures may be smaller, but the quality of their work must remain the same.

In small LIC hospitals, the medical superintendent is often the sole medically qualified person. It is common for them to be mired in administrative functions, restricting their availability to provide clinical care. Therefore, a health officer surgeon who has performed a thousand caesarean sections may be nominally supervised by a doctor who has performed very few.

CHAMPIONS OF TASK SHIFTING

Task shifting is supported at the highest level. *DCP3: Essential Surgery states*, "task sharing has been widely demonstrated as safe and can save lives while countries make long-term investments in their workforce." It discusses the physical impossibility of expanding access to surgery at an acceptable rate if we rely solely on medically qualified providers."[3]

WHO Resolution WHA68.15 acknowledges workforce shortages and embraces task sharing. It stresses the importance of professional standards, core competencies, monitoring, evaluation and safety.[4]

The Lancet Commission on Global Surgery 2030 states: "We endorse task sharing as a means to expand the surgical workforce. We understand that in many instances task shifting is an accepted form of surgical and anaesthesia care delivery in which there otherwise would be none."[5]

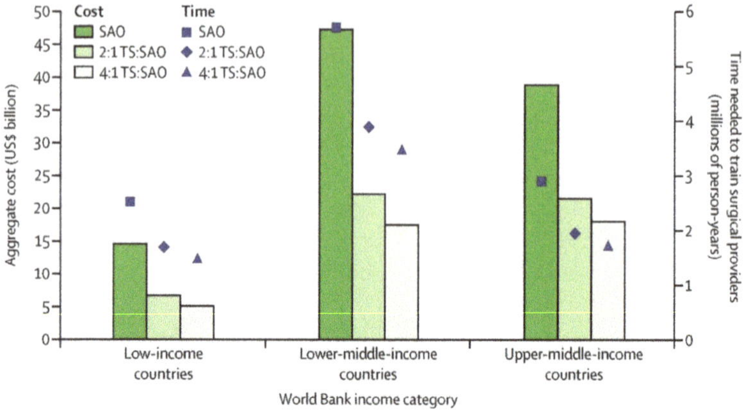

Figure 34. Cost and time required to scale up the surgical workforce: (physician) SAO-only model versus task-sharing SAO model. Reprinted from Meara, JG, Leather, AJ, Hagander, L et al. "Global Surgery 2030: Evidence and Solutions for Achieving Health, Welfare, and Economic Development." *The Lancet* 386, no. 9993 (2015): 569–624. Lancet special credit: Reprinted from *The Lancet*, Meara, JG, Leather, AJ, Hagander, L et al. 'Global Surgery" 2030: Evidence and Solutions for Achieving Health, Welfare, and Economic Development." *The Lancet* 386, no. 9993 (2015): 569–624. With permission from Elsevier.

However, it also states: "Although GPs[ii] and associate clinicians might function independently in this scenario, we believe a specialist provider should always be available to give assistance, either locally or remotely."

In many LICs, the specialist provider is not available or is not available in rural areas.

Cost and speed of upscaling

Mathematical modelling of the time and cost of upscaling — comparing scenarios where only medically qualified SAO providers are deployed with those where task sharing is implemented alongside them at 2:1 and 4:1 ratios — shows that task sharing is both quick and economical (**Figure 34**). Task sharing reduces the time taken by 40% and the cost by even more. Real-life data is also available; for example, a study in Mozambique found task sharing was three times more cost-effective than using only medically qualified SAO providers.[6]

[ii] General practitioners / primary care doctors.

TASK-SHARING OUTCOME DATA

A notable exception to the lack of quality data in LMICs is the effort to obtain quantity and quality data about surgery performed by health officers, although the number of publications is still small by Global North standards.[7] The single-handed status of many SAO providers makes randomised studies of emergency care all but impossible.

Observational and cohort data from numerous countries demonstrates that health officers and general practitioners can provide safe, skilful surgery and anaesthesia, with most studies reporting hard outcome measures, such as maternal mortality ratio (MMR).[8,9] A randomised study of elective hernia repair showed a significantly lower recurrence rate for patients operated on by health officer surgeons compared to doctors.[10]

It is possible there is publication bias, with studies reporting positive or significant outcomes more likely to be published. But the general safety, application, and quality of procedures performed by health officers is well documented. They consistently achieve outcomes comparable to or better than those of medically trained colleagues.[11,12]

It should come as no surprise to learn task shifters often become highly skilled surgeons. We know outcomes are associated with operative volume and many health officers have performed thousands of caesarean sections and hernia repairs and hundreds of emergency laparotomies. This dwarfs the number done by newly appointed consultants in HICs and, if they are clever and properly trained, we should expect good results.

There is less data available on anaesthesia, which may reflect greater acceptance of anaesthesia being performed by other cadres, or, sadly, less interest. A single study from South Africa in 2022 highlighted concerns about sedation by non-physician anaesthetists.[13] However, details about the type of sedation and providers' qualifications were unclear and the scientific rigour of the study was debated.[14]

Training of health officer SAO providers can often be of good quality. Some new programs have established clear goals and competencies at the outset, and the need to answer critics has ensured high-standard training. Sometimes the efforts invested in their training schemes were not made available to their medically qualified colleagues. For example, the health officers in the randomised hernia repair trial all derived from a single training programme that the doctors did not have access to.[15] This phenomenon explains some of the unexpected but pragmatic situations seen, whereby astute doctors seek training from health officers as they are the people with the skills.

"It gave young professionals like me the skills, confidence, and drive to serve communities through life-saving surgical care. I was proud to be part of this journey. The two-year training was intense, demanding, and transformative. It built in us strong decision-making, resilience under pressure, and a deep sense of purpose."

—Hassan Ahmad Sheriff, emergency surgical officer (Sierra Leone)

LACK OF ACCEPTANCE

In countries such as Mozambique, where health officers have been providing care for decades, there is acceptance and appreciation of the crucial role they play. Elsewhere, even when they are demonstrably providing excellent care, evidenced by measurable differences in indices such as MMR, they are still resented by some.

In fee-for-service systems, doctors may feel their income and status is threatened by new cadres who may have better training and higher surgical volumes. Over time, communities observe that certain health officers deliver more skilful and affordable care than doctors, aggravating these concerns. Given the investment doctors have made in their careers, it is understandable that some may feel threatened.

The world over, regulation has failed to keep pace with other cadres performing tasks traditionally done by doctors. In places, regulation is so inadequate that rogue providers operate unchecked for years.

Doctors may also be asked to supervise cadres with greater knowledge and skill than they have themselves. It is a testament to their professionalism that many manage this situation well, giving and receiving support with mutual respect as they struggle together to manage rural hospitals. However, the dynamic is inherently uncomfortable, and some cannot handle it. Jealousy, undermining, and badmouthing are common in certain countries, and systemic respect may be lacking.

Lack of respect towards health officer SAO providers can also come from visiting expatriate staff, particularly those with limited training or poor understanding of the local setup. They may lack insight as to why they are a doctor and the health officer with superior skill is not.[16]

LACK OF RETENTION

We have been unable to find longitudinal studies on health officer SAO provider retention. On the ground, one sees problems that often stem from a systemic lack of respect. Schemes of service and career progression are often lacking. Although health officer SAO providers may be the most knowledgeable, skilful and diligent people in their hospitals, their pay does not reflect this. Some go years without being paid, which encourages corruption as people sell their skills to survive.

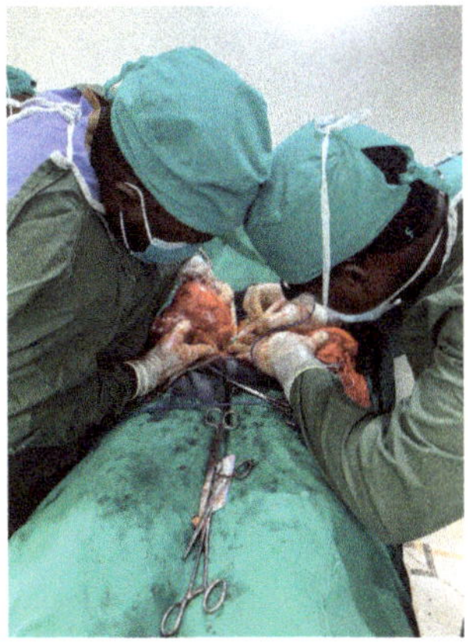

Figure 35. New Hope Hospital, Sierra Leone: Surgical Officer (R) and Doctor (L) working closely together. Photo: author's own.

Health officer SAO providers often work in remote, rural areas, where working conditions are poor and resources are inadequate. They may be the sole provider for miles around and permanently on duty, which quickly becomes wearing. Unsurprisingly, morale is often low, and housing and transport are also cited as issues.

Poor or absent supervision is common and the most important predictor of health officer SAO providers leaving their role. Given they are there because there are insufficient doctors, inadequate support should not come as surprise, but having no-one to refer to when you are stuck is terrible. Postgraduate education and opportunities to stay up to date are often unavailable or inaccessible for single-handed SAO providers who cannot take leave to attend.

> The challenges for health officer SAO providers can be so bad that highly skilled people leave the workforce for five years just to gain an MBChB. Only then are they able to fully use the knowledge and skills they already have.

There was hope, supported by some evidence, that health officer SAO providers tend to stay in underserved rural areas. Given the time-sensitive nature of their interventions, this makes their work even more effective. However, data from Malawi, Mozambique, and Tanzania show that many do leave, either to pursue further training, seek higher income, or move into less stressful work such as management or data collection.[17]

The financial gains a country can expect from training health officer SAO providers are significantly reduced if they leave. Creating an enabling environment for them should therefore be a priority for all countries with fewer than 20 SAO providers per 100,000 population, yet this this looks unlikely to happen.

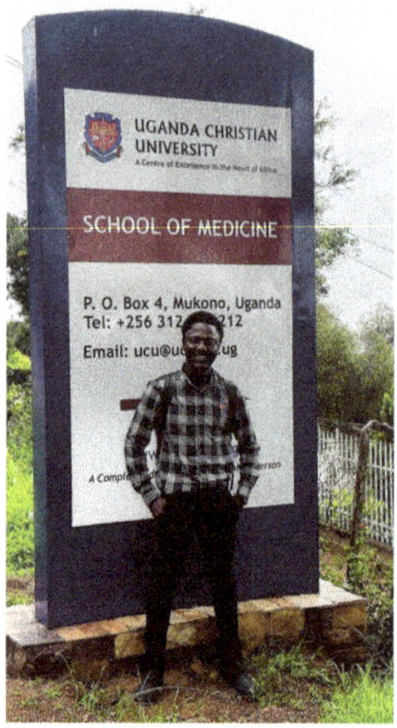

Figure 36. Anthony Abbot Kamara, Sierra Leonean health officer SAO provider, renowned for his skill as a surgical trainer, currently completing five years of medical school in Uganda. Photo: Anthony Abbot Kamara.

EXPLORE FURTHER

1. Global Health Workforce Alliance. *Task Shifting: Global Recommendations and Guidelines.* World Health Organization, 2008. https://www.who.int/workforcealliance/knowledge/resources/taskshifting_guidelines/en/.
2. World Health Organization. *Optimizing Health Worker Roles to Improve Access to Key Maternal and Newborn Health Interventions Through Task Shifting*. World Health Organization, 2012. https://iris.who.int/bitstream/handle/10665/77764/9789241504843_eng.pdf.
3. Asemu, Yohannes Molla, Etienne Nsereko, Dan Ian McIsaac, and M. Dylan Bould. “Nonphysician Sedation Providers in Africa: What Counts and What Is Being Counted?” *Anesthesia & Analgesia* 135, no. 2 (2022): 246. https://doi.org/10.1213/ANE.0000000000006037.

CHAPTER 12
RESEARCH IN GLOBAL SURGERY

ACADEMIC GLOBAL SURGERY has grown rapidly over the past 20 years (**Figure 37**). A MEDLINE search for "surgery" and "low- and middle-income" before 2008 returned only a handful of publications annually. After 2015 — the year global surgery became "a thing" — we see an abrupt rise in publications. However, before we get too excited by this explosion of interest, it's worth noting that these numbers remain

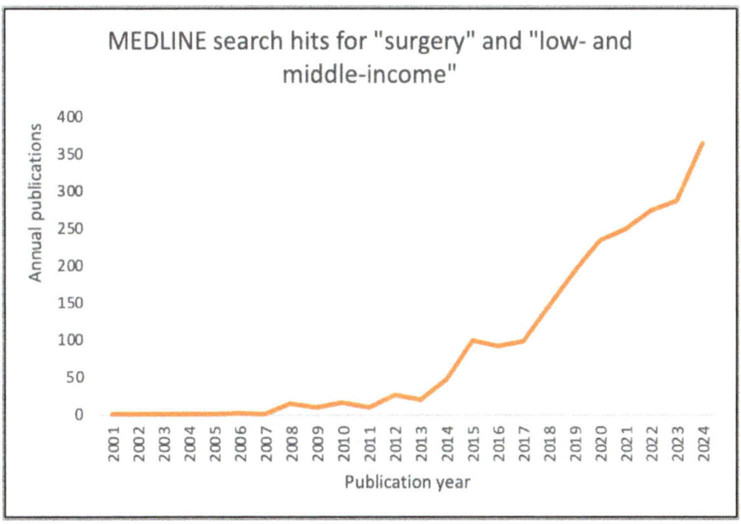

Figure 37. Number of MEDLINE search results for "surgery" in combination with "low- and middle-income countries."

an order of magnitude lower than the number of publications seen on topics of more interest to HICs. A search for "surgery" and "robotic," for example, found 4590 publications in 2024.

Research from 2005 onwards has tended to focus on system and capacity issues, increasing our understanding of global inequities and unmet need. This data was essential for informing both *DCP3: Essential Surgery* and the Lancet Commission: *Global Surgery: 2030*.

The 10-90 Gap in global health research funding:

- **10% of funding is allocated to diseases with the highest global prevalence in LMICs**
- **90% is allocated to conditions affecting populations in HICs**

Surgical research does not reflect the distribution of surgical disease. A "10/90 gap" has been described, whereby diseases rarely seen in HICs remain largely uninvestigated. Surgeons in LMICs routinely face clinical dilemmas for which there is little or no research evidence to guide them.

Even with a disease that is truly global, such as appendicitis, evidence usually focuses on the presentation and management in an HIC context. When research questions are solely framed for and tested in HICs, wider interpretation can be difficult. There is a tendency to consider findings universally applicable, when in fact they specifically apply to HICs and sometimes even favour certain racial groups, ages, or other demographics. How well do the conclusions apply in other settings?

Even if knowledge is relevant, it may not fit with the experience of those working in LMICs or be practical to implement. Hence locally applicable research and knowledge that meets the needs of those in LMICs is urgently needed.

".......it raises the question whether we should repair the (typhoid) perforation or treat such patients with a stoma. To answer this question, I am leading a 5-year audit ....hoping to come up with locally evidence-based answers."

—Darwin Nyirenda, surgical resident (Malawi)

SYSTEMIC PROBLEMS

This systemic bias is not just a surgical problem. There are profound problems in global health research generally. The academic knowledge system is heavily weighted to benefit HICs. Biases exist throughout the system, from generating ideas, obtaining funding and knowledge production, right through to publication, dissemination of knowledge and its application.

LMICs often lack research capacity, training and infrastructure, leading to the assumption that they cannot contribute as primary or equal partners. Outsiders feel they must come in and carry out research for them, with the expatriates who hold the funding dictating the research questions.

Knowledge systems and medical publishing are not immune to the structural prejudices and biases affecting all of society.

This mirrors the surgical camp model of service delivery: keeping the skills and resources in the hands of those from HICs. Surgical teams in LMICs become the passive recipients, or even the subject matter. Less credibility may be given to the knowledge of those in LMICs, as racism and colonialism make it difficult to learn from people deemed "lesser" and in need of help. In global health research, this is described as "epistemic injustice."[1]

EXPLOITATION

There may also be outright exploitation. Doctors in HICs, under pressure to publish for career advancement, may see LMICs as an untapped and potentially uncontrolled resource that they can benefit from. Properly conducted studies benefit everyone, but a lack of oversight and due process can allow unethical practices to develop. For example, an (unpublished) observational study on blood-borne virus prevalence in obstetric patients with no funding to help positive patients access care, so the impoverished, illiterate participants were not told their results.

The Belmont Report was issued in 1979 following revelations about the notorious Tuskegee syphilis study, in which disadvantaged rural, black participants were not told their results or offered treatment. It outlines three ethical principles that are still not always followed by global health researchers:[2]

1. **Respect for persons:** Demands that subjects enter research voluntarily with adequate information. If study subjects are impoverished, uneducated, or speak different languages, the same duty of care still applies and great lengths and inventive

solutions must be found to fully inform them, whatever the financial implications. It is not sufficient to just obtain consent; researchers must be certain participants have understood and are able to say "no."

2. **Beneficence**: Researchers must not only protect participants from harm but also make every effort to secure their wellbeing and maximise possible benefits to them.
3. **Justice**: Demands fairness in the distribution of benefits and burdens; an injustice is considered to have occurred when a participant is denied a benefit they are entitled to.

"There are significant ethical issues regarding research and medical trials conducted in Africa. Local populations have sometimes been used as human subjects without informed consent, raising serious concerns about exploitation."

—Anthony Abbot Kamara, surgical officer (Sierra Leone and Uganda)

GLOBAL HEALTH RESEARCH PARTNERSHIPS

Significant power and resource mismatches can make for iniquitous working relationships. Global North countries often provide the funding and technical, educational, logistic and even human resources. Because the North holds the resources, they hold the power, choosing the subject and where and when the study is conducted. In this situation, it is easy to see how negative consequences can outweigh any beneficial research outcome.

Thankfully, examples like the one above are few and far between, and there is increasing recognition that entrenched colonial attitudes and power imbalances have regularly resulted in accidental, suboptimal research practices; exploitation; failure to credit the efforts of local staff; and authorship malpractice.

Good partnerships actively consider how power dynamics favour certain interests and voices and marginalise others, especially the already disadvantaged.

This recognition has led to the development of both new research partnerships and more formal establishment of existing looser arrangements. A global health research partnership is any global health research project which involves collaboration between individuals or institutions in two or more countries. This usually involves at least one party from the Global North i.e. a HIC and a partner or partners from the Global South, i.e. an LMIC.

Good partnerships jointly agree on the research agenda and share the benefits of research equally, always guided by principles of fairness, equity, and justice.

> **"Identifying publishing gaps which are already known but may not have been systematically documented due to low research capacity in LMICs is not enough. Collaborators must adopt implementation research methods that ultimately lead to tangible change in the areas needed to make the greatest impact in LMICs."**
>
> **—Antia Eseenam Agbeko, vascular surgeon and deputy director, NIHR Research Hub (Ghana)**

The National Institute for Health and Care Research (NIHR) Equal Partnerships Guide

The UK's NIHR funds considerable global surgery research. Similar bodies operate in other countries, but we mention it as an example. Their online *Equal Partnerships Guide* describes the causes of inequity, explains how partnerships can be made as equal as possible (albeit still usually structurally unequal), and offers links to other insightful resources.[i]

NIHR Global Health Research Unit on Global Surgery

The NIHR Global Health Research Unit on Global Surgery (GSU) has been successful in building local research capacity in LMICs, via education, funding and genuine collaboration.[ii]

By training local research leads and funding capacity building, GSU brings surgeons, researchers, and policymakers together to set local research agendas. Its Delphi projects prioritise research topics and address the mismatch between clinical guidelines developed in HICs and LMIC realities.

The GSU's studies therefore focus on specific clinical concerns in LMICs. The best-known are the FALCON and ChEETah trials, conducted across seven LMICs (see text boxes).[3,4] These demonstrate

i NIHR Equitable Partnerships Guide: https://www.nihr.ac.uk/equitable-partnerships-guide

ii NIHR Global Health Research Unit on Global Surgery: https://www.globalsurgeryunit.org/

that, by growing local research expertise, large-scale trials into clinical problems affecting surgical teams in LMICs are perfectly possible. In fact, both studies completed *ahead* of schedule.

FALCON

- Surgical Site Infection reduction strategies in LMICs
- Largest RCT in surgical history
- No benefit for triclosan-coated sutures
- No benefit for 2% alcoholic chlorhexidine vs. 10% povidone–iodine in clean-contaminated, contaminated, or dirty wounds

ChEETah

- Largest cluster RCT in surgical history
- Found routine change of gloves and instruments before abdominal wound closure reduces Surgical Site Infection in LMICs

GlobalSurg is a collaborative network of more than 5,000 clinicians across over 100 countries that conducts research via open, grassroots cohort studies involving short, defined periods of collaborative data collection on surgical issues.[iii] Collaborators submit their own patient data via an online portal. Outcomes are published with all contributors receiving PubMed-citable attribution.

Lip-service

Most organisations are now genuinely trying to address the transgressions of the past. However, concerns remain that some merely pay lip service to the idea of partnership. Desmond Jumbam's biting satire "How (Not) to Write About Global Health," published in *BMJ Global Health* in 2020, calls out "partnerships" in which the lion's share of work is conducted locally while the vast majority of credit goes to the HIC researchers.[5] There are even cases where HIC researchers expose LMIC partners to risks and fail to recognise this. For example, data collectors travelling to remote sites by motorbike, while HIC partners use four-wheel drive vehicles.

AUTHORSHIP

Authorship is rightly contentious. HIC partners have typically taken the key authorship positions, regardless of the actual workload. The sense

iii GlobalSurg: https://globalsurg.org

of entitlement some expatriates feel about owning the spoils of research in LMICs can lead to extraordinary behaviour. An expatriate doctor once blocked research addressing a significant local need at the hospital where he worked after potential collaborators explained they could not agree to parachute him in as automatic first author on all publications. Despite his short-term position at the facility, he felt its resources were his and placed personal gain above the needs of a deprived population.

Recent analyses confirm that HIC-affiliated researchers — often male and of high seniority — dominate senior authorship in global surgery studies.[6] Gift authorship of HIC colleagues and inadequate recognition for LMIC investigators remain widespread. Gender and regional inequity are significant, especially in collaborative work where HIC researchers set publication terms.

ACADEMIC INSTITUTIONS INVOLVED IN GLOBAL SURGERY

Many academic institutions are involved in global surgery. The following English-speaking examples provide a reference point, but do search for similar activity at your local institutions (**Table 9**).

And many more

In addition to academic units, individuals and small groups often lead projects and collaborations. To get involved or learn more, try searching online for your local organisations, centres, or initiatives related to global surgery — many publish updates, calls for collaboration, and details of ongoing work on their websites or social media channels.

SPENDING CUTS

Global health research currently faces severe threats from government funding cuts in the UK, US, and other countries. Beyond the humanitarian impact, these cuts are likely to represent poor value for the global economy, as the burden of untreated disease is a drain on economies.

On 25th February 2025, the UK cut overseas aid to its lowest level as a percentage of national income since records began.

Institution	Country	Activities / Focus	Website
Blavatnik Institute Global Health and Social Medicine (Harvard)	USA	Program for Global Surgery and Social Change; surgical systems, advocacy, capacity building, fellowships	https://www.pgssc.org/
Global Academic Surgery Committee (Society of University Surgeons)	USA	Promotes global surgical care and education, sets guidance, international partnerships	https://www.susweb.org/
Stanford University Centre of Innovation in Global Health (CIGH)	USA	Collaborations, observer programme, bidirectional, sustainable partnerships, training in research	https://surgery.stanford.edu/about/global-surgery.html
King's Global Health Institute (King's College London)	UK	Primary research, policy, cost-effectiveness, partnerships (Sierra Leone, Somaliland, DRC)	https://www.kcl.ac.uk/kghi
NIHR Global Health Research Unit on Global Surgery (Birmingham)	UK	Hubs in Mexico, India, Nigeria, Ghana, Rwanda, South Africa, Benin; multicentre RCTs, cohort studies, audits, education, infrastructure empowering partners to design and deliver research	https://www.globalsurgeryunit.org/global-surgery-our-teams/university-of-birmingham/
Edinburgh University (GSU Principal Partner)	UK	Data-driven research, leadership, education, scholarships for postgrad LMIC students	https://www.globalsurgeryunit.org/global-surgery-our-teams/university-of-edinburgh/
Oxford University Global Surgery Group (OUGSG)	UK	Clinical, research and educational support for underserved, capacity building for LMICs, advocacy	https://www.globalsurgery.ox.ac.uk/

Table 9. Examples of anglophone academic institutions involved in global surgery. DRC, Democratic Republic of the Congo.

EXPLORE FURTHER

1. The NIHR Global Health Research Unit on Global Surgery (GSU). https://www.globalsurgeryunit.org/global-surgery-about-us/. — *Extensive educational materials and training opportunities for global surgery research.*
2. U.S. Department of Health, Education, and Welfare. *The Belmont Report: Ethical Principles and Guidelines for the Protection of Human Subjects of Research.* April 1979. https://www.hhs.gov/ohrp/sites/default/files/the-belmont-report-508c_FINAL.pdf.
3. National Institute for Health Research. *Equitable Research Partnership Guide.* Version 1.1, March 2021. Published May 1, 2020. https://www.nihr.ac.uk/equitable-partnerships-guide.
4. Jumbam, Desmond T. "How (Not) to Write about Global Health." *BMJ Global Health* 5, no. 7 (2020). https://doi.org/10.1136/bmjgh-2020-003164.

CHAPTER 13
INNOVATION IN GLOBAL SURGERY

by Vijna Boodhoo, Noel Aruparayil and Lesley Hunt

NECESSITY IS the mother of invention, and low-resource environments are a hotbed of innovation, as enterprising teams adapt to deliver care despite equipment and financial constraints.

FRUGAL AND REVERSE INNOVATION

Frugal innovation maximises the ratio of value to resources, "doing more with less, then evaluating, and scaling up." Reverse innovation refers to any innovation that is first adopted in the Global South; the "reverse" label is an ethnocentric and potentially patronising term.

CONTEXT-SPECIFIC AND USER-CENTRED INNOVATION

Teams in the Global South are drawn to medical technology from HICs. However, devices designed and tested in HICs may fail when transplanted or donated to LMICs ending up in equipment graveyards.

Innovations are more likely to succeed if they are context-specific and user-centred. Co-developed innovations therefore work better than imposed ones. Engaging users from the start of the innovation cycle, understanding their unique realities, barriers, and facilitators ensures innovation responds to need. Local stakeholders are best placed to identify and organise any training needed, and to collaborate with maintenance staff and engineers, driving local production of parts and, ideally, the device itself.

Devices specifically designed for low-resource settings address explicit needs, avoid consumables, and minimise maintenance and repair. Lifebox® pulse oximeters and headlights are good examples; they put their success down to design that focuses on core functions, minimum standards, durability, and affordability (see chapter 9, page 94).[i]

> **"*Jugaad* — the Indian art of inventing out of nothing, just to get on with life."**
>
> **—Sushil Maslekar**

AFFORDABILITY

Extreme affordability is essential. Surgeons in ultra-low resource settings prepare autologous blood for transfusion by filtering it through surgical gauze. Commercial low-tech autologous transfusion devices exclude air and achieve better filtration but, although a fraction of the cost of HIC systems, still cost $200 per use and effectively price themselves out of the market they are trying to help.

LOOKING AT THE WORLD DIFFERENTLY

The dominance of Global North perspectives is restrictive and great innovations don't necessarily come from new technology; they also arise from looking at the world differently. The example, par excellence, is low-cost hernia mesh. Commercial mesh is beyond the budget of most patients in LICs. Inspired by a colleague, rural Indian surgeon Dr Ravi Tongaonkar pioneered mesh made using the processes used in mosquito net manufacturing, rather than those used to make medical devices. He then tirelessly pursued rigorous scientific

> **The Aravind Eye Care System delivers affordable, high-quality eye care using an assembly line model boosting surgical productivity tenfold. Surgeons perform six to eight operations per hour. All patients receive equal high-quality care. Half are treated for free or at minimal cost. The in-house Aurolab manufactures lenses at 2.5% of import prices, improving access for all.**

i https://www.lifebox.org/

testing, and the product's non-inferiority has since been widely demonstrated in LICs.[1,2]

The Association of Rural Surgeons of India (ARSI) Karad Consensus encourages rural innovators in India to partner with academic institutions to formally study, publicise, and scale up their cost-saving and quality-improving innovations.[3] Gasless laparoscopy, for example, gained wider implementation thanks to ARSI and the rural surgeons of India.[4]

"I invariably returned humbled, inspired, and educated by the versatility, innovation, and dedication of rural surgeons....The steel of the rural surgeon is tempered in the furnace of want, deprivation, and necessity, and these have inculcated in them the strength and qualities of ingenuity, innovation, courage, and determination to face and meet all odds."

—T.E. Udwadia, "Father of Laparoscopic Surgery in India"

"LEAPFROGGING"

This is where intermediary technologies are effectively "skipped." For example, LICs skipped the landline phase of telecommunications and went straight to mobile services, which are quicker and cheaper to set up. Secure, user-friendly platforms then rapidly took off because they solved a need. Telemedicine, once cumbersome and requiring travel to a facility, can now be undertaken by anyone with a smartphone, even while the patient is on the operating table.

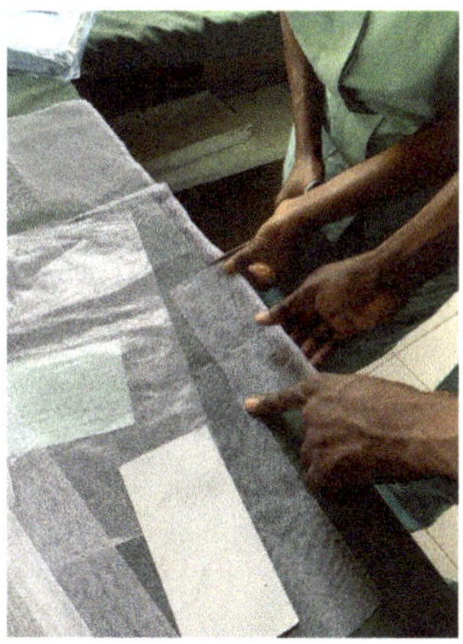

Figure 38. Dr Ravi's mesh being prepared at Hatfield Archer Memorial Hospital, Sierra Leone, as part of the SWIFTSS (Surgical teams Working in aFrica Together for Safer Surgery) Affordable Mesh Hernia Initiative. An example of South-on-South development. Photo: author's own.

Hospitals struggling with unreliable electricity and high fuel costs are bypassing fossil fuels and jumping directly to alternative energy. As hospitals in HICs transition to electronic patient records after decades of using reliable paper systems, facilities in LMICs struggling to establish retrievable paper systems move directly to electronic records.

.... AND "PIGGY BACKING"

Digital advances allow medical systems to integrate with generic consumer devices. For example, ultrasound probes, cystoscopes, capnographs, and vision testing equipment link to laptops, tablets, and mobiles, removing the need for expensive bespoke stacks requiring separate maintenance.

INNOVATION IS MORE THAN JUST "STUFF"

Innovation can be misconstrued as referring solely to devices, but improving access to surgery also requires creative solutions in education, training, financing, infrastructure, health systems, and service delivery. The critical shortage of surgical, anaesthesia, and obstetric (SAO) providers in LMICs has led to innovation in education and training.

Three-dimensional printed simulation models are heralded as great value in LMICs. But, in practice, their effectiveness depends on the quality of the accompanying tuition, making them unlikely to be more useful than models produced by other means. On the other hand, some low-cost models, such as the LaApSi appendicectomy trainer, harness the power of computerised learning to provide trainees with continuous formative feedback, enabling meaningful learning, even at a distance from the trainer.[5]

Virtual reality has struggled to find a role in SAO training in LMICs. But with advances in AI-supported surgical safety, this is likely to change. Cheap models, programs and devices rely on the willingness of inventors to part with their intellectual property free of charge.

The uneven power dynamic between a HIC trainer and the LMIC trainee can make evaluation of innovative training challenging, as feedback is likely to be positive even when sustained learning is unproven.

EVIDENCE-BASED INNOVATION

Efficacy and safety evaluation underpin good innovation and are most effective when conducted throughout the innovation process. Because innovators and users in LMICs often lack the research capacity to generate such evidence, building that capacity is essential, as

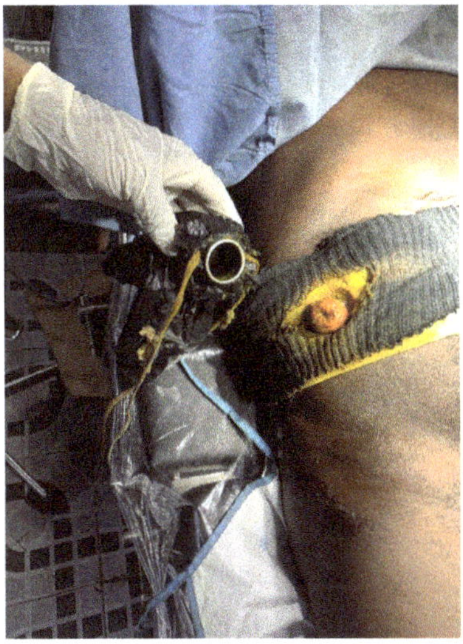

Figure 39. Sierra Leone. It is not just the staff who are innovative! We thought this petrol cap and foam stoma bag was good, until we saw Figure 40. Photo: author's own.

publication plays a critical role in disseminating successful innovations and securing their implementation funding. The IDEAL (Idea, Development, Exploration, Assessment, and Long-term study) framework is a standard for evaluating innovations, but it can be problematic in LMICs, and modifications have been proposed to ensure that evaluation is context specific.[6]

REGULATORY CHALLENGES

Regulation is complex and LMICs may lack regulatory frameworks or use frameworks descended from those in HICs. This can be problematic, especially in countries where access to essential surgery is unevenly distributed. Well-resourced areas want to follow gold standards, which can inadvertently block pragmatic care for their poor neighbours.

The ARSI Karad Consensus highlights creative workarounds and novel innovations by rural surgical teams, which make surgery possible despite severe constraints in infrastructure.[7] However, even after proving effective in low-resource settings, lifesaving innovations can be blocked by regulations shaped by HIC standards. For example,

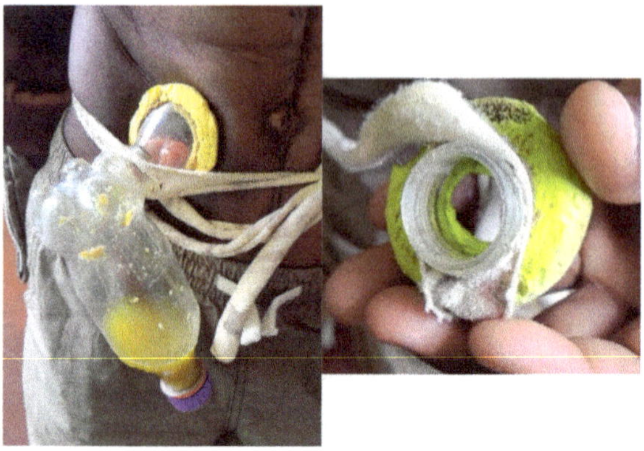

Figure 40. Malawi: This is extremely clever. It is challenging to get a seal and the inset photo shows how this was achieved. Photo: Dominik von Malsen.

Unbanked Directed Blood Transfusion (UDBT) is prohibited in India, posing a threat to the lives of people in impoverished areas where there is no blood bank.

SUPPORT FOR INNOVATORS

The Innovation in Global Surgery (IGS) group identifies needs, conducts research, and develops context-appropriate solutions for low-resource settings. Its biennial International Congress (ICIGS) allows multidisciplinary collaboration to promote surgical innovation. [ii] The World Health Organization (WHO) also provides generic support for healthcare innovation, as outlined on its WHO Innovation Hub. [iii]

Innovation hackathons have become popular, bringing together clinicians and engineers to generate low-cost innovations. Diverse teams of clinicians and engineers intensively tackle defined healthcare problems over one or two days, with the aim of developing prototype devices. They are often convened by trainee and medical student groups, who are likely to be freer of entrenched concepts and can hopefully provide fresh eyes on old problems.

---

ii https://www.surgicalinnovations.org/

iii WHO Innovation Hub: https://www.who.int/teams/digital-health-and-innovation/who-innovation-hub

INNOVATIVE FINANCING

> **"…. working as a scrub technician in high school, I observed failed attempts to surgically remove thrombus. I came up with my first design in my senior year of college. During medical school, I built some prototypes using the tip of a No. 5 latex surgical glove and a urethral catheter."**
>
> **—Thomas Fogarty, surgeon and inventor of the Fogarty catheter**

The control and treatment of communicable diseases, particularly HIV/AIDS, were partially funded by innovative financing solutions, and global surgery has also started to attract financial innovators. WHO's Unitaid was established in 2006 to create a better market to buy necessary drugs at scale and is funded by a small levy on airline tickets.[iv] This levy — still collected by Cameroon, Chile, Congo, France, Madagascar, Mali, Mauritius, Niger, and South Korea — raises about €160 million a year.[v]

In 2006, musician Bono and US activist Bobby Shriver started RED. When customers purchase RED-branded products, a corporate contribution is activated for the Global Fund, creating money and publicity. As of 2025, RED has raised US$785 million.[vi]

Several governments and the Gates Foundation fund the Advance Market Commitment (AMC), which incentivises manufacturers to develop vaccines specifically for LMICs by guaranteeing the price and quantity of an initial purchase.[vii]

NARROW THE GAP

We can no more invent our way out of the crisis in global surgery than we can operate our way out of it. However, innovation can narrow the gap faster than just relying on the "trickle-down" of existing methods from rich to poor countries. The most inspiring innovators are in the Global South.

[iv] "Unitaid" stands for "Everyone united to help," derived from the French phrase ,"*tous unis pour aider.*"

[v] Unitaid: https://unitaid.org/

[vi] RED and ONE Campaign: https://www.red.org/

[vii] GAVI — the vaccine alliance: https://www.gavi.org/?gad_source=1&gclid=EAIaIQobChMIpc_BhNTFjAMVQtkWBR1f_BvxEAAYASAAEgLpNvD_BwE

EXPLORE FURTHER

1. WHO Innovation Hub. World Health Organization (2025). WHO Innovation hub. [online] www.who.int. https://www.who.int/teams/digital-health-and-innovation/who-innovation-hub.
2. GASOC courses. Global Anaesthesia Surgery Obstetric Collaboration (GASOC) Global Frugal Innovation Skills course. https://www.gasocuk.co.uk/innovation-course.
3. The Aravind Eye Care System: Innovation in the Delivery of Care. https://aravind.org/
4. Global Surgery Student Alliance Hackathon Toolkit. https://www.globalsurgerystudents.org/toolkits.

CHAPTER 14
NATIONAL SURGICAL, OBSTETRIC AND ANAESTHESIA PLANS (NSOAPS)

BY THIS STAGE, we hope readers are convinced of both the need for LMICs to scale up surgery and the gains they can achieve by doing so.

National Surgical, Obstetric and Anaesthesia Plans (NSOAPs) offer a logical way to achieve this, and if countries want to up-scale quickly, an NSOAP is an absolute prerequisite. Clear identification of workforce and infrastructure gaps should enable efficient deployment of trainers and capacity building. Good NSOAPs also provide accountability for both money and quality of care. This transparency encourages partnership with HIC institutions and funders.

A concerted effort by all stakeholders is required, including the ministry of health, professional societies, individual healthcare providers, and the private sector. The process of producing an NSOAP serves to bring these bodies together. NSOAPs are locally owned, country-specific, and part of a national health strategy.

The World Health Organization (WHO) likes a toolkit and, starting in 2009, it published the *Integrated Management for Emergency and Essential Surgical Care* (IMEESC) eLearning toolkit.[i] This provides information for policymakers, managers, and service providers and sets minimum standards for emergency surgery, obstetrics, and anaesthesia at district hospital level.

---

[i] WHO IMEESC toolkit https://www.who.int/publications/i/item/integrated-management-for-emergency-and-surgical-care-(-imeesc)-toolkit

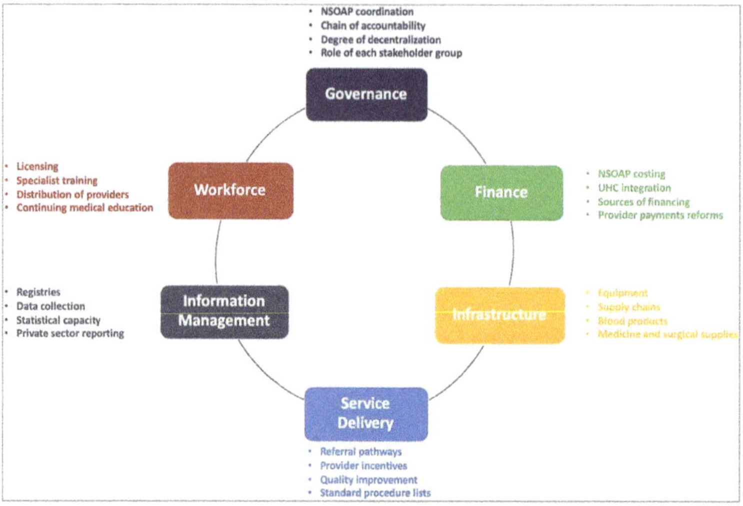

Figure 41. The six domains of NSOAPs. NSOAP, National Surgical, Obstetric and Anaesthesia Plan. UHC, Universal Health Coverage. Adapted from: Reddy CL, Peters AW, Jumbam DT et al. "Innovative financing to fund surgical systems and expand surgical care in low-income and middle-income countries." *BMJ Global Health* 2020;5:e002375. doi:10.1136/bmjgh-2020-002375. Adapted from Citron et al. Can J Anesth 66, 263–271 (2019). https://doi.org/10.1007/s12630-018-01269-5. Creative Commons CC-BY-NC 4.0 Licence 6115310947922.

In partnership with the Harvard Medical School Program in Global Surgery and Social Change (PGSSC), WHO released *Surgical Care Systems Strengthening: Developing National Surgical, Obstetric and Anaesthesia Plans* in 2017.[1] This publication sets out a three-step process for NSOAP design and provides case studies and feedback from countries already developing them.

THE SIX DOMAINS AND THREE STEPS OF NSOAPS

NSOAPs have six strategic domains: governance, finance, infrastructure, service delivery, information management and workforce (**Figure 41**). Assessment of the six domains can be broken down into three steps:

Step 1 Establishing the baseline

Effective NSOAPs are data-driven and clearly describe current service and knowledge gaps in the country. Data can be collected against the Lancet Commission on Global Surgery's (LCoGS) six core indicators (see chapter 7, page 57). This baseline assessment should also include a plan for ongoing monitoring during implementation.

Step 2 Facility assessments

Ideally, countries would assess all healthcare facilities, but financial constraints usually prevent this. NSOAPs therefore use systematic sampling, focusing on the readiness of district hospitals to provide safe surgery. Facility assessments can be conducted using the WHO/PGSSC Surgical Assessment Tool (SAT), which examines infrastructure, workforce, service delivery, information management, and financing. [ii]

Step 3 National planning

Stakeholder engagement and consensus-building establish a set of goals and measurable targets. These are written into a formal national plan, establishing a strategic framework for surgical development as part of national health policy. Goals and targets should cover five domains: infrastructure, workforce, service delivery, information management, and finance.

WHO and PGSSC's *Surgical Care Systems Strengthening* report provides practical case studies from countries that have launched NSOAPs.[2] PGSSC also maintains a database tracking the progress of plans in nearly 50 countries.[iii]

A few examples of NSOAPs are presented here.

ZAMBIA

A 2010 Ministry of Health audit showed that Zambia would not achieve its infant and maternal mortality Millennium Development Goals (MDGs).[3,4] The primary barrier was lack of access to essential surgery at district hospitals; three-quarters of Zambians could not access timely, safe and affordable surgical care. Women died for lack of caesarean section. The Zambian delegation led negotiations that culminated in the adoption of WHA 68.15, committing UN member states to upscaling surgery. Zambia then developed the first ever NSOAP, which

---

ii WHO/PGSSC Surgical Assessment Tool (SAT): https://cdn.who.int/media/docs/default-source/integrated-health-services-(ihs)/csy/surgical-care/who_surgical_assessment_tool.pdf?sfvrsn=739788e4_7

iii PGSSC tools for NSOAPs examples and dashboard: https://www.pgssc.org/national-surgical-planning

was signed off in 2017 and included in the National Development Plan to coordinate funding and policy.

District hospitals were found to be suffering from a lack of equipment (stuff) and surgical workforce (staff). The ambitious plan aimed to increase the national SAO workforce from 1.1 to 3 per 100,000 population by 2021.

ETHIOPIA

In 2015, Ethiopia had insufficient SAO providers, weak supply chains, and lacked surgical leadership and monitoring. Surgical hospitals had terrible infrastructure: 72% had no running water, 59% had intermittent electricity, and only 33% had a reliable oxygen supply. Using the authority provided by WHA 68.15, the Federal Ministry of Health developed the *Saving Lives Through Safe Surgery* (SaLTS) initiative, a national surgical planning effort, with a *National Surgical Workforce Expansion Plan and Anaesthesia Roadmap.*

A clear financial plan attracted implementation funds from key HIC partners, with funding to build and renovate operating theatres, build oxygen plants, and train biomedical engineers. A national structure was established to collect 15 hospital-level performance indicators. SaLTS was formally launched by the Ministry of Health in 2016.[iv]

BRAZIL

Facility assessments are particularly important where access to surgery is unevenly distributed. SAO workforce density was 48 per 100,000 in Southeast Brazil, but only 11 in parts of Amazonas. Seventy-five percent of Brazil's 95,169 SAO providers are concentrated in the largest cities, where less than half of the population lives.

A forward-looking medical team undertook targeted assessments in poorly served regions, establishing whether minimum standards were being met and identifying the barriers to meeting them. They found a lack of manpower and infrastructure, and profound travel barriers that often made free healthcare inaccessible.[5]

[iv] Saving Lives Through Safe Surgery (SALTS) Ethiopia: https://www.moh.gov.et/en/initiatives-4-col/Saving_Lives_Through_Safe_Surgery

THE SOUTH PACIFIC REGION

The South Pacific region is diverse, with rich countries alongside poorer neighbours and small island states. In October 2015, an international symposium organised by the Royal Australasian College of Surgeons (RACS) responded to WHA 68.15 and the LCoGS.[6] All countries present agreed to prioritise access to safe, affordable surgical and anaesthetic care, and a collaborative working group with representatives from 18 countries was established, meeting by teleconference.

Fourteen countries began data collection and data mining. Australia, New Zealand and five other countries reached the target of two-hour Bellwether access for 80% of the population, while in Papua New Guinea and the Solomon Islands, only 20% of the population could reach care in two hours.[7] There was huge variation in surgical volume, with seven South Pacific countries performing less than 1600 procedures per 100,000 population annually. Only four countries had achieved the LCoGS benchmark of at least twenty SAO workforce per 100,000 population with Timor-Leste having only 0.9.

The South Pacific region has achieved impressive data collection, highlighted many of the difficulties and discrepancies associated with this process, and made a clear plan.

NIGERIA

Nigeria identified a shortage of SAO providers, with only 1 per 100,000 population, and paediatric surgeons in especially short supply.[8] Surgical volume was low, and two-thirds of Nigerians were found to be exposed to the risk of impoverishing or catastrophic expenditure from surgery. Although most Nigerians could reach a hospital within two hours, the staff and stuff to provide essential surgery was not necessarily there.

A Nigerian National Surgical, Obstetrics, Anaesthesia & Nursing Plan (NSOANP), known as the *Strategic Priorities for Surgical Care* (StraPS) was created in 2018.[9] Between 2019 and 2023, they planned to:

- Expand surgical care to cover 75% of the population and 50% of children
- Increase SAO providers to 5/100,000 population
- Increase the density of paediatric surgeons to 0.25/100,000 children

- Double surgical volume
- Train family physicians and general duty doctors to provide Bellwether Procedures and the Essential Paediatric Surgery Package
- Train general duty doctors and diplomates to provide anaesthesia at secondary and primary level hospitals and improve the nurse anaesthetist service

StraPS implementation was projected to cost about US$16 billion, with transparent monitoring and integration into the national strategic health plan.

RWANDA

By 2017, Rwanda was the first country to complete baseline assessments of every district hospital.[10] It will come as no surprise to learn that they found a gap in workforce and training. Their NSOAP focuses on expanding specialist, non-specialist, non-physician and ancillary SAO providers. The structure of the Rwandan plan helps us understand the key domains of NSOAPs: infrastructure, service delivery, workforce, information management, finance, and governance (Figure 41).

Infrastructure

Rwanda has an adequate geographic distribution of hospitals; almost 100% of the population lives within two hours of a hospital that ought to be capable of Bellwether Procedures. However, in practice, many operating theatres were not working. A key priority was renovating operating theatres to ensure reliable lighting, electricity, water, sterilisation, operating tables, and essential operating and anaesthetic equipment — alongside improvements in pharmacy, laboratory, blood bank, radiology, and the supply chain.

Service delivery

In 2017, surgical volume was 786 procedures per 100,000 population at district hospital level, but only a quarter of these performed Bellwether Procedures. Rwanda proposed that each district and provincial hospital should have one surgeon, one obstetrician, and one anaesthetist. Quality of care was to be improved through monitoring, WHO Safe Surgery and standardisation.

. . .

Workforce

Surgical workforce shortage was assessed to be the biggest problem; in 2017, there was one provider per 100,000 population. At district level, only 25 SAO providers served 42 hospitals. The NSOAP's top priority was training SAO providers of diverse cadres to proficiency with the bellwether and other essential procedures. Retention strategies included financial and other incentives for serving in district hospitals and attractive packages for graduating residents to practise in rural settings.

Information management

The NSOAP included regular data collection against the six LCoGS indicators, a longer set of indicators for the entire plan and registration and monitoring of all SAO providers. Developing research capacity was also prioritised.

Finance

Although most of the population had some form of health coverage, there were substantial out-of-pocket (OOP) costs for patients having surgery. The 2017 NSOAP proposed to increase Ministry of Health funding for surgical and obstetric care at district hospitals and build partnerships with overseas organisations to support NSOAP implementation.

Governance

To ensure accountability and progress, the priorities of the NSOAP and related hospital initiatives were to be shared with all staff, with a designated local person responsible at each facility. A national coordinator was to oversee provincial committees and the domains of the plan. The total cost for the Rwandan NSOAP was estimated at US$70 million spread over 5 years.

SUMMARY

The examples above show that, although NSOAPs are tailored to an individual country's needs, the similarities outweigh the differences. The king of all needs is a shortage of trained SAO providers, closely followed by infrastructure problems. If done well, context-specific, locally driven, well-resourced, measurably tracked, equitably implemented, and flexibly managed NSOAPs can be invaluable for scaling up surgery. Achieving this requires honesty in addressing problems and a strong commitment from both national governments and international partners.

NSOAP STAKEHOLDERS

We use the term "NSOAP stakeholders." Who are they and what are their roles?

Healthcare workers on the ground are the most important. Good NSOAPs include them from the outset, as strong local engagement is critical. In some countries, the SAO providers themselves are the ones who trigger the NSOAP process.

Professional societies, such as surgical, obstetric, anaesthesia, and nursing associations, are natural advocates and champions for NSOAPs. However, in the most surgically deprived parts of the world, these societies are new, underfunded, or non-existent. In the example above, RACS advocated to help its poorer South Pacific neighbours. Similarly, the College of Surgeons of East, Central and Southern Africa (COSECSA) has influenced health ministries in its region to prioritise surgical planning.

Without national ministry of health engagement, NSOAPs will never be incorporated into national health policy and are doomed to fail. Ministries of health and finance should be involved from the get-go, as NSOAPs compete for money with other services. If surgery is to be prioritised, national ministries need to provide proper leadership to the process and be heavily involved with data collection and monitoring.

WHO is charged with supporting and channelling efforts beyond the mandate of WHA 68.15, facilitating global and regional partnerships, and supporting ministries with data collection and reporting. It sets priorities for funding organisations and, by supporting NSOAPs, helps countries obtain external funding. The World Bank also supports and shares data collection.

Partnerships with the private sector, not-for-profits, donor organisations, foundations, and industry are all required for successful NSOAPs. Partners provide technical support, human resources, and money, with international organisations playing a key role. For example, Harvard's PGSSC provides intellectual resources and practical backing for many countries,[v] while the Global Surgery Foundation has instruction manuals, videos, and information, and works with groups and governments wishing to develop NSOAPs.[11]

CHALLENGES

NSOAPs present challenges for funders because surgical systems require wide-ranging, medium-term investment. Funding projects that promote integration of surgical, obstetric, and anaesthesia care into stronger health systems may not be as immediately attractive to donors as camps fixing cleft lips.

NSOAP planning is gaining momentum worldwide, but having a plan does not guarantee implementation. There is the concept of "shelf documents," where the necessary steps are taken to please external stakeholders, but without real commitment to change.

Unfortunately, it appears many NSOAPs are at high risk of becoming shelf documents. Reference may be made to NSOAPs being implemented, in some countries, yet those on the ground see nothing happening.

Our intention was to write a few paragraphs about the results beginning to accrue from some of the earlier NSOAPs, but internet and medical literature searches show precious little so far. Tanzania has been able to describe improvement in the physical status of its primary health facilities and compliance with some safe surgery practice.[12]

Money is the obvious barrier. Although the budgets needed are substantial, they represent good value when viewed on a per-capita, per-year basis, and are unlikely to be prohibitive if there is genuine will to make it work. For example, when the Tanzanian NSOAP was developed in 2018, the cost of implementation over seven years was estimated at US$600 million, which is only US$1.7 per capita per year (**Figure 42**).[13]

Implementation of the first ever NSOAP in Zambia has been slow. A new strategy to leverage funding to support surgery into existing health programmes, at cross-cutting points, is now being tried, and pilot programmes are underway to generate evidence of impact and cost-effectiveness.

---

[v] https://www.pgssc.org/

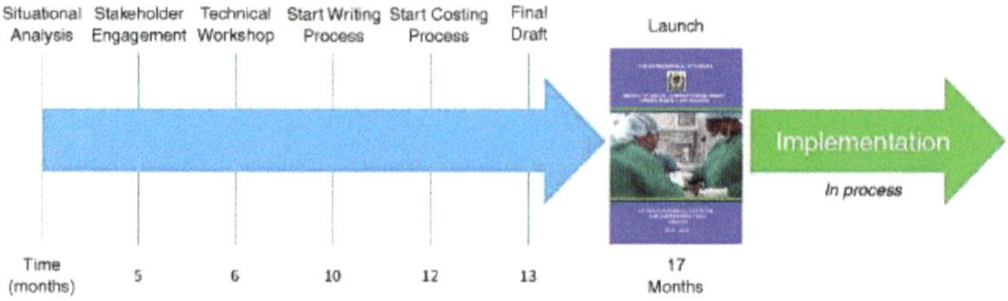

Figure 42. The timeline for the Tanzanian 2018 NSOAP. Adapted from: National Surgical, Obstetric, and Anesthesia Plans Supporting the Vision of Universal Health Coverage. Alexander W. Peters, Lina Roa, Emile Rwamasirabo, Emmanuel Ameh, Mpoki M. Ulisubisya, Lubna Samad, Emmanuel M. Makasa, John G. Meara *Global Health: Science and Practice* Mar 2020, 8 (1) 1-9; DOI: 10.9745/GHSP-D-19-00314. Reproduced under Creative Commons Licence. https://doi.org/10.9745/GHSP-D-19-00314.

Data collection and monitoring is also very problematic and increasingly supported by international professional societies such as RACS, the World Federation of Societies of Anaesthesiologists and research partnerships.

Ethiopia was an early adopter of NSOAPs in Sub-Saharan Africa. Five years on they reported the challenges they were having with data collection and quality indicators, making it hard for them to understand what progress has been made.[14]

A GLIMMER OF HOPE

In 2021, WHO published the *Action Framework for Safe Affordable Surgery in the Western Pacific Region* (2021–2030), identifying short, medium, and long-term actions to deliver safe, affordable surgery that can be incorporated into national health planning. Four operational shifts were agreed: [15]

1. Championing health beyond the health sector
2. Working backwards from a shared vision for access to safe and affordable surgical care
3. Ground-up systems strengthening and redesigning of existing surgical care systems
4. Driving country impact by developing and strengthening information and monitoring systems

The wealth of data in this document is extraordinary, contrasting with the paucity elsewhere. This allows for effective targeting of resources to the areas in need.

EXPLORE FURTHER

1. World Health Organization. *Surgical Care Systems Strengthening: Developing National Surgical, Obstetric and Anaesthesia Plans*. World Health Organization, 2017. https://iris.who.int/bitstream/handle/10665/255566/9789241512244-eng.pdf.
2. Program in Global Surgery and Social Change. "NSOAP Website and Dashboard." https://www.pgssc.org/national-surgical-planning.
3. Global Surgery Foundation NSOAP Manual: UNITAR. *National Surgical, Obstetric and Anaesthesia Planning Manual*. Edition 2020. Geneva, Switzerland: United Nations Institute for Training and Research (UNITAR). DOI: 10.5281/zenodo.398286.
4. Global Surgery Foundation. "Event Recordings: Special Educational Online Series on the NSOAP Manual & Process." https://www.globalsurgeryfoundation.org/events/nsoap-series.

CHAPTER 15

HUMANITARIAN SURGERY — LESSONS FROM HAITI AND OTHER DISASTERS

THE OXFORD ENGLISH Dictionary defines humanitarian as "concerned with or seeking to promote human welfare."[1] By this definition, all altruistic organisations involved in surgical care and capacity building in LMICs could be considered humanitarian.

However, the term "humanitarian organisation" is understood to mean groups responding to the acute needs of populations in crisis, caused by natural or man-made disasters or armed conflict. "Humanitarian surgery" therefore denotes surgical teams responding to crises, differentiating them from long-term care providers and development agencies.

> **MSF is currently working in 70 countries.**
>
> **International Medical Corps (IMC) delivered US$4.5 billion worth of services and training last year.**

For some, working in LMICs conjures images of Médecins Sans Frontières (MSF) or the International Committee of the Red Cross (ICRC), providing emergency surgery in war zones and during disaster relief. These organisations have a high profile as they often work in newsworthy locations, and their work has a certain edgy glamour. They are experts at working in fast-changing and insecure environments, and the heroism of some of their staff is awe inspiring.

Humanitarian organisations seek to follow four key principles:

1. **Humanity** — relieve human suffering wherever it is found

2. **Impartiality** — respond solely on need without discrimination
3. **Neutrality** — avoid favouring one side in a conflict or engaging in political, racial, or religious matters
4. **Independence** — responses are free from political, economic, or military objectives

Additionally, they always respect the sovereignty of recipient states, abiding by local rules and medical regulations.

Trauma surgery is often key in the first days after a disaster, leaving the general healthcare needs of the population temporarily unattended. However, those needs quite quickly begin to exceed those of the acutely injured. Rapid restoration of other services, particularly maternal care and communicable disease surveillance and prevention, is therefore essential.

WHERE DO DEVELOPMENT AND LONG-TERM AGENCIES FIT IN?

Long-term care providers are organisations and individuals supporting day-to-day healthcare in resource and educationally poor areas, such as running mission hospitals in deprived areas. **Development agencies**, on the other hand, focus on teaching, training, and system-strengthening, building capacity so local staff can care for their own population. Many agencies work in medium- or long-term partnerships with local institutions.

Although long-term care and development organisations have different priorities, there is some overlap with humanitarian organisations. Natural disasters are magnified when they occur in poor countries already struggling to meet the day-to-day needs of the population. In well-resourced countries, humanitarian teams often go in and out quickly, handing back responsibilities to local services once the immediate crisis is over. But in poor countries, they may find nobody to hand over to, and disasters can thereby cause long-term harm.

Hence, humanitarian and development teams often work together, and humanitarian organisations are not solely involved in disaster response. They also support local structures in the medium and longer term, providing workforce training and system-strengthening to help countries withstand future knocks. Both the US International Medical Corps

(IMC) and MSF are renowned first responders, who switch to long-term support and training when needed. The ICRC also maintains field hospitals where needed and supports local institutions and capacity building in post-conflict areas. These facilities often serve as first missions for those new to the organisations.

ORGANISATION OF HUMANITARIAN ACTORS

The key lesson from previous disasters is coordination is the key to effective response. **Who** is doing **What**, **Where**, **When**, and for **How Long**?

RAPID SITUATIONAL ASSESSMENT

After major disasters, time is of the essence. Humanitarian teams must deploy before complete information about the situation is available. Immediate needs are usually met by local teams, boosted by the first international responders. However, some needs can be overlooked, and a comprehensive rapid situational assessment is essential to establish priorities.

> **"We brought antibiotics, dressings, plasters, IV fluids, anti-tetanus injections, suture material, local anaesthetic, Ketamine, basic surgical tools, and a small sterilisation kit from Islamabad.**
>
> **The civil administration and Pakistan Army restored electricity in 3–4 days. Tents were provided, water reservoirs established, and helicopters used to bring aid and evacuate the injured.**
>
> **We contacted Major Majid, the coordination officer at the hub, and were given two tents in the military ground. A field hospital was set up and electricity arranged. Under ketamine, we performed debridement, drainage, back slabs, reductions, salvage amputations, and suturing. After resuscitation, transfers were promptly arranged by military helicopter."**
>
> **—Qaiser Jalal, surgeon and Muzaffarabad Diaspora, talking about the 2005 Pakistan earthquake**

CLUSTERS

The UN uses the cluster approach to improve coordination among humanitarian actors during an emergency response.[i] Humanitarian organisations form clusters for each of the main response sectors (see

---

i https://www.humanitarianresponse.info/en/coordination/clusters

text box). Aid is given out via the cluster, with the WHO leading the health cluster and coordinating emergency medical teams (EMTs).

Each cluster carries out its own rapid assessment, setting priorities and ensuring each organisation has clear goals. This is monitored and corrective action taken where needed. Problems and contingencies are common, as damaged infrastructure causes access issues and communication networks may be down. The unexpected is expected.

The cluster approach was first used after the 2005 Pakistan earthquake. Nine clusters were operational within 24 hours, providing leadership, accountability, and technical capacity. In contrast, the response to the Haiti earthquake in 2010 was chaotic. The Pan American Health Organization (PAHO), a regional office of WHO, later analysed these failures and published *Health Response to the Earthquake in Haiti January 2010 - Lessons to Be Learnt for the Next Massive Sudden-Onset Disaster* (2011).[2,3]

Humanitarian Response Clusters

- Protection
- Camp coordination and management
- Water sanitation and hygiene
- Emergency shelter
- Nutrition, food security
- Telecommunications
- Logistics
- Early recovery
- Health

(and Education and Agriculture)

SO, WHAT HAPPENED IN HAITI?

In January 2010, a massive earthquake struck Port-au-Prince, Haiti's capital. It would be hard to find a worse location for such a disaster.

There were 22 major earthquakes in 2010, causing 227,000 deaths. 98% of those deaths occurred in Haiti. Port-au-Prince's dense population and weak infrastructure meant there was little capacity to respond to a disaster. Even prior to the earthquake, Haiti had been described as "a republic of NGOs," with these organisations and faith groups already providing three-quarters of the country's healthcare. Half the population had no access to basic services and 80% lacked clean water and sanitation. Local organisations were corrupt and lacked governance.

Haiti had never invested in disaster preparedness or risk reduction, but had just lurched from one crisis to the next. This is quite logical. Why prepare for future mass casualties when you are too poor to meet the day-to-day medical needs of your population?

Because the earthquake struck the capital, the Haitian government, main hospitals, blood transfusion service, and NGOs, as well as WHO teams and UN peacekeepers already on the ground, were all directly hit. The very organisations who would normally control a disaster situation lost buildings, vehicles, staff and connectivity themselves.

Global mass media and 24-hour news mean the modern response to natural disasters is usually very generous. After the earthquake, the global healthcare sector responded on a hitherto unknown scale. Haiti saw the highest number of foreign field hospitals of any disaster, and teams arrived quickly due to Haiti's proximity to the USA. There was much disquiet about the sheer number of teams involved.

The number of injured and the dire state of pre-existing services resulted in a massive gap between need and locally available resources. This health vacuum meant foreign teams provided significant assistance. For instance, hospital ships — often underutilised in disasters — worked at full capacity, providing short-term, secondary and tertiary services. Huge numbers of highly competent organisations provided great care.

So why was there such criticism?

Chaotic

The healthcare response appeared to be something of a free-for-all, and, in some cases, the quality of care was not what it should have been. The organisation was chaotic and information and coordination were lacking. Decisions were not always evidence-based and lessons from previous disasters were not heeded. Problems with language, administration, customs, security and the availability of escorts all hampered the aid response.

Coordination requires effective national authorities equipped to assume leadership and the authority to establish and implement relief and recovery priorities. Lack of governance and high levels of corruption were the norm in Haiti and national authorities were unable to exercise control over NGOs.

. . .

Too many teams

The number of foreign medical teams has increased exponentially over the past 20 years. There was a "proliferation of actors" in response to the Indian Ocean Tsunami in 2004 and this included some incompetent organisations. After the tsunami, 180 agencies registered with the UN in Banda Aceh, Indonesia, but estimates suggest about 200 more organisations were there but failed to register.[4] Some teams were considered a burden and got in the way of constructive efforts.

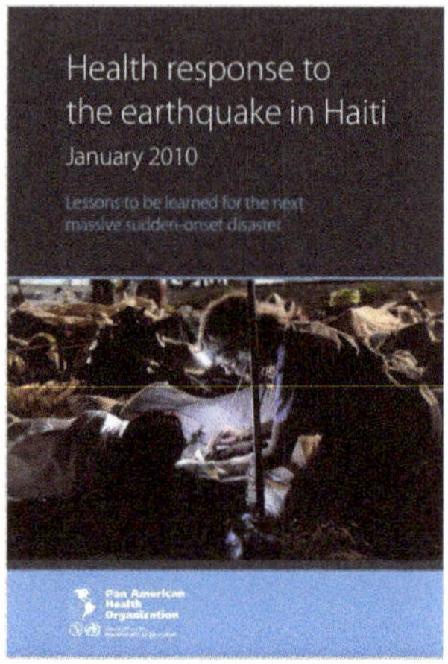

Figure 43. Pan American Health Organization. *Health response to the earthquake in Haiti,* January 2010. Available from: https://www.paho.org/en/documents/health-response-earthquake-haiti.

In Haiti 2010, 396 organisations registered with the health cluster alone, and many more did not register.[5] After the 2004 tsunami and in Haiti 2010, some organisations came and left quickly — seventy-six agencies left Haiti within two weeks. There were some groups with doubtful competence, and a few even had questionable motives. Several unqualified and unprepared voluntary teams were able to bypass the overwhelmed coordination mechanisms. The transient nature of some efforts led to a lack of postoperative care; there were "too many doctors and not enough nurses." Patients were sometimes discharged quickly, without adequate follow-up or rehabilitation, and not all organisations considered the local context — poor living conditions, lack of community healthcare and the profound problems associated with returning if complications occurred.

OVERLOOKING THE LOCAL HEALTHCARE COMMUNITY

After disasters, the earliest and usually most effective responders are relatives and neighbours, quickly followed by local medical teams and NGOs already on the ground. These efforts are frequently overlooked as the media focuses on external organisations, who can generate publicity.

Local healthcare workers have even been wrongly criticised for their absence from public hospitals. On the first night after the earthquake, Haiti's University Hospital treated 1,500 trauma patients, using all the hospital's consumables. Local staff then joined external agencies and private clinics because they still had supplies. The diaspora also often provides unseen care as they are absorbed into local facilities.

One of the lessons of disaster management is to strengthen and empower local government to enable a rapid handover of responsibility. External bodies can help temporarily, but a country's own government must set ongoing priorities. Wherever possible, local staff should lead, manage, and coordinate the deployment of international EMTs.

Coordinators may be nominated by the host country or provided by WHO. Coordination cells mobilise, register and assign EMTs and provide logistical support. After its 2016 earthquake, Ecuador successfully deployed 22 national and seven international EMTs within hours of the impact.

A Rapid Health Assessment after the 2015 earthquake in Nepal found that hospitals in the worst area were destroyed, but their staff retrieved equipment and set up field hospitals in the grounds. Five major hospitals in surrounding areas benefited from an influx of staff from the damaged hospitals, providing enough people to deal with incoming casualties. Preparedness measures taken by Nepal meant local staff largely coped, with WHO supporting with supplies.[6]

> **"Opening lines of communication — roads and telephone — were imperative. A strong command-and-control system existed directing resources to the required area and ensuring safety of the whole supply chain of men and material. I can surely say no one died of hunger or a preventable cause."**
>
> **—Qaiser Jalal, a surgeon from the Muzaffarabad diaspora, describing the 2005 Pakistan earthquake**

Economic impact

The economic impact of disasters jeopardises future healthcare. The financial cost of the 2010 earthquake exceeded Haiti's annual GDP, setting the country's economy back to its 2001 level, with half the population living in severe poverty.

Critics say that the international community focuses too much on mortality rates and not enough on the needs of survivors. Aid funding may be linked to death tolls, encouraging inflated figures to circulate. In Haiti, the reported mortality figure suddenly increased on the first anniversary of the disaster. The official count was 220,000 dead and 300,000 injured, but this was thought to include double counting of bodies and missing persons. Higher reported mortality may also boost fundraising within the humanitarian community.

Counting the injured can be difficult and failure by some medical teams to collect data was a real problem in Haiti. There may even be attempts to milk the suffering of victims to get more aid. After an African petrol tanker fire, for example, a mission doctor described the room holding the victims as a vision of hell from a Hieronymus Bosch painting. People with horrific burns were not getting treatment, not even analgesia. Local mission hospitals offered to transfer some the injured to their facilities, but this was denied. The motive for keeping them all together, without care, appeared to be to maximise the visible suffering to attract more aid contributions.

COMPETENCY ISSUES AND TRAINING

Surgical teams in HICs tend to be specialised and dependant on technology. In contrast, the burden of disease in low-resource settings is wider and technology less available. These problems are magnified in disaster relief situations, where access to support may be limited.

> **"Volunteers are well served by evaluating not only the personal benefit they derive from participating but also the overall impact of the mission on local healthcare and public health priorities."**
>
> **—PAHO report: *Health response to the earthquake in Haiti* (2010)**

There are excellent courses available to upgrade skills prior to joining humanitarian relief operations (see Appendix B), but organisations also have concerns about the ongoing learning and continuing professional development of their workforce beyond initial training and between deployments.

HUMANITARIAN SURGERY INITIATIVE

The Humanitarian Surgery Initiative (HSI) is a collaboration between MSF, Stanford University's Centre of Innovation in Global Health, the London School of Economics, and the Royal College of Surgeons of England. It aims to help specialised surgeons, who may struggle in LMICs and disaster situations, by understanding their training needs, optimising existing digital platforms and online learning and developing new technology-enabled training. [ii]

Knowledge and understanding of the burden of surgically treatable conditions during humanitarian crises is limited by a lack of systematic data collection and research. HSI also aims to develop these themes, building a network to support training, standards, and capacity building.

Faculty of Remote, Rural and Humanitarian Healthcare (FRRHH)

The Royal College of Surgeons of Edinburgh's (RCSEd) FRRHH aims to improve health outcomes in remote, austere, and life-threatening environments. It is addressing competency standards for healthcare organisations and personnel in such settings.[iii]

> **The reading list suggested in the FRRHH "Introduction to Humanitarian Healthcare" includes journalistic as well as medical texts opening our eyes to the wider picture in humanitarian crises and attitudes towards LMICs.**

RCSEd's online course Introduction to Humanitarian Healthcare will benefit anyone interested in global surgery, especially those considering disaster relief organisations. It gives a comprehensive description of the key elements and agencies involved in humanitarian responses.[iv]

QUALITY FRAMEWORK

Foreign teams have been known to take over local facilities, displacing staff doing good work with limited resources before the foreign teams arrived. Strong government institutions can guard against this, as was seen in Pakistan. However, where government bodies are dysfunctional, this behaviour goes unchecked, and ongoing damage has been inflicted on local health institutions after disasters. International NGOs poach staff with higher salaries, thereby weakening the country's recovery efforts.

---

ii https://www.rcseng.ac.uk/about-the-rcs/international-affairs/humanitarian-surgery-initiative/

iii https://www.rcsed.ac.uk/faculties/faculty-of-remote-rural-and-humanitarian-health care

iv https://services.rcsed.ac.uk/events-courses/introduction-to-humanitarian-healthcare-online-course

In some countries, humanitarian organisations operate in an unregulated free market. The *World Disasters Report 2005* of the International Federation of Red Cross and Red Crescent Societies described the humanitarian sector as "the world's largest unregulated industry."[7]

A few bad apples can overshadow the quality and professionalism of the majority. In Haiti, some foreign teams caused harm by misguided short-term efforts, failure to arrange adequate postoperative care and even people doing surgery they were not adequately trained for. The incompetence and unethical behaviour of a minority underlined the need for a quality framework with minimum standards and recorded outcomes.

Discussions after Haiti made headlines in the medical, and sometimes mainstream press, but the humanitarian health community was already regularly reflecting on and upgrading its disaster response. As far back as 1991, the UN General Assembly adopted resolution 46/182, which established new arrangements for humanitarian responses, strengthening coordination and disaster relief funding.[8]

The WHO's 2013 *Classification and Minimum Standards for Emergency Medical Teams (EMT) and Field Hospitals* sets guiding principles and minimum standards for clinical care and support. An EMT knowledge hub allows receiving countries to see the operational and technical capabilities of the international teams. It can support credible smaller organisations adhere to standards and weed out those who are harmful or merely an encumbrance.[9]

A WORD ABOUT AMPUTATIONS

Of particular interest to surgical teams is the discussion around amputations. After the 2005 Pakistan earthquake, some EMTs appeared to view high numbers of amputations, done in difficult field conditions, as "heroic." In Haiti, there were approximately 1500 amputations and 200 more amongst patients evacuated to the Dominican Republic. Concerns were also voiced about the level of amputations. Many were above above-knee, perhaps because that was all the expatriates in some teams knew how to do.

> **WHO's *Classification and Minimum Standards for EMTs* stipulates that a second opinion must be sought before all amputations, and that they must all be officially registered.**

Amputations are unavoidable for non-viable limbs, or for the life-threatening gangrene that can develop when treatment of compound fractures is delayed. Organisations that reviewed the number of amputations in the aftermath of Haiti concluded that, in some cases, additional amputations were the only pragmatic solution where facilities for the complex care necessary to save limbs were not available.

One of the principles of triage is to maximise benefit to the whole injured population. This means that additional amputations can also be justified in circumstances where need massively outstrips capacity. Complex care for one patient, for example, could lead to additional delay and the death of others. The scale of the triage in Haiti was almost unimaginable. As many as 37,000 people are thought to have survived the initial impact but subsequently died from their injuries. However, in the aftermath, it became evident the PAHO/WHO amputation guidelines were not followed by all volunteer organisations.

Interestingly, the high number of amputations resulting from earthquakes may have contributed to increased visibility and greater social acceptance of people with disabilities in some parts of the world. Additionally, the negative publicity about amputations in Haiti also attracted investment in rehabilitation assistance and learning.[10]

EMERGENCY ROSTERS OF EXPERTS

Organisations such as MSF, ICRC, IMC, UK-Med, and the International Rescue Committee (IRC) maintain rosters of medical staff, including surgical teams, able to deploy for humanitarian emergencies. Organisations usually need people who can deploy rapidly for missions of two to twelve weeks.

EXPLORE FURTHER

1. Royal College of Surgeons of Edinburgh. "Introduction to Humanitarian Healthcare Online Course." https://services.rcsed.ac.uk/events-courses/introduction-to-humanitarian-healthcare-online-course.
2. Pan American Health Organization. "Health Response to the Earthquake in Haiti, January 2010." https://www.paho.org/en/documents/health-response-earthquake-haiti.

3. Schuller, Mark, and Paul Farmer. *Killing with Kindness: Haiti, International Aid, and NGOs*. Rutgers University Press, 2012.
4. World Health Organization. *Classification and Minimum Standards for Emergency Medical Teams.* World Health Organization, 2021. Licence: CC BY-NC-SA 3.0 IGO. https://www.who.int/publications/i/item/9789240029330.
5. Polman, Linda S. *War Games: The Story of Aid and War in Modern Times*. Viking, 2011.

CHAPTER 16
GLOBAL SURGERY ORGANISATIONS AND FUNDING SOURCES

SINCE THE EXPLOSION of interest and publication of seminal documents in 2015, most surgical, obstetric and anaesthetic organisations in HICs have become interested in global surgery on some level. Interest ranges from superficial endorsement to genuine commitment and funding.

From 2015 to 2020, most speciality meetings and forums included sessions about global surgery issues, and for a while it felt as if the tide had turned, and global surgery would be seen as the most important issue facing surgeons in HICs. However, since the COVID-19 pandemic, this initial enthusiasm appears to have waned.

This chapter provides an overview of key global health and global surgery organisations, and examples of what professional bodies in HICs are doing.

NGOS, IGOS, INGOS AND MONGOS

The United Nations (UN) defines a non-governmental organisation (NGO) as "a not-for-profit, voluntary citizens' group that is organised on a local, national or international level to address issues in support of the public good." The term encompasses a highly diverse range of organisations, from multibillion-pound international charities such as Oxfam and Médecins Sans Frontières (MSF), to small community organisations, professional associations and lobby groups.

Intergovernmental organisations (IGOs) are made up of the governments of member states, for example, the UN, the World Health Organization (WHO) and the World Bank.

Big international NGOs are sometimes referred to as INGOs, and where national governments have set up bodies addressing the same problems as NGOs, we get Government Organised Non-Governmental Organisations, or GONGOS!

NGOs by Numbers

- Over 3 million NGOs worldwide; 2 million in India alone
- Top 10 international NGOs receive more than 1/3 of total funding
- Most NGOs spend 10–20% of their budget on fundraising
- Salary disparities up to 3–4 times local rates in some LMIC regions

The World Association of Non-Governmental Organisations (WANGO) lists over 54,000 NGOs in 190 countries, but estimates suggest there are over 3 million, with more than 2 million working in India alone.[i]

Roles and functions

NGOs are task-focused, working towards a specific vision or mission. They are almost always altruistic, aiming to improve human experience by supporting specific causes.

NGOs are hugely influential in international development, bringing in much-needed charitable funding and working in close collaboration with governmental organisations. The UN and World Bank channel a lot of development aid to teams on the ground via NGOs. Some large NGOs even have official associative status with the UN.

In global surgery, NGOs fulfil two main roles. The first is operational delivery: their primary purpose is direct service provision or the creation and implementation of improvement projects. The second is advocacy: defending and promoting the global surgery agenda and influencing the policies of IGOs.

Funding and resource challenges

The NGO system is not something one would design if starting from scratch. The need to keep chasing funds takes up a significant part of the budgets of some organisations, with most spending 10–20% of their income on fundraising activities. The shifting priorities of donors leaves

---

i https://www.wango.org/

organisations in a semi-permanent state of uncertainty, and small NGOs lack financial sustainability.

Funding models often favour large, professionalised NGOs based in HICs, who have been criticised for monopolising resources. More than one-third of funding goes to the top ten organisations. There is logic to this, as these bodies have proven track records and the ability to deliver at scale, but it nonetheless ingrains capacity imbalances.

Small organisations, especially those based in the Global South, struggle to pitch for funding against the big boys.

Partnership and local impact issues

Funding allocations now often require NGOs to have formed local partnerships. However, some organisations have been criticised for only paying lip service to this process. They may develop plans internally without meaningful involvement from local partners, who are brought in later merely to formalise agreements and increase the chances of securing funding.

With their dependence on fundraising, branding is commercially important for many NGOs. As well as resulting in a lot of T-shirt production, this can restrict partnership options on the ground. Money trickles down to LMICs — but control, not so much — and partners may be treated more like subcontractors. Some NGOs fail to discuss concerns raised by local partners in their annual reports, or convey these concerns back to funding bodies. This selective reporting (or "reputational risk management") is likely done out of fear of losing income or reputation.

Many NGOs can pay higher wages than local structures in LMICs, so that salaries can be three to four times those affordable locally. This can pull staff from local employment, destabilising hitherto functional local bodies. Local facilities sometimes report significant staff losses when NGOs move into an area in the aftermath of a disaster.

When NGOs move in to support government hospitals, there can even be differential salaries amongst staff doing the same job. The justification for this is that NGOs demand the highest standards, and higher pay incentivises staff to deliver those standards. But unfortunately, the resulting wage gaps can disincentivise locally paid employees, undermining the very institutions that NGOs aim to support.

Governance and accountability concerns

Not unreasonably, some HIC organisations may have doubts about corruption and mismanagement that prevent them from fully sharing responsibility with their LMIC partners. However, it should not be forgotten that NGOs based in HICs have also had serious issues with governance. The UK government, for instance, has *twice* suspended funding to Oxfam due to allegations of sexual exploitation and bullying.[1]

Small NGOs can also suffer a lack of effective governance. They may not abide by the rules governing other employers or operate effective boards of directors. Even organisations receiving significant donor aid have given board membership to friends and family members. This can distort priorities, and the agenda of the NGO may not match that of those they are purportedly trying to help. Boards may also be "unconscious-incompetent," i.e. failing to seek out appropriate expertise and thereby unwittingly making poor decisions.

Weak governance can undermine both the effectiveness and legitimacy of the NGO sector. When organisations do not operate transparently and ethically, both donor and local trust is eroded.

Criticisms and unintended consequences

NGOs have also been criticised for doing too *good* a job, as this can absolve local governments and institutions from assuming proper responsibility for their peoples' needs. In situations where all NGOs are forced to exit an area, governments may struggle to fill the void, or can only do so in ways that disadvantage part of the population, such as the loss of girls' education where NGOs were previously the sole providers.

Other organisations have been described as "self-serving." The aid sector is a multibillion-pound industry, and individuals whose livelihoods depend on their NGO may be disincentivised from fully achieving its aims, since doing so could put themselves out of a job. This "self-serving bias" can mean continuing the work takes precedence over the original goal, such as when training organisations continue to deliver programmes themselves rather than supporting local training faculty.

MONGOs

The term MONGO was coined as a derogatory term meaning "My Own NGO." This can mean organisations not playing by the rules, but it more often refers to well-meaning but misguided ones. Most dynamic and highly functional organisations began with a single person's idea and passion; however, poorly conceived organisations may inadvertently cause harm or squander resources.

The response to the Indian Ocean Tsunami in 2004 was the most generous and immediately funded humanitarian response in history. But unfortunately, there was also said to have been a second "tsunami" of aid organisations, some with little experience or competence. Items such as outdated medicines, broken toys, and assorted debris from HICs ended up in some of the world's poorest regions, sometimes blocking more meaningful help getting through.

Lack of oversight of NGOs is a major concern. The humanitarian sector reviews and reflects on disaster responses, steadily getting its house in order and setting standards. However, much of the global surgery space remains entirely unregulated. Anyone can set up a surgical NGO, surgical camp, or teaching organisation without their credentials being checked by a body that necessarily understands them. White saviourism is a significant issue in global health initiatives in LMICs (see chapter 22, page 273).

Linda Polman and other authors' accounts of the entitlement culture among some INGO staff make for difficult but important reading.[2,3,4] High salaries, per diems, and danger-and-discomfort bonuses sometimes fuel lavish lifestyles, and even prostitution, amid poverty and suffering.

UNITED NATIONS ORGANISATIONS

For surgical teams, understanding the UN ecosystem is useful and may occasionally open doors to influencing policy, accessing programme funding, or sharing materials. WHO, the United Nations Population Fund (UNFPA), the United Nations Children's Fund (UNICEF), and the United Nations Institute for Training and Research (UNITAR) play overlapping roles in expanding surgical access and advancing the Sustainable Development Goals (SDGs; see chapter 7, page 63).

WHO

WHO is the key UN agency for global public health. Established in 1945 and headquartered in Geneva, it formulates health policy for current and emerging threats such as climate change and pandemics, advocates for marginalised communities, conducts research and data collection, and disseminates health information. It also maintains the Central Emergency Response Fund (CERF) for urgent humanitarian responses and the Contingency Fund for Emergencies (CFE) for rapid responses to outbreaks and natural disasters.

The UN gives project grants for all aspects of human wellbeing aligned to the SDGs. Health organisations can access funds if they meet specific eligibility criteria. Generally, eligible applicants are government bodies, large NGOs, and academic institutions with proposals aligned with WHO priorities who can demonstrate capacity for effective intervention. Funds support national, regional, or global development aims, with pooled resources allowing cross-cutting programmes, like those required to up-scale surgery. Recipient countries may also pool WHO funding with money from other sources.

WHO also provides technical assistance, such as training workshops, expert advisory services, and resources for monitoring and evaluation, to help organisations deliver projects effectively. It facilitates partnerships between countries and organisations for knowledge exchange and collaborative effort.

WHO supports the Global Initiative for Emergency and Essential Surgical Care (GIEESC), convening over 2,300 multidisciplinary stakeholders from 140 countries to share knowledge, advise on policy, and develop educational resources. [ii]

WHO is funded by UN member states, each contributing an agreed percentage of GDP.[5] This covers less than 20% of the budget, with the remainder coming from voluntary contributions by those member states able to pay more, along with intergovernmental organisations, philanthropic foundations, the private sector, and others. Governments provide approximately 72% of WHO funding, with 17% more coming from multilateral contributions, which are also predominantly governmental. The lion's share of both streams comes from OECD (Organisation for Economic Cooperation and Development) countries.

The UN Foundation was founded in 1998 by philanthropist Ted Turner to demonstrate the value of the UN and the value of investing in it. In its first 25 years, it mobilised more than US$2 billion. The WHO Foun-

---

[ii] Global Initiative for Emergency and Essential Surgical Care: https://www.who.int/initiatives/who-global-initiative-for-emergency-and-essential-surgical-care

dation is an independent foundation affiliated with WHO, which marshals donor resources.

Health funding and the wider economic funding that support access to healthcare are both subject to the political imperatives and colonial biases of donor countries. Concerns about the politicisation of humanitarian aid, as well as the failings of foreign aid generally, are covered by many authors. See Explore Further at the end of this chapter for examples.

UNFPA

UNFPA was originally called the United Nations Fund for Population Activities. It changed its name but kept the acronym and both names are still sometimes used.[iii] Its mission is to ensure every pregnancy is wanted, and every woman safe in childbirth, giving it a major role in increasing access to essential surgery. The fight against excess maternal mortality is data-driven, with UNFPA advocating directly with governments and supporting training, data collection, and monitoring. It publishes the annual *State of World Population* report and the *Orange Results Book*. Funding comes from voluntary contributions by donor governments, intergovernmental organisations, the private sector, foundations, and individuals.

> **"African countries continue to experience modern colonialism. We may appear independent, but we often remain under the indirect influence of Western powers who exploit our resources and potential."**
>
> **—Anthony Abbot Kamara, SAO provider and renowned surgical trainer (Sierra Leone)**

UNICEF

UNICEF was created in 1946 to provide emergency food and healthcare to children and mothers in countries ravaged by World War II.[iv] In 1950, its mandate broadened, and it became the United Nations Children's Fund, but it also kept the original acronym.

UNICEF operates in 190 countries, protecting children's rights and providing education, health, and nutrition services. Surgically, it works to prevent maternal, newborn, and child deaths. Maternal deaths affect the life chances of surviving children and increase child mortality. UNICEF is heavily involved in strengthening health systems to achieve

iii The United Nations Population Fund: https://www.unfpa.org/

iv The United Nations Children's Fund: https://www.unicef.org/

universal health coverage (UHC), including surgical care. It is well known through news coverage as a major health provider in crisis situations and is the world's largest vaccine supplier.

UNITAR

UNITAR supports surgical and anaesthesia learning through its online platform, SURGhub.[v] Educational material is developed by a variety of partners, and front-line learners can access content from anywhere and earn UNITAR certificates.

UNITAR partners with the Royal College of Surgeons of Ireland, the Global Surgery Foundation (GSF), and Harvard's Program in Global Surgery and Social Change (PGSSC), with whom it published the National Surgical, Obstetric and Anaesthesia Planning (NSOAP) manual.[vi]

THE WORLD BANK GROUP

The World Bank consists of five organisations working under one umbrella. Its mission is to reduce poverty and promote sustainable development through knowledge, finance, and expertise:[vii]

The World Bank was established in 1944 to help rebuild Europe and Japan after World War 2.

1. The International Bank for Reconstruction and Development (IBRD) provides financial products and advice to help MICs and creditworthy LICs reduce poverty and respond to regional and global challenges.
2. The International Development Association (IDA) gives grants and low-interest loans, helping LICs invest and build safer, more prosperous communities.
3. The International Finance Corporation (IFC) drives economic development by encouraging private sector growth in developing countries.

---

[v] https://unitar.org/sustainable-development-goals/people/our-portfolio/surghub-united-nations-global-surgery-learning-hub

[vi] UNITAR, Harvard PGSSC and GSF NSOAP Manual available here: https://www.globalsurgeryfoundation.org/nsoap-manual

[vii] World Bank information websites: https://www.worldbank.org/ext/en/who-we-are and https://www.worldbank.org/en/topic/health

4. The Multilateral Investment Guarantee Agency (MIGA) offers political risk insurance (guarantees) for projects in developing countries.
5. The International Centre for Settlement of Investment Disputes (ICSID) provides facilities for conciliation and arbitration of international investment disputes.

Describing these organisations only in financial terms understates the extent to which the World Bank uses its financial power to shape global health policy. It supports countries working towards UHC by strengthening health systems to allow quality care regardless of ability to pay. The Bank collects and collates a wealth of freely available data on myriad health indicators. Its *Disease Control Priorities* (*DCP*) publications were pivotal in establishing the economic and moral imperative for scaling up surgery in LMICs, and *DCP3: Essential Surgery* (2015) provides a blueprint for developing surgical services.[6]

History and Third World Debt

However, the World Bank is not without controversy. World Bank and International Monetary Fund (IMF) policies have been criticised for subjugating and exploiting poor countries.

The organisation has been dominated by a few economically powerful countries, who provide most of its funding and choose its leadership, thereby creating an obvious conflict of interest. It has been accused of cronyism and bias, such as giving more money to countries occupying the rotating seats on the UN Security Council than to others in need.[7] The Bank continued to invest in fossil fuel projects up to 2022, despite its pledges to go green.

Historically, World Bank leaders publicly framed debt obligations as a powerful incentive for impoverished countries to modernise their agriculture and industry. However, aid for this development was inadequate, and punitive import tariffs on goods from developing countries restricted progress. From 1968 to 1981, its annual loans increased from US$2.7 to $12 billion, setting the scene for the "Third World debt crisis."[8]

The Bank then loaned more and more money to developing countries, hoping they could service their debts via economic growth. There was undoubtedly waste and embezzlement by some regimes, but the price of commodities exported from the Global South, such as minerals and food, dropped and international policies aimed at controlling oil prices then resulted in a sudden increase in interest rates.

Until the appointment of Jim Yong Kim, (Partners in Health and Harvard), World Bank leaders were people with financial and business, rather than humanitarian, backgrounds.

The Bank was slow to recognise that debtor countries were insolvent, so debt spiralled, leading to financial disaster. In 1986, Third World debt exceeded US$1 trillion. Rich countries profited and the World Bank added to its reserves.

To be eligible for debt relief and loan readjustment, the World Bank required structural economic adjustments, including privatisations, removal of food subsidies, increased taxation, and opening of markets to international competition. These strategies failed in countries that were not politically and economically mature enough, such as most of Sub-Saharan Africa. In the late 1980s and 1990s, a succession of countries went into financial meltdown, including many that were not amongst the world's poorest, such as Mexico and Brazil.

The suggested remedies made life worse for the poor. Social spending reduced as LMICs focused everything on exports to service debts. Deregulation to promote development ignored sustainability, going for quick growth without improving lives. There was insufficient effort to stop corruption and focus on results rather than just issuing more loans.

The World Bank was criticised for going too fast with free-market policies in countries who were not ready and failing to consider how these policies might worsen inequality. Projects failed to help the poor but did expand government bureaucracy.

Debt repayments made it impossible for willing countries to provide aid effectively. After the 2004 Indian Ocean tsunami, some affected countries had their debts wiped, but Sri Lanka was still servicing a bill of US$493 million annually, and Indonesia paid US$1.9 billion to the World Bank in 2006.

Public opinion in HICs turned, with multiple campaigns, such as Jubilee 2000, calling for debt cancellation. In 1996, the World Bank and IMF launched partial debt relief for 41 countries, wiping out 80% of debt, but the actual relief was still tiny compared to the World Bank's profits.[9] It tried to win over NGOs and detractors via soft loans for microcredit. However, poor countries still paid back more than they borrowed, and debts continued to crush social budgets. The rich retained influence over indebted countries and the World Bank and IMF faced a legitimacy crisis.

In 2005, the G8 Summit in London agreed to write off US$40 billion in debt for 18 Heavily Indebted Poor Countries (HIPC), and 20 more countries qualified for relief if they met targets on reducing corruption and liberalising their economies.[10]

The "Third World Debt Crisis" is still far from resolved. In 2024, the World Bank warned urgent action is needed to prevent record debt repayments from crushing LICs.[11,12] Rising interest rates have led to escalating costs of servicing current debts, especially those held by private lenders. This continues to draw funds away from health, education, and climate initiatives.

SOURCES OF FUNDING FOR GLOBAL SURGERY

PHILANTHROPIC ORGANISATIONS AND FOUNDATIONS

Anyone can set up a foundation, and there are no universal naming systems or criteria. Foundations range from major funders, through small groups focusing on niche areas, right through to the frankly bogus and fraudulent. Many large, competent foundations combine funding from philanthropic partners with global health expertise, and some specialise in improving access to surgery.

Significant global health and, increasingly, global surgery funding comes from wealthy philanthropic donors. The Bill & Melinda Gates Foundation alone has made thousands of individual grants and donated more than US$1.8 billion to global health, and other foundations contribute millions of US dollars annually.[13]

Other philanthropic funders work directly with smaller groups to support global surgery projects; for example, the Kletjian Foundation works with surgeons in Boston USA.[viii] Some donors fund causes allied to their business activities. For example, the Novo Nordisk Foundation reinvests profits from its anti-obesity and diabetes medications in initiatives to reduce global health inequalities;[ix] the Aga Khan Foundation

---

[viii] The Kletjian Foundation: https://kletjianfoundation.mystrikingly.com/#whom-we-support

[ix] Novo Nordisk Foundation: https://www.novonordisk.com/content/dam/nncorp/global/en/partnering-and-open-innovation/pdfs/the-next-era-global-health.pdf

focuses on sustainability, linking living conditions and nutrition to health;[x] and the Wellcome Trust supports health research, reflecting its founder's pharmaceutical background.[xi]

Myriad small and medium-sized charities fund capacity building and direct care in LMICs. Among direct care organisations, certain conditions are better funded than others, with ophthalmology and cleft lip and palate surgery particularly well supported.

The Global Surgery Foundation

GSF brings together clinical expertise, UN contacts, governments, and international partners on a common platform.[xii] Its SURGfund uses a catalytic funding mechanism, whereby seed corn investment enables small organisations to gain traction and attract mainstream investment. Catalytic funding often targets issues that would otherwise not be addressed. The GSF supports training and education, policy and planning, project implementation, research, and infrastructure i.e. Staff, Stuff, Space, Systems, and Social Support.

Government aid

Governments support international development. For example, prior to 2020, when it merged with the Foreign, Commonwealth and Development Office, the UK Department for International Development (DFID) supported global health through direct grants and collaborations, and via the Tropical Health and Education Trust (THET) partnership scheme. In New Zealand, the International Development Cooperation supports global surgery capacity building, with a particular focus on the Pacific Islands.

However, recent cuts in overseas development budgets by numerous Global North governments are likely to have devastating effects in LICs. Many organisations get at least part of their funding from governmental sources, and cuts are biting quickly. This will increase pressure on private donors as everyone now scrambles in a smaller pot.

Professional bodies

Many professional bodies in HICs make regular small grants, often

---

[x] The Aga Khan Foundations: https://the.akdn/en/what-we-do/developing-human-capacity/health

[xi] The Wellcome Trust: https://wellcome.org/

[xii] The Global Surgery Foundation: https://www.globalsurgeryfoundation.org/

themed to support their particular aims and interests. For example, the Royal College of Surgeons of Edinburgh and the Royal College of Surgeons of England offer small grants and travelling bursaries. Trainees and medical students can look out for these, but the application windows often close relatively quickly, so be sure to monitor actively and ensure you are on relevant mailing lists.

> **"Everyone is at risk of non-renewal of their contracts due to funding cuts. There are ongoing layoffs. We don't know what's going to happen in the coming months."**
>
> **—Sandi Gangha, emergency surgical officer employed by PIH in Sierra Leone, June 2025**

Salaries and self-funding

The average salary of a doctor working for WHO is about £100,000 annually, often enhanced by additional reimbursements.[xiii] People working for small and clinical organisations on the ground in LMICs tend to get paid much less. Salaries may be in line with local pay, although there is always a tendency for expatriates to be paid more than local staff. Some organisations do not pay salaries but cover major expenses such as flights and often provide free accommodation or a stipend.

Self-funding to work in global surgery is common. The pragmatic solidarity that has proven effective in many settings, and in some cases laid the foundation for more formal partnerships, is usually self-funded. Some organisations offer volunteers the option to either have their expenses reimbursed or to self-fund, if they can do so. Sometimes the organisation will arrange the travel and related logistics, and the volunteer donates the cash equivalent back to the organisation, as this can be the most tax-efficient way of making the donation.

Novel funding organisations in global health

Innovative funding mechanisms for global surgery are emerging and are discussed in chapter 13 (see page 133).

[xiii] Glassdoor: https://www.glassdoor.co.uk/Salary/World-Health-Organization-Doctor-Salaries-E11724_D_KO26,32.htm

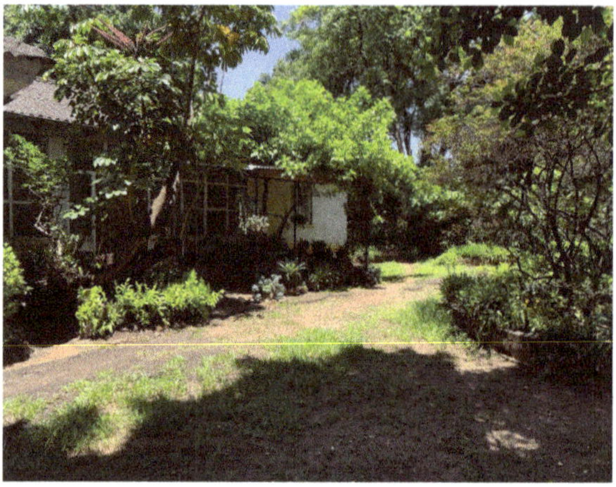

Figure 44. House available for use by volunteers in Malawi.
Photo: author's own.

FUNDRAISERS

Most large, many medium, and even some small NGOs employ professional fundraisers. Grants are available from multiple sources, and application windows are often short, so it can pay to have someone continuously looking. Writing grant applications is a time-consuming skill that must be learnt, and training is available. Many funders are happy to work with applicants to strengthen submissions.

Individual volunteers often fundraise for smaller organisations. This invaluable contribution is a way for those, as yet too inexperienced, or with life circumstances making it difficult to contribute on the ground, to support equitable access to surgery.

TRAINING INSTITUTIONS

The response of surgical, obstetrics and anaesthetic colleges in HICs to global surgery varies from large-scale formal commitment and innovation, backed by meaningful financial support, to a tokenistic, "put something on the website saying we support global surgery." In terms of output, some efforts appear to be all talk while others are involved in meaningful long-term partnerships and education programs. Examples below reflect typical activities in English-speaking countries. Readers should also look into their own colleges' initiatives.

. . .

Royal College of Surgeons of Ireland (RCSI)

RCSI is very active in global surgery.[xiv] Its Institute of Global Surgery supports training in surgery, obstetrics, and anaesthesia in LMICs, with numerous projects and grants, often involving substantial funding.

RCSI provides low-cost training in LMICs, pan-African paediatric surgery e-learning courses, and anaesthetic and surgical training across East, Central, and Southern Africa. It also supports initiatives such as SURG-Africa and KidSURG, which provide support and supervision platforms for rural surgeons in Malawi, Zambia, and Tanzania, as well as the UNITAR Global Surgery Learning Hub, an online repository for surgical care educational resources. The college is also involved in disease-specific projects and perioperative nursing education, and has developed a deep, wide-ranging collaboration with the College of Surgeons of East, Central, and Southern Africa (COSECSA).

As well as clinical materials, the RCSI has an extensive portfolio of global surgery education with undergraduate, Masters, PhD, and continuous professional development (CPD) courses. It also facilitates short clinical exchanges at ST5–8 (middle to late residency), medical student electives, and global surgery internships.

Royal College of Anaesthetists UK (RCoA)

RCoA's Global Partnership raises the profile of anaesthesia among international bodies and decision makers.[xv] It develops projects, products and services that share good practice, and strengthen the workforce in LMICs, and works in partnership with education providers to develop standards and deliver high-quality training, meeting local needs. It supports members based outside the UK and has established local country champions.

RCoA actively promotes safe anaesthesia in LMICs, attempting to replicate the knowledge and safety improvements that prevent anaesthesia-related deaths in HICs. As part of this effort, it contributes to curriculum, examination, syllabus, and question bank development for the College of Anaesthesiologists of East, Central, and Southern Africa (CANECSA).

The college's work with SAFE courses is discussed in chapter 9 (see

xiv https://www.rcsi.com/surgery/global-surgery

xv https://www.rcoa.ac.uk/about-us/global-partnerships

page 93). This includes the e-SAFE educational tool developed and funded by the RCoA and the Association of Anaesthetists (formerly AAGBI) to support anaesthesia training and related issues in LMICs.[xvi] While other organisations labour over how to deliver e-learning in regions with poor internet connections, the anaesthetists kept it simple and placed over 100 interactive e-learning materials on USB sticks, which are available free to anaesthetic teams worldwide.

RCoA actively supports the training of advanced trainees and early-years consultants from LMICs via the Global Fellowship Scheme (GFS), allowing them to undertake subspecialty training in the UK, with sponsorship for GMC registration and post-training certification.[xvii]

Royal College of Obstetrics and Gynaecology (RCOG)

RCOG advocates for sustainable, long-term improvements in women's healthcare, guided by the experience and views of its international members.[xviii] It provides support, training, and resources to help change attitudes and influence policy locally and nationally, amplifying the voices of its international members.

Collaboration between RCOG, the American College of Obstetricians and Gynecologists (ACOG), the International Federation of Gynecology and Obstetrics (FIGO), as well as public health organisations and charities, resulted in the shared statement: *Childbirth: A Bill of Rights*, published in September 2021. The statement calls for all countries to provide safe, inclusive, accessible, affordable, and respectful maternal care. [14]

RCOG's network and its Centre for Women's Global Health connect experienced clinicians worldwide and offer projects and opportunities for involvement.[xix] It advocates for investment in the workforce, including improving medical curricula and promoting task shifting and sustainable donor funding by both government and bilateral donors to achieve the UN SDGs. RCOG promotes access to contraception and safe abortion, campaigns against female genital mutilation and promotes services for neglected gynaecological conditions.

The college also has a lot of freely available online resources that can be

---

xvi https://e-safe-anaesthesia.org

xvii https://www.rcoa.ac.uk/training-careers/working-anaesthesia/international-training/global-fellowship-scheme

xviii https://www.rcog.org.uk

xix https://www.rcog.org.uk/about-us/global-network/centre-for-womens-global-health/

adapted to meet the needs of individual countries, as well as a wealth of educational material and skills-training facilities in London.

Royal College of Surgeons of England (RCS England)

The RCS England Global Surgery Policy Unit is a collaboration between RCS England and the London School of Economics and Political Science (LSE) to expand access to safe, affordable surgery through policy research, capacity-building partnerships, advocacy, and engagement in LMICs. [xx] Its mandate includes developing health policy and influencing decision makers and donors. It also aims to train and empower future health leaders and create platforms and opportunities to encourage exchange of expertise.

RCS England runs a SAFE OR programme developed in partnership with the Association of Anaesthetists, the Association for Perioperative Practice (AfPP), Lifebox®, RCOG, and the World Federation of Societies of Anaesthesiologists.[xxi] The programme aims to improve patient safety and surgical care through multidisciplinary teamwork and the implementation of the WHO Surgical Safety Checklist. Training includes a Train the Trainer component, one of the few skill acquisition programmes delivered this way.

The Humanitarian Surgery Initiative (HIS) is discussed in chapter 15 (see page 154).

Royal College of Surgeons of Edinburgh (RCSEd)

In 2015, RCSEd established the Global Surgery Foundation (GSF), a charitable body tackling inequality in surgery, by focusing on the surgical workforce. This foundation recently evolved into Global CARE.[xxii]

GSF awarded small grants and partnered with local providers and organisations to build sustainable capacity in LMICs, with projects such as training scholarships in Malawi, NOTSS training in Rwanda, plastic and reconstructive surgery in Ethiopia, and trauma care training in Haiti. As Global CARE, they will continue to fund projects in LMICs, provide individual training scholarships for LMIC surgeons and dentists and develop targeted education and training programs.

[xx] LSE's Global Surgery Policy Unit: https://www.lse.ac.uk/lse-health/research/GSPU/

[xxi] RCS England's SAFE OR Program: https://www.rcseng.ac.uk/about-the-rcs/international-affairs/safe-or-programme/

[xxii] https://www.rcsed.ac.uk/the-college/what-we-do/global-care

The mandate of RCSEd's Faculty of Remote and Rural and Humanitarian Healthcare (FRRHH) is to "improve the health outcomes of individuals living and working in remote, rural, austere and life-threatening areas of the world." [xxiii] It addresses competency standards for organisations and personnel delivering healthcare in difficult environments and provides an excellent online course, Introduction to Humanitarian Healthcare.[xxiv]

American College of Surgeons (ACS)

ACS's Operation Giving Back (OGB) initiative was originally developed to help the college's fellows participate in humanitarian medical missions. However, since 2016, ACS has shifted its priorities developing its Health Outreach Program for Equity (ACS-HOPE) programme, building on the foundation established by OGB.[xxv] Through ACS-HOPE and its expanded approach, ACS has partnered with COSECSA to develop surgical education and training collaboratives in Ethiopia, Rwanda, and Zambia, and provide scholarships for female scholars.

Additionally, OGB continues to provide tools supporting humanitarian outreach by ACS members, maintaining an online facility where volunteers can access and contact partner organisations offering opportunities. The ACS Pfizer Awards honour members whose altruistic work has made a sustainable impact or provides a model for others.

Royal Australasian College of Surgeons (RACS)

RACS exemplifies both working in partnership with regional neighbours and the importance of robust data collection in guiding meaningful change. Through partnerships, it provides training, medical education, capacity building, and aid to fifteen countries in the Asia-Pacific region, supporting local healthcare and assisting with data collection. Projects include trauma care in Myanmar, training and empowering of local faculty in Timor-Leste, and critical care capacity building in Papua New Guinea. It funds and facilitates scholarships and exchange programs for the surgical workforce in regional LMICs. The online RACS *Global Health Deployment Guidebook* focuses on profes-

[xxiii] RCSEd Faculty of Remote Rural and Humanitarian Healthcare free courses: https://www.rcsed.ac.uk/faculties/faculty-of-remote-rural-and-humanitarian-healthcare
[xxiv] RCSEd's Introduction to Humanitartian Healthcare online course: https://services.rcsed.ac.uk/events-courses/introduction-to-humanitarian-healthcare-online-course
[xxv] https://www.facs.org/for-medical-professionals/membership-community/acs-hope/international-programs

sional standards and behaviours as well as providing practical information.[xxvi]

The Lancet Commission on Global Surgery (LCoGS) holds the Australasian College up as an example of good practice. The data collection achieved against the LCoGS indicators is largely thanks to the college actively supporting its less affluent neighbours.[xxvii]

PROFESSIONAL AND SPECIALITY ASSOCIATIONS

It has become politically incorrect for SAO professional organisations in HICs *not* be involved in global surgery. The scale and impact of these efforts range from token gestures to genuinely meaningful involvement. Listing every international activity is not practical, so representative English-speaking examples are highlighted below. Readers are encouraged to explore their own specialty organisation's website for further information.

International Federation of Gynecology and Obstetrics (FIGO)

FIGO, an alliance of 130 national obstetrics and gynaecology societies, collaborates to improve and protect the rights of women and girls worldwide, especially in Sub-Saharan Africa and Southeast Asia, where the need is greatest.[xxviii] Focussing on education, research implementation, advocacy and capacity building, they support projects, run programs and events, and have an extensive knowledge hub with an online education platform.

The World Federation of Societies of Anaesthesiologists (WFSA)

The WFSA is a global alliance of anaesthetists that works with the national and speciality societies making up the organisation, and other bodies who share its aims, to advocate for the importance of anaesthesia and systems strengthening via partnerships with providers in LMICs.

They fight for universal access to safe anaesthesia and eradication of

---

[xxvi] Global Health Deployment Guidebook. Royal Australasian College of Surgeons; 2021. Available from: https://www.surgeons.org/-/media/Project/RACS/surgeons-org/files/global-health/Global-Health-Deployment-Guidebook.pdf

[xxvii] https://www.surgeons.org/about-racs/global-health

[xxviii] International Federation of Gynecology and Obstetrics: https://www.figo.org/

avoidable deaths, through the Safer Anaesthesia From Education (SAFE) programme and other educational resources and toolkits. They offer funding for individuals from LMICs to travel for education and have numerous volunteer opportunities available.[xxix]

International surgical associations

A few international surgical associations with altruistic and educational aims exist, such as the International College of Surgeons, the International Surgical Society and the International Federation of Surgical Colleges. The latter represents the Global South at the international surgical table with an agenda to decolonialise global surgical education and research, i.e. the flow of educational materials designed for HICs being applied in LMICs and the flow of research rewards the other way.[xxx]

Overarching surgical organisations have not achieved the same cohesion as the obstetricians and anaesthetists. Surgical specialisation in HICs often leads to professional silos, which can hamper a united international voice for surgery. International specialty organisations, such as the International Council of Ophthalmology, have been able to advocate and influence development.

Surgical associations have not achieved the same level of unity or collective influence as obstetric and anaesthetic organisations.

British Association of Urological Surgeons (BAUS) and Urolink[xxxi]

Of the UK speciality organisations, pride of place goes to the vision of BAUS and its membership. Urolink is a shining light for others to emulate. In 1990, the BAUS council set up a working party to propose Urolink (Urology Overseas Links). The aim was to "promote and encourage the provision of appropriate urological expertise and education worldwide with particular emphasis on the materially disadvantaged."[15] Thus, 25 years ahead of everybody else, BAUS was encouraging its members to contribute actively and effectively in LMICs.

[xxix] World Federation of Societies of Anaesthesiology: https://wfsahq.org/about/
[xxx] https://theifsc.org
[xxxi] Urolink: https://www.baus.org.uk/professionals/urolink/urolink_home.aspx

UROLINK

PROMOTING UROLOGICAL CARE AND EDUCATION WORLDWIDE

Global Code of Conduct

Urolink is a Committee of the British Association of Urological Surgeons (BAUS) which aims to encourage and support the establishment of links with individual departments and organisations in low or middle-income countries (LMICs) and to facilitate professional visits to work with colleagues in resource-poor settings.

Urolink's core values

At Urolink, everything we do is guided by our core values:

Respect: We treat everyone with dignity and respect and champion the rights and contributions of all to achieve a fairer world.

Accountability: We are accountable to those whose lives we hope to help, to those we work with and to those who support us.

Courage: We are bold and inspiring in our actions and words in promoting global urological care and education.

Collaboration: We work with others to maximise our impact, respecting diversity and difference in the pursuit of common goals.

Innovation: We are creative and agile, always learning, and prepared to take risks to accelerate change.

Integrity: We act with honesty and conviction and our actions are consistent with openness, equality and human rights.

Figure 45. The Urolink code of conduct, reproduced by kind permission of Urolink. We strongly recommend, regardless of your specialty, viewing the Urolink website: https://www.baus.org.uk/professionals/urolink/urolink_home.aspx.

Urolink supports links with individual departments and organisations in LMICs and facilitates professional visits to work with colleagues in resource-poor settings. Underpinning this was the belief that the most fruitful connections are based on individuals forming enduring links with overseas counterparts. Decades on, almost every international organisation, policymaker and funding organisation agrees.[16]

BAUS's small-scale, bottom-up approach was also supported at the top. Urolink is not just a group of like-minded individuals, but a formal committee of BAUS. Their activities have received support and promotion from the *British Journal of Urology International*, which featured the work of Urolink members and their global initiatives.

Urolink is also ahead of other UK groups in establishing core values and clear codes of conduct (**Figure 45**), while huge swathes of activity in LMICs fail to match their values and continue to be unregulated.

Other speciality organisations

Interest from UK specialty organisations varies considerably; some lack any visible global surgery presence. While this does not mean individual members are not engaged or interested, it does mean that word of mouth and personal contacts are the only way to find out what is going on. In other cases, web resources are available, and some examples are provided below.

ENT UK, the professional membership body for UK ENT surgeons, has established Global Health ENT UK to advance sustainable care in LMICs and raise awareness of ENT conditions worldwide.[xxxii] They provide educational resources, in-country courses, camps, and a database of members and opportunities, aiming to increase organisational links and partnerships and assist with equipment and technology.

The British Association of Paediatric Surgeons (BAPS) highlights global surgery issues and hosts a range of activities on its website, including its members' projects, postgraduate educational activities, and links to resources.[xxxiii]

Ordinary members of the Association of Coloproctology of Great Britain and Ireland (ACPGBI) recently established Cololink to emulate Urolink. The fact that, more than two years on, this is still a WhatsApp group with no web presence or formal standing is indicative of how far ahead the urologists are.

Similarly, the British Orthopaedic Association are just starting out with international mentoring in a limited way, and UK ophthalmologists support initiatives such as Vision 2020. The Association of Surgeons of Great Britain and Ireland has focused on sustainability, an issue of huge relevance in LMICs, as many of these countries are suffering the worst effects of climate change, to which surgical teams in HICs are contributing.

TRAINEES AND STUDENT ASSOCIATIONS

The Global Anaesthesia, Surgery and Obstetric Collaboration (GASOC)

Established in 2015, GASOC is a trainees' organisation, founded in the UK, with an international membership.[xxxiv] It encourages its members to engage responsibly in global surgery and helps them make an impact. The hope is their interest in global surgery will continue after completion of training and they can become future leaders in the field.

---

xxxii https://www.entuk.org/about/groups/global_health/default.aspx
xxxiii https://www.baps.org.uk/events/global-surgery/
xxxiv GASOC: https://www.gasocuk.co.uk/

They collaborate with organisations internationally to share knowledge and experience and provide real networking opportunities for those who want to become involved.

GASOC have championed innovation harnessing new technologies, designed and implemented small-scale research and collaborated with bigger projects. They provide innovation training, courses and hackathons, and have regular educational webinars. They also support various prizes and offer small travel grants.[xxxv]

The GASOC annual conference is a friendly forum that is valuable for trainees and others interested in getting started in global surgery but not really knowing where to begin. It is a good opportunity to meet like-minded peers and hear about opportunities for involvement. Additional signposting and resources are hosted on its website.

Global surgery Amsterdam

This is a mixed group of surgeons, surgical residents, research candidates and medical students promoting global surgery issues, and organising summer schools and ad hoc training, with expertise and interest in burn care.[xxxvi] They have developed free online materials, such as Basics of Burn Care and Open Fracture Care — both issues of great importance in LMICs.[xxxvii]

Medical student organisations

Many people first get inspired as medical students, and the student elective is no small part of this. At first sight, what can students possibly do to help? Well, "something" is the answer. As individuals from HICs, we all have contacts and privileges that can be harnessed to help.

> **"I organised an observership in Cameroon in my first summer. My medical school allowed selected students to do paediatric placements abroad, so I organised a placement in South Africa, and used my final-year elective to do a placement in Madagascar.**
>
> **I co-established the Oxford Electives Conference to prepare students practically and ethically for electives in low-resource settings."**
>
> **—Helen Please, surgical resident and Past President of GASOC, talking about activities at medical school**

---

xxxv Hackathon: An event, typically lasting several days where people meet and collaborate to solve a problem or identify new opportunities.

xxxvi Global Surgery Amsterdam: https://globalsurgeryamsterdam.com/

xxxvii Basics of Burn Care: https://globalsurgeryamsterdam.com/basics-of-burn-care-book/; Basics of Open Fractures: https://basicsofopenfractures.org/

The Global Surgery Student Alliance (GSSA) working in the USA, is affiliated with the International Student Surgical Network (InciSioN).[xxxviii] Students can find ideas for getting involved on the GSSA and InciSioN websites.[xxxix] Although aimed at medical students, the *GSSA Toolkit for Trainee Experiences in Global Surgery* is a useful read for everyone.

These organisations offer toolkits for specific activities, such as hackathons, as well as an online lecture series and signposting to additional resources, all with a strong emphasis on safe involvement.

EXPLORE FURTHER

1. Polman, Linda. *The Crisis Caravan: What's Wrong with Humanitarian Aid*. Picador, 2011.
2. British Association of Urological Surgeons (BAUS). Urolink. https://www.baus.org.uk/professionals/urolink/urolink_home.aspx.
3. "GSSA Toolkit for Trainee Experiences in Global Surgery." Global Surgery Student Alliance. 2025. https://docs.google.com/document/d/1-5L_WAJAMnTP4UNkqtvKtDKhXcW-Fu8ZmXCn_MDZnD4/edit?tab=t.0.

[xxxviii] Note: This InciSioN should not be confused with Incision, the more widely known surgical training platform.

[xxxix] https://www.globalsurgerystudents.org/; https://www.incisionuk.com/resources

CHAPTER 17
FROM POLICY TO PRACTICE: MODES OF DELIVERY

THIS CHAPTER EXAMINES THE EFFICACY, ethics, and evolution of global surgery initiatives. Understanding common approaches, their benefits and limitations, helps us in our pursuit towards meaningful involvement.

SURGICAL CAMPS

Short-term surgical missions (aka camps) have been very popular with expatriate teams, often targeting specific conditions such as cleft lip, cataracts, or groin hernia.

How camps work

A few weeks before the camp begins, a team member or local partner identifies potential patients. Upon arrival, the team screens them, makes their selection, and operates on these patients, usually over a period of one to two weeks. Camps can efficiently deliver elective surgery for a number of patients and may focus on the quantity of procedures, as this is perceived to be what donors want.

The charities usually pay for the operation, perioperative care, patient transport and feeding, and sometimes even gifts or bonuses for the patients. Teams bring their own consumables — and sometimes hardware — but the surgery usually takes place within existing facilities. Local teams may get to assist, but some groups are entirely self-contained, flying out everybody from surgeon to theatre runner.

Camps help individual patients who could not otherwise afford surgery. Specialist camps targeting complex procedures also provide expertise that is not available locally, for example, complex fistula or reconstructive surgery. Some camps leave lasting legacies, including valuable hardware for local teams. The short duration of camps appeals to expatriates who can only commit a small amount of time.

"I took part in hernia camps in Nepal and Ghana, gaining great understanding of how healthcare in LMICs works and how to integrate with teams locally. However, I became increasingly dissatisfied with the impact this model had on host hospitals, putting a strain on the system, using beds and operating theatres that could have been used for the normal day to day work. Often, the hernia camps wanted to provide training or exposure for the surgical officers. Visiting doctors would be frustrated by apparent lack of engagement. The reality was those who would have gained most from training were struggling to manage the volume of pre- and post-operative patients generated by the visiting team and were unable to attend the operating theatre as a result. The benefits to me outweighed those to the hospitals I was visiting."

—Jen Watt, post-CCT surgeon (London UK), relating experience as a surgical registrar

Criticisms

Surgical camps receive a lot of criticism due to a flawed underlying premise. They imply that universal access to essential surgery can be achieved by foreign teams attempting to "operate their way out of the problem." Moreover, such camps keep skills and resources in expatriate hands instead of building local capacity.

DCP3: Essential Surgery found camps wanting: "Short-term surgical missions by outside surgeons appear beneficial only if no other option is available; otherwise, suboptimal outcomes, unfavourable cost-effectiveness, and lack of sustainability limit their usefulness."[1]

Camps place temporary stress on surgical infrastructure, with local teams sometimes having to wait to do their emergency cases as the expatriate team is occupying the theatre. Camps can also divert attention and resources away from those who are struggling long-term to provide services, thereby distorting local healthcare economies.

Local teams providing emergency surgery are often poorly paid but may be able to supplement their income with elective work. One might

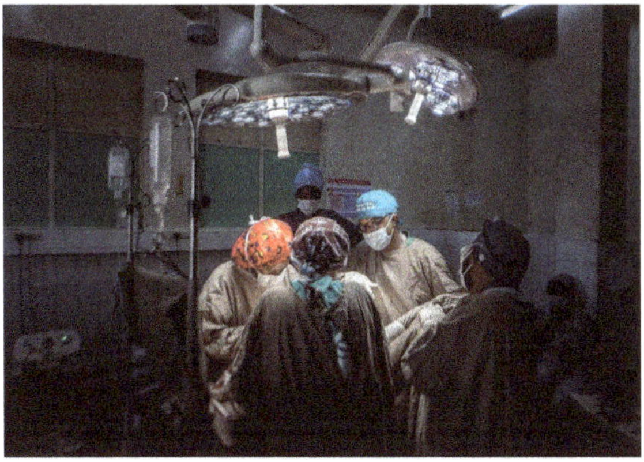

Figure 46. Dr Raymond Nyirenda and team operating in Blantyre, Malawi. The lights were donated by Operation Smile (https://www.operationsmile.org). Photo: author's own.

expect the well-resourced camp teams to do the more difficult cases, but they may cherry pick, either because quantity is their metric of success, or because they are mindful of complications and wisely avoid the challenging cases. But, by creaming off the easier cases, they risk taking valuable income from local providers.

Camps can also distort health-seeking behaviour. This can work both ways; if camps get good clinical results, people get the impression that international providers provide a better service and therefore delay seeking care until the next camp.

The opposite can also happen, with camps producing unsatisfactory results. Some expatriate volunteers have failed to maintain proper standards, picking cases they would like to try rather than those they are trained for. They may also mistakenly believe there is no-one competent locally. The poor outcomes seen after some camps can have a detrimental effect on future care-seeking behaviour. For example, fistula rates twenty times higher than those seen in the USA have been described after camps repairing cleft palate.[2] Camps have also been known to leave partially treated patients and complications for local providers to salvage.

Lastly, camps are also a notoriously expensive way of delivering surgery. Simply providing a fund for patients to have surgery by local providers would likely help many more people than deploying travelling surgical teams.

CHANGING BEHAVIOURS

In response to these concerns, many camps have changed their modus operandi, with the USA leading efforts to make them more sustainable. Some now foster long-term relationships, training, and sponsorship programmes, becoming integrated into local communities and building genuine partnerships and pragmatic solidarity.

Many camps donate unused materials and pay rent to host hospitals, providing income that can support development. To demonstrate sustainability, camps increasingly include teaching components. This can vary from genuinely working to upskill local teams and eventually phase themselves out, to adding token training sessions to the main show, just to tick the sustainability box.

Other organisations recognise that there is local expertise to do the high-volume elective surgery they favour, but that the barrier to delivery is affordability. They therefore employ local teams to do the surgery for free, bolstering rather than damaging local providers. Some organisations still take the easy cases for themselves but fund local providers to operate more challenging cases. There is undeniably some irony in this, but the argument is that the transient presence of the foreign teams does not lend itself to cases where there is a risk of complications.

"I teach bowel anastomosis in the standard fashion: easy to teach and reproducible. We do stoma reversals one day a week, with the procedure performed by a local registrar under direct supervision of me (consultant GI-surgeon). A short-term mission came for one week. Five elective stoma reversals were chosen. So far so good. BUT: the visiting surgeon was specialised in laparoscopic and upper GI surgery and not open stoma reversal. The operations were done by the visiting surgeon, with a local registrar as first assistant (no training opportunity). The anastomosis was done in a different way than we have been teaching. One patient developed a colonic fistula and abscess, requiring re-operation and eventually died of complications.

Why does a short-term mission do a procedure already done regularly as a real teaching operation for the local registrars? Time/theatre space could have been used better for other operations (AV-fistulas, transurethral prostatic resections, and obstetric fistula repair), where local expertise was limited, so this probably made more sense...."

—Dominik von Malsen, surgeon and international medical educator (Blantyre, Malawi)

TRAINEES IN SURGICAL CAMPS

DCP3: Essential Surgery lists papers that laud the benefit of short-term missions for the intensive exposure of expatriate trainees. This includes procedures commonly performed in HICs. It goes on to say, "the benefits to surgical residents in HICs clearly cannot come at the cost of delivery of unsatisfactory care in LMICs," and one should add, "or at the expense of local trainees."

Pragmatic solidarity is a social justice approach focused on practical support to communities through real actions, while seeking to change the underlying conditions that lead to poverty and injustice. As Paul Farmer put it, "taking a stand by the side of those who suffer the most."

The poor outcomes achieved by some camps could be related in part to expatriate trainees using camps as a "practice ground." It is difficult for expatriate trainees to operate during camps without straying into serious ethical difficulty, but what about assisting? Sometimes assistants are genuinely in short supply, but when local trainees are available, they should do the assisting.

However, there may be roles trainees can take on, such as perioperative care, which frees up time for local staff to receive training. Camps that state the duration and rate of their follow-up have reported higher complication rates, raising concerns that others may be under-reporting. So, another role for trainees might be to help develop practical strategies for outcome measurement, including collecting data and patients' contact details for later telephone follow-up.

Today's trainees are tomorrow's surgeons and anaesthetists and hooking them into global surgery at an early age could be a good thing. Camps are an easy first foray into low-resource settings, introducing individuals to the needs of LMICs. There are people making highly meaningful contributions whose first experience was a with a camp. One option is to go as a self-paid observer or helper, enabling local trainees to benefit from the camp.

SELF-CONTAINED MOBILE PLATFORMS

Self-contained mobile surgical platforms carry their entire infrastructure with them, on ships, planes, trains, or automobiles.

Mercy Ships, for example, have two fully functional US hospitals on ships, which dock in African ports, often for many months.[i]

These fulfil a different role to surgical camps. Their high-end facilities allow them to take on complex surgery, which may not otherwise be available locally for decades. Despite the complex nature of the work, the prolonged sojourns of the ships mean they have also contributed to training opportunities for local providers.

PARTNERSHIPS

The UN Sustainable Development Goals focus on partnerships to build local capacity and strengthen health systems, and this is reinforced in WHA 68.15 (see chapter 7, page 61). Two principles underpin this partnership model.

Firstly, equal partnerships and balanced relationships emphasise and uphold equal rights, equal access to resources and human worth. Secondly, partnerships offer the means to sustainably address development and manage projects efficiently, as those in LMICs can make their unmet needs visible to HIC partners. Without this, there is a substantial risk that inaccurate analysis leads to well-meaning but potentially misguided projects.

This contrasts with the donor-recipient model of development, where the donor holds the power, chooses the project, provides the money, and sets the rules of engagement. This dynamic is inherently colonialist and patronising; the donor perceives they know what is best for the "weaker" partner who needs to be guided in a paternalistic manner.

The Austrian "Appear" programme attempts to disrupt the entrenched colonialist power dynamic. The funding call is open to Global South institutions who then select suitable Global North partners, rather than the other way around.

https://oead.at/de/kooperationen/internationale-hochschulkooperationen/austrian-partnership-programme-in-higher-education-research-for-development-appear

Bona fide partnerships are long-term, institutionalised relationships between facilities and organisations in HICs and those in LMICs. They often grow from less formal relationships and friendships between individuals, which are then strengthened and

i https://www.mercyships.org/

formalised over time. They are proven to be an effective, sustainable and financially efficient model of capacity building, with a reciprocal exchange of skills, knowledge, experience and ideas.

True partners co-develop plans and projects together but are driven by the specific needs and requests of the LMIC partner, to which the HIC institution responds. Partnerships collaborating with front-line services typically focus on strengthening systems and building the health workforce by improving human resources, developing clinical pathways and operating policies, and providing education and training for health workers.[ii]

> **"My experience is that the most successful and impactful global health work continues to be centred around work 'on the shop floor'. Projects that arise from the realities of local healthcare practise, informed by population need, and inspired by the desire of individuals to do better, tend to be crafted in such a way that they work. And the reality is that when motivated individuals work collaboratively with each other, these projects make a big difference to real people."**
>
> **—Mark Szymankiewicz, consultant surgeon and founder of SWIFTSS**

The argument for partnership is strong, and since funding now often depends on it, nearly every global surgery organisation claims to work in partnership and espouses the benefits of collaboration. Though, in reality, some so-called partnerships can be superficial — like the "partnership" you might have with your hairdresser: they do the work and offer suggestions, but ultimately, you control the style, pay for it, and get the admiration. When all the ideas come from and are imposed by HICs, they will stifle innovation from the Global South.[iii]

Partners in Health (PIH)

In the 1980s, the global health establishment regarded quality care for marginalised communities as "unsustainable." A small group of social justice and global health advocates set out to disprove this. PIH's model of training local people to provide healthcare, treating everyone with dignity and providing world-class care changed the narrative. Two of PIH's founders, Dr. Paul Farmer (later Professor of Global Health at

---

[ii] NHS Managed Educational Partnerships: https://global.hee.nhs.uk/wp-content/uploads/sites/24/2023/11/MEP-brochure-January-2023.pdf

[iii] North South Research Partnership: https://www.eadi.org/fileadmin/user_upload/EADI/03_Publications/EADI_Policy_Paper/EADI_policy_paper_Carbonnier_Kontinen_FINAL.pdf.

Harvard) and Dr. Jim Kim (later President of the World Bank), have played a pivotal role in the global surgery story.

PIH establishes long-term relationships with sister organisations in impoverished areas, bringing modern medicine to those most in need and creating pragmatic solidarity between the world's leading institutions and the world's poorest, sickest communities. PIH works with government partners in Haiti, Kazakhstan, Lesotho, Liberia, Malawi, Mexico, Peru, Rwanda, and Sierra Leone, following its Five Ss approach to health system strengthening (see text box). They employ over 17,000 staff, 98% of whom come from local communities. PIH adopt a pragmatic "whatever it takes" approach, extending support beyond medical care and providing food and cash when needed to allow people to access care.

These few paragraphs describe what PIH does but cannot convey the magnitude of what the handful of individuals who started the organisation have achieved over the last 40 years. They challenged received wisdom whenever it worked against the poor and refused to accept the narrative that people cannot be helped due to cultural or educational barriers. They exposed the raw truth: poverty is the barrier to good healthcare and everything else is just excuses.

PIH is responsible for WHO overturning its decision to block treatment for MDR TB in poor countries, by proving the treatment was both effec-

Pragmatic Solidarity: Building Specialised Services in Kilimanjaro

"Six years ago, KCMC Regional Hospital appointed its first sub-specialist colorectal surgeon. I have the privilege of working with him for about a month each year. The first few visits were about building trust and understanding what I can offer. Equipment is always needed, and leg stirrups, fistula probes, etc., were easily sourced and donated. Many challenges are similar to the NHS: data collection, owning outcomes, and fair and challenging discussions at M&M meetings. Many patients don't have insurance, so pay for treatment, adding a layer of complexity to decision-making. Two more surgeons have now been appointed, and we are looking at methods of distant mentorship and being able to virtually attend European professional meetings. We plan to develop workshops for benign ano-rectal problems."

—Mark Chapman, UK consultant colorectal surgeon, talking about Kilimanjaro Christian Medical Centre, Kenya

tive and pragmatic.[iv] They were significant players in the movement to treat HIV/AIDS in LMICs, again providing evidence this was pragmatic.

Although the founders of PIH are physicians and programme managers, they played a huge role in calling out inequity in surgery. Their landmark paper, "Surgery and Global Health: A View from Beyond the OR," was the first to describe surgery as "the neglected stepchild of global public health."[3]

Dr Agnes Binagwaho, the Rwandan Minister of Health and Dr Paul Farmer co-founded the University of Global Health Equity (UGHE) in Rwanda. The curriculum pairs medical education with human rights and social justice, and the UN has applauded it as a high-quality health sciences institution, helping to move the centre of gravity to LICs.

PIH's Five Ss Approach

Staff: enough well-trained, qualified staff

Stuff: tools and resources for delivery and administration

Space: safe, appropriate facilities with power and water

Systems: leadership, governance, information and financing for best practice and quality

Social support: necessities allowing patients to access care.

UK GLOBAL HEALTH PARTNERSHIP SCHEME

The UK government-funded Health Partnership Scheme (HPS), formerly the Tropical Health and Education Trust (THET), harnessed expertise in UK institutions to respond to the needs of colleagues in LMICs. They supported 191 partnerships, with a focus on systems strengthening. Over 2,000 NHS staff volunteered overseas and trained 93,000 health workers in 30 African and Asian countries, the majority of whom went on to train others.

"Our goal is to improve surgical outcomes for patients in Sierra Leone. Local processing of mesh furthers quality of care in an environment that empowers our team and the patients we serve."

—Anthony Abbot Kamara, SWIFTSS lead (Sierra Leone)

These partnerships facilitated knowledge and skills sharing between

iv Multi Drug Resistant Tuberculosis.

NHS institutions and African hospitals and provided specialist international development expertise. THET suffered knockbacks with cuts to overseas aid, and HPS similarly faces great uncertainty.

> **Decisions made in HICs led to "a disorderly patchwork of small-scale, insufficient quality, short-term, and unsustainable health professional training initiatives that have focused only on a few diseases, created unnecessary gaps or overlaps in resources, and failed to help meet long-term national health workforce needs."[5]**

TRAINING PARTNERSHIPS

Training programmes are common and typically described as "partnerships." Ideally, training follows a National Surgical Obstetric and Anaesthesia Plan (NSOAP; chapter 14, page 135). Where an NSOAP does not yet exist, joint planning is essential from the outset. Where HIC actors have driven training, it has not always been aligned with local priorities or integrated into national health strategy. HIC partners often select and directly fund training partners, cutting LMIC governments out of the equation. This can hinder investment in the infrastructure and resources of local schools and teaching hospitals.

Initiatives may be short-term and tend to be classroom-based, with training duration determined more by the availability of funding and trainers than by the needs of local institutions or the time necessary to achieve competency. Against this background, Cuba, Denmark, Finland, and four USA-funded initiatives — the Medical Education Training Partnership Initiative (MEPI), the Nursing Training Partnership Initiative (NEPI), the Rwanda Human Resources for Health (HRH) programme, and the Global Health Service Partnership (GHSP) — have developed innovative programmes focused on increasing human resources.

Rwanda's HRH programme is a seven-year collaboration between US academic institutions and the Rwandan Ministry of Health that has been extensively described.[4] Analysis of the four US programs led to new recommendations for Best Practices for Training Initiatives in LICs, which emphasise alignment to local priorities with joint planning, and coordination, funding flexibility and, most importantly, host country ownership.[5] For training to be effective, it should build local institutional capacity via sustainable partnerships and communities of practice.

A key lesson of these best practices is to not attach too many restrictions to how funds are spent. Allowing the recipient country to decide where money is spent may sound obvious but has rarely happened. With proper systems in place to ensure accountability, countries like Rwanda have in recent years been allowed more direct control of funds, with local governments and/or academic institutions serving as the primary recipients. Rwanda has used these funds for infrastructure and equipment in health professional schools and teaching hospitals, as well as for teaching.

Best Practices for Training Initiatives in LICs:

1. Align training with local priorities
2. Ensure joint planning and coordination
3. Maintain flexible funding arrangements
4. Prioritise host country ownership

In other countries, some training partnerships have fallen short due to lack of proper quality controls. Where LMICs are not equal partners, they have been unable to address poor quality training, even when they have alerted the HIC "partner" to it.

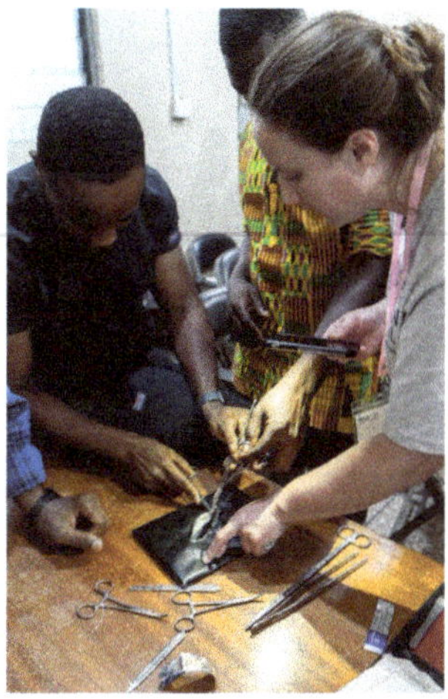

Figure 47. Techiman, Ghana: Jen Watt teaching with the SWIFTSS (Surgical teams Working in aFrica Together for Safer Surgery) ultra-low-cost hernia model. Photo: Mark Szymankiewicz.

Reflections garnered from the Rwandan HRH training project reinforce what bona fide trainers know: healthcare training should be competency-based. Counting the number of "training episodes delivered" or number of "trainees attending" is largely meaningless, and yet it continues to be the main metric collected by some partnerships. Low quality training only compounds existing problems for LMICs.

The MEPI, the HRH Program and GHSP have established teaching hospitals where trainees can witness high-quality healthcare and governance. This is so important in countries where poor quality care risks being accepted as normal.

Allowing recipient countries to make the major decisions about how funding is spent enables them to specifically design teaching programmes to meet their own needs, for example, preparing SAO providers for practice in remote and under-resourced facilities.

Good training partnerships strengthen the teaching and mentoring skills of local faculty, including clinicians in rural areas who mentor trainees on placement. Visiting faculty can serve as "force multipliers" training local clinicians who become faculty, exponentially expanding the pool of educators.

Both abrupt cessation and indefinite continuation of training partnerships work against sustainability. Ideally, partnerships fade out as and when the HIC partners become unnecessary, with local institutions assuming responsibility for sustaining and expanding training and absorbing graduates into the workforce.

Ad hoc short courses and unfamiliar trainers are likely to be no more effective at addressing problems than surgical camps. Relationships are fundamental to good training, just as they are in HICs. By prioritising LMIC ownership, the Rwandan HRH programme is credited with helping Rwanda develop one of the highest quality health systems in Africa. It eschews quick wins, in favour of long-term capacity strengthening and structural change.

TELEMEDICINE PROGRAMMES

Advances in mobile communications increase opportunities for LMIC teams to get advice from international experts via telemedicine. A review of telemedicine publications found that plastic surgery was the most represented specialty, followed by ophthalmology and general surgery.[6]

Telemedicine is useful for patient assessment and management advice, intraoperative consultations and things like ultrasound scanning, which can be performed live with remote expert radiological support. The cases where telemedicine support is requested are usually challenging, as local teams are used to dealing with the more common things. Telemedicine organisations appoint fully trained staff, familiar with the patient's country, but some include opportunities for trainees to work alongside consultants.

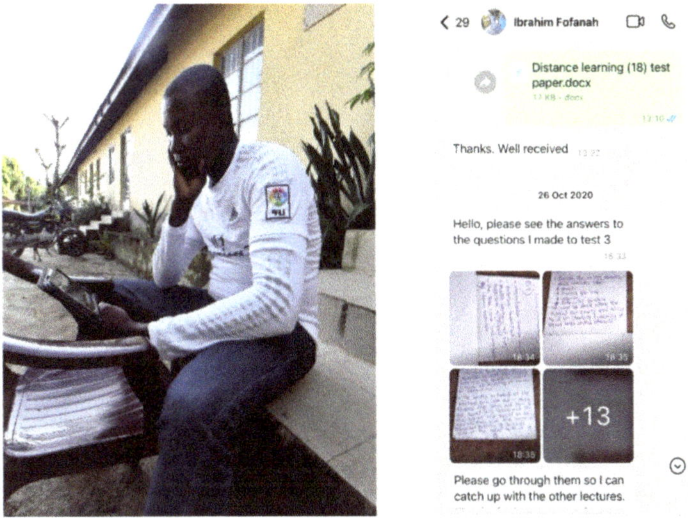
29
Ibrahim Fofanah
Distance learning (18) test paper.docx
Thanks. Well received
26 Oct 2020
Hello, please see the answers to the questions I made to test 3
+13
Please go through them so I can catch up with the other lectures.

Figure 48. Emergency Surgical Officer Ibrahim Fofanah studying video lectures in Sierra Leone during the COVID-19 pandemic. Low bandwidth meant downloads took several hours and could only be completed overnight. Tests between modules were completed remotely and reviewed with the trainer via WhatsApp calls. A bespoke e-learning platform would be nice, but the relationship is what matters most. Photo: author's own.

Social media use in Africa is growing faster than anywhere in the world, with an estimated 384 million social media users at time of writing. WhatsApp is the dominant communications platform. While concerns about misuse are real and shouldn't be ignored, it works well as an informal telemedicine tool.

DISTANCE LEARNING PROJECTS

Some organisations provide distance learning platforms, and international trainers with in-country (or equivalent) experience have successfully managed to teach remotely. Projects are dogged by low bandwidth and unreliable networks, the high cost of platforms, and particularly concerns about the relevance and quality of some teaching. Necessity is the mother of invention and the explosion in online learning during the COVID-19 pandemic resulted in education for trainers, improving the quality of online offerings.

MISSION HOSPITALS

Mission hospitals, faith-based hospitals, charity hospitals, and private not-for-profit hospitals are common, particularly in LICs. Many were founded by religious missionaries and may still be operated by missionary organisations, though philanthropic individuals, groups, and foundations are often also involved. Although many are faith-based, they usually provide care to all in need, regardless of beliefs.

In many Sub-Saharan African countries, these facilities provide a significant proportion of available surgical care. For example, in Uganda the Catholic Church manages dozens of hospitals and hundreds of smaller facilities, and for the rural poor this may be the only care available.

Heavy dependence on externally funded mission hospitals can leave national health systems vulnerable, and increasingly the mission hospitals themselves face financial difficulty. Some organisations provide free care; however, most pursue some degree of cost recovery, providing subsidised but not free care.

Many mission hospitals employ expatriate doctors to deliver day-to-day clinical care. The International Health and Tropical Medicine (IHTM) training programme in the Netherlands leads the world in producing graduates for these posts.

STANDALONE SPECIALISED HOSPITALS

Although relatively few in number, standalone speciality hospitals dedicated to treating specific conditions are significant because they have developed the world's best expertise directly in the countries where those conditions are prevalent. Many received support from external specialists at first and continue to host visiting experts, but they remain the premier facilities for the conditions they specialise in.

Evidence suggests that the best outcomes for complicated elective cases, such as obstetric fistula, are achieved in these facilities. They also appear cost-effective, because quality surgery is normally financially efficient. Centres like this have therefore become beacons for training. The best-known is the Addis Ababa Fistula Hospital (see chapter 3, page 23),[7] which has trained hundreds of surgeons and nurses working across Africa.

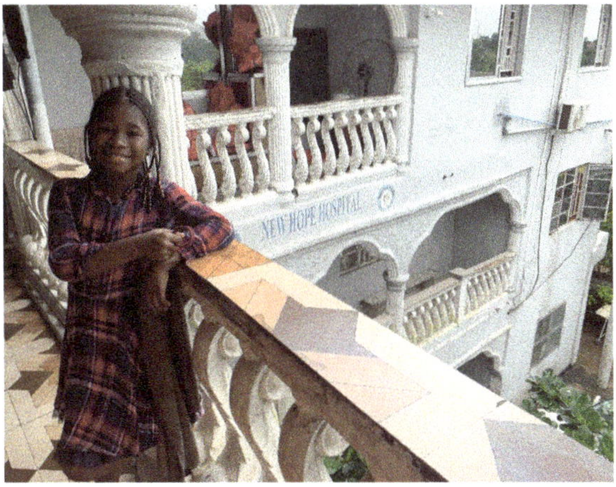

Figure 49. New Hope Hospital, a private hospital in Makeni, Sierra Leone, provides affordable surgery to those in need, free educational facilities for local providers and pro bono care for community members in crisis. Photo: author's own.

ALTRUISTIC PRIVATE FACILITIES

Thousands of private for-profit and not-for-profit hospitals provide surgery in LMICs. They are often small and deeply embedded in local communities. Models of practice vary. Some run efficient services, allowing them to turn enough profit to offer free or heavily subsidised care to patients who cannot afford it. Others, working in communities where the whole community is poor, provide heavily subsidised care to all.

The Jan Swasthya Sahyog (JSS) model of surgical care in the Bilaspur district, Chhattisgarh, India is an exemplar.[v] Founded by a small group of altruistic people, this non-profit, community-based hospital provides surgical services to a low-income rural Indian population, combined with extensive prevention-focused community support. Through innovation and evidence-based care, JSS provides high-quality, low-cost care. This comes at the price of great self-sacrifice from the team. A huge and largely overlooked issue in global surgery is how to support highly successful teams like those at JSS.

---

v https://www.jssbilaspur.org/

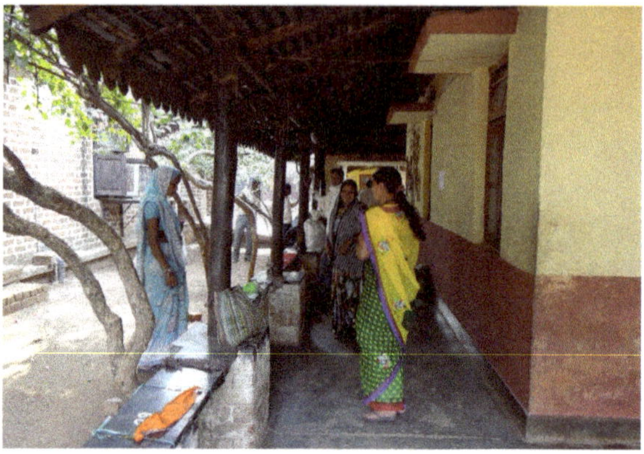

Figure 50. Patients attending outpatients at JSS mark their places in the queue. Photo: author's own.

Aravind Eye Hospitals (see chapter 13, page 128) is a large Indian institution that quickly became world-leading because its production-line system enables high-volume, über-efficient care. High-volume surgeons usually become experts, and high-quality care with minimal complications is key to this efficiency. In turn, this allows Aravind to provide free or heavily subsidised care for half of its patients.

EXPLORE FURTHER

Please see Appendix A (page 291) for examples of organisations in global surgery.

1. OeAD. *Austrian Partnership Programme in Higher Education and Research for Development (APPEAR).* https://oead.at/de/kooperationen/internationale-hochschulkooperationen/austrian-partnership-programme-in-higher-education-research-for-development-appear.
2. Davidson, Kief, and Pedro Kos, dirs. *Bending the Arc.* Decoy Productions, Impact Partners, Scout & Scholar, 2017. 1h42m. https://www.pih.org/bending-the-arc.
3. Dodson, Jude. *Building Partnerships of Equals.* UK Collaborative on Development Research, 2017. https://www.ukcdr.org.uk/wp-content/uploads/2017/11/Building-Partnerships-of-Equals_-REPORT-2.pdf.
4. Jan Swasthya Sahyog. https://www.jssbilaspur.org.

CHAPTER 18
MOTIVES, SKILLS AND READINESS

THIS CHAPTER HOPES to prompt you to consider your own unique situation, maximising the chance of finding a role where your contribution is helpful and reducing the risk you inadvertently become part of the problem.

MOTIVATION

This section discusses some commonly cited motives, which can, of course, be multifactorial.

SOCIAL JUSTICE

"I want to change the world" sounds a bit 'beauty-pageant contestant', but when we hear an inspiring presentation, read an incredible memoir or watch a film about people who have done just that, it triggers a wish to make our own little contribution. Being inspired by somebody else, especially someone you can relate to, is powerful.

Most of us have an inherent or learned sense of social justice and when you go somewhere where people are not getting a fair crack at life, the wish to do something about it grows and becomes a motivator for change. It is also natural to feel pity and want to help, but this needs to be pragmatic and not just handwringing.

Faith can also be a powerful motivator.

. . .

Giving back

The desire to "give something back" is probably an extension of the reason many people get satisfaction from training others. We appreciate those who trained us and want to help the next generation. Retirement can be an opportunity to give back at the end of a career. Training at home is satisfying, especially when those you worked with become highflyers, but we know if we had not been there, somebody else would have filled our shoes. This is not the case in LMICs.

Giving back is also something we might do to honour the many opportunities we ourselves have had.

Diaspora may feel they perhaps have it easier than some compatriots back home and many do a lot of work in their home countries, both clinically and raising funds and awareness. Much of this work is done quietly and unsung.

> **Leaving a legacy can also be a motivator. This could be seeing those you trained take over, or helping them set up something sustainable, such as a hospital or new service.**

Challenge and excitement

Some may have reached a career point where they have done it all and need a new challenge. Give thought to whether this is a professional challenge, or simply a challenge per se.

Most people find the inherently risky nature of our work sufficient, but others seek adventure and maybe an edgy experience. Others would simply like to experience new places and cultures. If excitement is attractive, think about how this is best achieved and whether non-work-related travel might be more appropriate.

Professional development

Articles about working abroad usually espouse the personal and professional benefits, such as greater resilience and cultural awareness. Getting a better understanding of the lives of others can improve us as humans, employees and supervisors.

> **"…. it is crucial to recognise that many foreign visitors do not come to Africa solely for philanthropic reasons."**
>
> **—Anthony Abbot Kamara, SWIFTSS lead, Sierra Leone**

For those who might feel over-cosseted, experiencing a challenging work environment can be a strong motivator. In modern practice, dependence on diagnostic technologies and long hours at computer screens leads some junior doctors to yearn for clinical exposure. Working in a low-resource setting is likely to strengthen clinical diagnostic skills and decision making, since diagnosis relies largely on history and examination. For some, this is appealing; for others, it may be daunting.[i]

> **Think not, "What can I get out of this?" but "What can I contribute?"**

There is a lot of talk about the benefit of developing leadership skills in LMICs, but considering the inherent power imbalances, this must be approached with extreme caution. Expatriates are often automatically afforded great respect, sometimes without having earned it. Less experienced individuals might flex their leadership muscles inappropriately, when their priority should be building listening skills and understanding.

For some, clinical work and surgery have proven less professionally rewarding than they had hoped. Global surgery offers avenues into research, public health, and epidemiology, and can also serve as a path into international organisations such as the WHO.

A "Global Surgery Experience"

> **Contemporary capitalism no longer requires we just obtain a lot of stuff; we now want *experiences*.**

Recent generations have learnt to appreciate the value of experiences in terms of self-development. Wanting a "a global surgery experience" is a natural response to this. If managed well, this could benefit the participant, the organisation and the host country. However, it also has the potential to be the latest form of colonialism, with global surgery framed as an opportunity for Global North residents.

Running away

It is not unheard of for people to go abroad because of unhappiness at home, such as relationship breakdown or professional disappointment. If working abroad has been a long-held ambition, and the change at home facilitates this, then this should be seen as an opportunity, not a doubtful motivation. Not being able to face retirement or an "empty nest" are relatively common motives, which can be put to good use.

---

i Thanks to Miss Sammy Conroy for items in this section.

However, there are other things, such as heart-ache, that going abroad cannot fix. Meeting new people and volunteering both have the potential to improve personal morale, but self-awareness is important so that we don't simply move our unhappiness to a different environment or treat volunteering as a 'last-ditch dating agency'.

Escaping an unsatisfactory job is another motivator that also cuts both ways. You may return from your experience with renewed vigour. On the other hand, you might just find out the hard way that you and your job just aren't compatible.

Boredom

Escaping boredom and monotony are common reasons for taking sabbaticals and making life changes that align with the need for new professional challenges. Retirees may fear boredom and seek additional responsibilities. Their wealth of experience makes them attractive to many organisations; however, retirees must be mindful that unused skills rapidly degrade and knowledge moves on. Keeping up to date and continuing some clinical work at home is usually important if you are going to be useful abroad.

With constant challenges at work, it is unusual for trainees whose careers are progressing well to feel bored. If trainees are looking to global surgery or anaesthesia to relieve boredom, they should therefore also consider whether they are on the right training path.

Adventure

Some people seek hardcore adventure, travel, and cultural experiences. However, we should recognise that global health and surgery often involve routine clinical work rather than constant excitement. Those primarily seeking thrills might be disappointed to find themselves collecting data instead of climbing mountains.

Humanitarian work is sometimes seen as particularly exciting and, given the dangerous environments in which humanitarian organisations operate, it can be very exciting — though sometimes not in a good way. While some people are drawn to danger, drama, and being where the action is, these organisations need steady people working with them. If the thrill is the main attraction, adventure travel may be a better option.

. . .

Filling a career gap

Some trainees take a deliberate pause in training, e.g. the Out of Programme for Experience in the UK, specifically to gain experience in global surgery. Others may find an unanticipated training hiatus and these gaps, even early in a career, have been put to good use by some trainees.

Wanting to improve your surgical skills

Some perceive working in an LMIC as an easier way to acquire skills that are also taught at home, with publications in reputable journals even supporting this idea. It has been suggested that the poor patient outcomes from some surgical camps are because Global North trainees were given opportunities to practise. It is unlikely trainees set out to exploit vulnerable populations or deliberately block sustainable change by taking training opportunities from local trainees, it is more likely they are naïve and did not appreciate the situation.

That is not to say you cannot learn abroad. Everybody gains new knowledge and skills, often at a fast rate, but this must not be at the expense of local trainees or the local population. Today's trainees are tomorrow's trainers, and many organisations allow trainees to travel if they go with their mentor. This makes good sense, as in the fullness of time, once they have completed their training, they can travel as productive members of the team.

White privilege is powerful and easily abused:

Local doctors had to call out a situation where doctors doing their Netherlands International Health and Tropical Medicine residency were given priority over local trainees. Expatriate doctors have even afforded opportunities to perform operations to their visiting friends.

Wanting to get involved in research

Some people see research in LMICs as an untapped resource that they can take advantage of. Exploiting research opportunities for self-advantage without benefiting the trusting local population is abuse, but if your interest is in genuine research, there are manifold ethical and meaningful opportunities available (see chapter 12, page 117).

CV/Resumé embellishment

We have seen people latch onto a project, arrive without preparation, insist things are adjusted to fit their planned activity, take a few beach days, and return home. The only plausible motive for this is CV embellishment.

People often get away with it, but the HIC global surgery community is quite connected, so there is a risk that this type of sham becomes known to supervisors back home. Fortunately, there are authentic ways to contribute that also provide material for the CV. Many communities urgently need help with research, innovation, fundraising, publicity, and practical tasks such as website development. Interview committees rightly value the skills needed for this work.

Unable to find employment at home

A difficult truth is that there are people working in surgical care in LMICs who were driven there because they were not employable at home. This includes people who have been exited from, or could not get places on, training schemes in their own countries.

> **LICs can find themselves the "employers of last resort" for expatriates who could not obtain employment in their own countries.**

There are others that are competent but, for various reasons, came off the training or employment ladder for sufficiently long that they then found it difficult to return home. If this is your situation, seek advice from a trusted supervisor, or make contact back home to keep your skills in line with accepted practice. Engaging with a partnership organisation would be an excellent way to keep in touch with developments.

MAPPING YOUR SKILLS TO WHERE THEY'RE NEEDED

Humanitarian organisations

The minimum requirement for a doctor working with Médecins Sans Frontières (MSF) is two years' clinical experience, and we know of people who were recruited to challenging posts with only this level of experience.

For anaesthesia, MSF requires two years' anaesthetic experience, but the ability to anaesthetise a wide range of patients including children, trauma cases, reconstructive work, and maternal care, alongside the ability to ensure and maintain the proper functioning of equipment. Because it takes time to rotate through different specialties, UK anaesthetic training does not get people to that level in two years. Therefore, treat the two-year requirement as the *minimum*, not the expected standard.

Similarly, for obstetricians/gynaecologists, two years' experience in gynaecology is required, alongside the ability to be flexible and work under stress. For other surgical fields, the requirement is to be fully trained (i.e. post Certificate of Completion of Training (CCT) or Board Certified).

Humanitarian organisations want an ability to perform a broad range of surgery, including paediatrics and caesarean section, because of the need to meet the general healthcare needs of the affected population, as well as the trauma. A&E and orthopaedic experience is considered desirable.

Additionally, most humanitarian organisations require applicants to already have three months' experience working or travelling in LMICs.

LOOK AT THE APPLICATION FORMS

Some large NGOs have detailed application forms that itemise operative and other competencies, including the dates on which procedures were last performed. Even if you aren't applying immediately, completing these forms can be a valuable self-test, clarifying where you are at in terms of required skills. Old-school practitioners with wide-ranging early experience will usually meet most requirements. For others, this exercise can highlight areas for focused training.

PLAY TO YOUR STRENGTHS

A high level of competence in a single field is very valuable to many organisations. If you are a UK-trained orthopaedic surgeon with 25 years' experience teaching others how to manage lower limb trauma, you will be very useful in almost every LIC. Although, it is eminently possible to learn new skills specifically for working in LMICs, it makes sense to play to your strengths and search for opportunities where they can be put to good use.

Dr Mark Shrime, talking on the US podcast *ENT in a Nutshell*, advised medical students interested in global surgery: "Be the best student and or resident that you can be...." — highlighting that striving for the highest level of skill and knowledge in your field is exactly what is needed to be of constructive help in LMICs.[1]

Being very good at your day job, even in a niche area, is often very useful. If your last ten years' work has been thyroid surgery, you may hesitate to approach humanitarian organisations, but we met surgeons just wanting somebody to come teach them how to do challenging thyroidectomies really well.

People may go abroad with the aim of stretching themselves, but nobody wants to land in a post where they are completely out of their depth.

Skills trainees might not realise they have

For trainees, it can be less obvious what you have to offer, and some roles will be unsuitable. However, with openness and planning, there are many other roles that are possible. Forward-thinking organisations appreciate that trainees will be fully trained in the future, and if these people have already spent time in LMICs, so much the better.

Some skills are overlooked. For example, organisations want people to run journal clubs, collate educational materials, and assist with syllabus development. Doctors in HICs are trained in audit, service evaluation, and quality improvement, which are rare skills in LMICs and would be valuable in many settings.

Development of operating policy, algorithms, logbooks, competency assessments and portfolios are all also needed in LMICs. These tasks require bilateral and senior input, but generating the documents is often time consuming and a tech-savvy trainee would be a great addition to many teams.

"There is a significant need for complex operations in LMICs, which must be delivered by highly skilled personnel. Collaborations should explore how this need can be met and implemented within LMICs to ensure retention and thus contribute to equitable distribution of the surgical workforce."

—Anita Eseenam Agbeko, vascular surgeon and deputy director, NIHR Research Hub, Ghana

Some HIC skills and courses can be adapted for different environments. For example, teaching standard Advanced Trauma Life Support (ATLS) drills is silly when training single-handed surgical, anaesthetic, and obstetric (SAO) providers in rural areas without radiology and primitive labs. However, elements of ATLS are very valuable and can be developed into setting-appropriate training.

Computer literacy (e.g. Word, PowerPoint, Excel) is generally required for compiling, understanding, and presenting reports. In addition, many SAO providers in resource-limited settings are less familiar with the programs, and welcome support writing their own documents and publications and preparing their presentations.

A junior resident doctor devised a resuscitation course specifically for single-handed SAO providers in Sierra Leone, adapting HIC practice to suit their environment and working conditions.

Being out of your depth

All global surgery texts stress the importance of HIC trainees not working beyond their level in LMICs, yet this continues to happen. Inadequate local knowledge may lead to more skilled local providers being overlooked by visiting teams. Some HIC trainees may be arrogant or even cynically choose to practice procedures out of sight of the supervision and clinical governance processes of home, but inexperience is likely to be a key factor for many.

The **Dunning-Kruger effect** is the cognitive bias that makes those with low competence overestimate their knowledge and skills (**Figure 51**). It is well known to healthcare trainers and is why "works within their limitations" is part of competence assessments. Most of us pass through this phase without recognising it at the time.

We are all familiar with maximising our employability by stretching the CV, but if you're going to an LMIC, don't make exaggerated claims about your abilities.

However, inexperienced HIC trainees risk being in LMICs at the height of what Americans call "mount stupid," the point on the curve where someone most overestimates their ability. This may explain why it is relatively common to see people out of their depth yet failing to reach out.

There are cases where people with just one year of general surgery experience thought themselves ready to be trainers, and organisations failed to monitor this. Such people can come across as arrogant, but more likely they are simply going through this normal developmental process. Unfortunately for them, it is happening out of sight of the

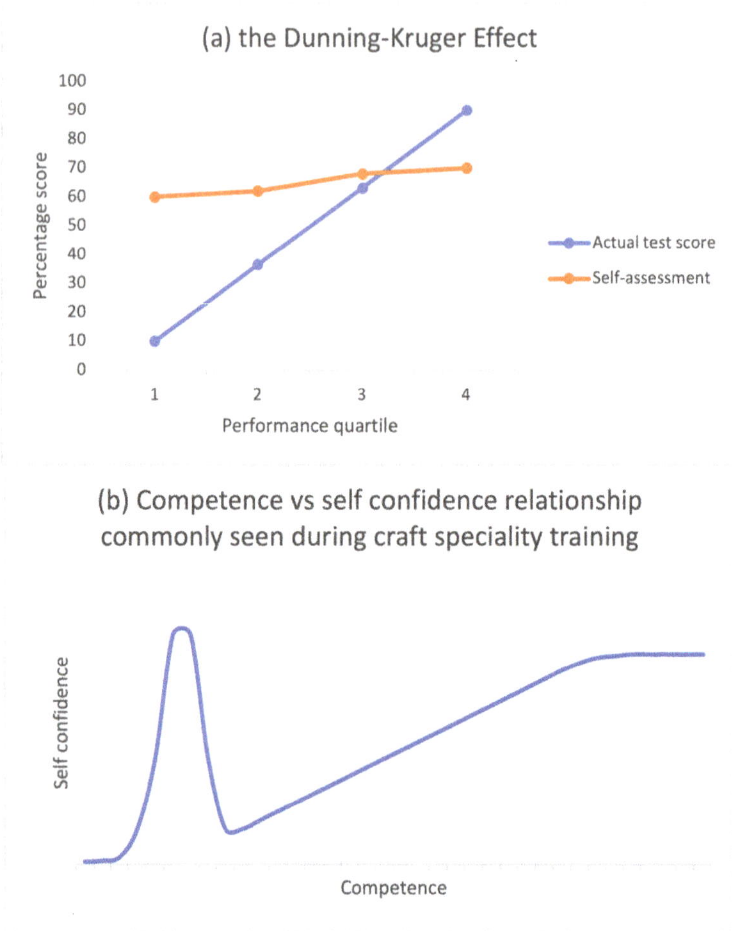

Figure 51. (a) Dunning and Kruger described the relationship between self-perceived performance and actual performance in an exam: lower-performing students overestimated their abilities, and vice versa. (b) In healthcare training, this effect commonly shows itself as a spike in self-confidence during the early years, followed by a return to appropriate confidence once the trainee has acquired enough knowledge to know when to call for help.

usual supervision safeguards, and in an environment, where being white affords unearned respect.

To safeguard against taking on situations beyond their capability, trainees should discuss their plans early with their educational supervisor, list current supervisors as referees, and ensure references and

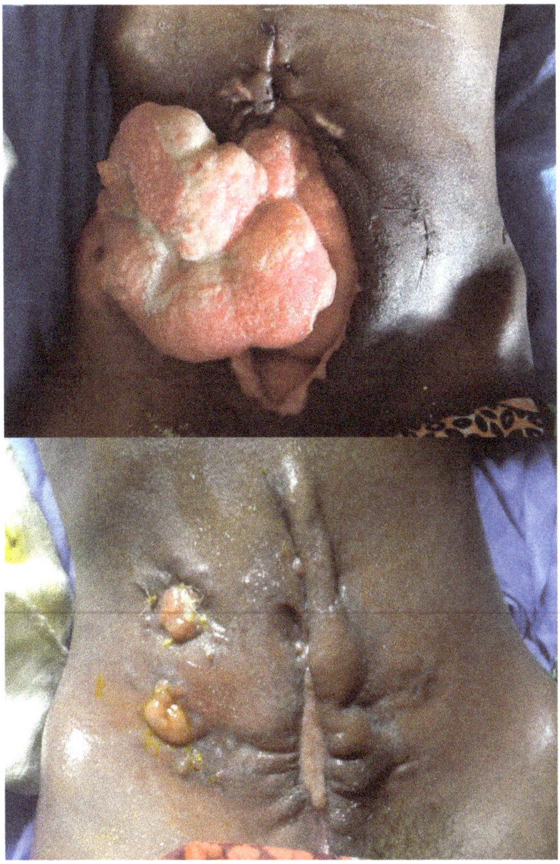

Figure 52. A health officer SAO provider returned from leave to find this patient (above). Expatriates had attempted surgery, got into trouble and did not seek help. The patient was left with an open abdomen and developed an enteric fistula. The local provider managed to "get the ends on the surface" and partially close the abdomen. Below: the same patient five weeks later. Photos: Peter Mboma.

competence assessments are properly followed up. The world is an increasingly small place, and accounts of inappropriate behaviour, such as self-taught surgery, could filter back home. Doctors registered with their home country medical council are also bound by its professional standards as well as those of the country they are visiting.

Interestingly, the Dunning-Kruger effect also works the other way, in that highly skilled people tend to focus on their areas of weakness and assume that others are more knowledgeable than they really are. If you provide some of the surgical or anaesthetic procedures listed in chapters 5 and 8, and particularly if you currently train others to do them, you have skills badly needed in the fight for universal access to essential surgery.

BEING REALISTIC ABOUT YOUR CIRCUMSTANCES

Career

Consider your long-term plans and career milestones. Twenty years ago, taking time off to volunteer impeded career progression, even implying a lack of direction or flakiness. Thankfully, times have changed, and appropriately planned volunteering is seen as positive. Nevertheless, trainees should reflect on what appointment committees are looking for. The two years you served in Congo, for example, might not be as attractive as the endovascular fellowship your rival undertook.

Emergency and general posts offer flexibility for those seeking to combine a career with global surgery, and there is some innovative thinking by employers seeking to fill these posts. By contrast, if you are one of only two sub-speciality providers in your hospital, taking time off will negatively impact your colleague.

Trainees should consider when they need to prepare for exams and selection processes. Some specialties weight selection criteria according to time from qualification, not time in training.

Family considerations

Do you have dependants to consider? Can the family manage on a reduced income?

Those who take children abroad extol the benefits to them in developing a sense of humanity, freedom from preconceptions and language development, but also acknowledge the challenges for children in making fresh starts and a cultural transition, particularly if moves are frequent.

Could some positions have negative implications for your children? Is there an international school within reach? Do you leave your partner and dependants and go abroad alone?

TIME

In theory, any amount of time is valuable, but in practice it is not like that. Very short stays in-country can be disruptive and burdensome for those on the receiving end. Lack of time therefore prevents effective contribution to certain projects. However, there are options where even a few weeks can work, and contributions that can be made from home, such as telemedicine, fundraising, or developing educational material. These can be done alongside your normal employment without loss of income.

MINIMUM TIME REQUIREMENTS

Many organisations stipulate a minimum commitment, with three to six months being typical for a first trip that involves either training or clinical commitments. Humanitarian organisations usually require six to eight weeks, but also need flexibility and the ability to deploy staff at short notice. The complexity of places, and the extent to which they differ from your normal working environment, will vary, but by general consensus, three months in-country is about the time it takes to get past being "unconscious-incompetent." Repeated trips to the same centre can, of course, still be meaningful when shorter; what matters most is building meaningful and sustained connections.

> **"I encourage people that there are also opportunities to be involved in work from home. I have been a committee member and past president of GASOC, in which UK trainees seek to advocate, innovate, and unite with those in low-resource settings including through journal clubs exchanging knowledge, projects, and an annual conference. There are many opportunities, particularly with increasing virtual learning and technological innovations."**
>
> **—Helen Please, surgical resident (Oxford, UK)**

Major humanitarian organisations have established strategies to enable experienced staff to hit the ground running, as this is so necessary in acute mass casualty situations. At the other end of the spectrum, it will take longer to build effective partnerships. The pragmatic solidarity that has been so effective in capacity building takes time, repeated visits and can take years to mature.

Adaptation period consideration

The first few weeks on the ground are likely to be less productive than you hoped. A common phenomenon is "rapid appraisal bias" (see chapter 22, page 277). People have caused lasting harm by sharing and attempting to impose their views at this early stage. Instead, take a breath, have patience, and observe a little longer — you will likely see things very differently with time.

> "I took a six-month sabbatical in Uganda, combining a supernumerary clinical role with educational endeavours, including a surgical training conference, and setting up a scholarship for East African surgeons to experience training in the UK. I am now building a more sustainable, relationship in Uganda, where I feel a longer-term connection. I have been appointed a trustee of the hospital and actively support a collaboration between a UK and Ugandan hospital, for which we have secured ongoing external funding."
>
> —Helen Please, surgical resident (Oxford, UK)

With hard work and strong local support, you gradually begin to grasp the real situation, understand clinical presentations, and learn how local systems work, allowing you to transition into being effective. This adaptation phase can be shortened somewhat by diligent study before travel, high-quality handover, or by shadowing an experienced colleague for the first weeks. However, stories abound of new arrivals beginning the day after the previous incumbent left, so it is best to factor in a period of low productivity at the start.

Options for those with limited time

Short volunteering trips by people unfamiliar with local conditions can be very disruptive to local providers and damage what has already been built up. If you only have limited time available, consider options such as surgical camps — albeit with an understanding of the concerns around this type of volunteering (see chapter 17, page 183).

If you want to pursue the more sustainable options, but do not currently have enough time to make this meaningful, consider going as an observer alongside someone already familiar with the environment, undertaking preparatory courses, or activities such as fundraising or preparing materials for the projects you support.

GETTING MORE TIME — TRAINING PATHWAY OPTIONS

UK

UK trainees have several options for gaining international experience, with similar schemes existing in other countries. In the UK, you can temporarily step away from your training through Out of Programme for Clinical Experience (OOPE), Out of Programme Career Break (OOPC) — both of which allow time away without shortening UK training time. Out of Programme for Research (OOPR) is also possible. You should discuss these options with both your educational supervisor and training programme director to determine the most appropriate path.

The gap between foundation and core training can also provide an opportunity. Unfortunately, for SAO trainees, this gap occurs too early in training to contribute meaningfully to many projects. However, a post such as working as a junior doctor in A&E in a MIC may be both enjoyable and relevant to future career aspirations.

USA

US residents can also typically request a leave of absence, apply for research years, or use international electives to gain overseas experience without losing their place in training. Some specialties run dedicated global health or international surgery tracks, and these can extend into a "chief resident year" depending on programme structure. Hardy and Hochman's *Global Surgery: How to Work and Teach in Low- and Middle-Income Countries* provides excellent information for US trainees.[2,3]

ELSEWHERE

Trainees from other countries should speak to their supervisors and training programme directors to establish how to take time away, without falling off the training ladder.

GETTING MORE TIME — CONSULTANT AND STAFF GRADE OPTIONS

Employers often see volunteering as a benefit to their organisation. Innovative job planning can facilitate overseas volunteering, and an overview is given here.

Many HICs offer generous employment break schemes (sabbaticals), especially in Australasia. These are often readily available and, although most do not allow individuals to work for rival employers, exceptions may be made for humanitarian work overseas.

The ageing workforce in HICs has forced employers to introduce measures such as "retire and return" options. This includes managed or phased retirement with flexible working patterns, which can make humanitarian work possible. There can be financial implications, of course, so pension advice should always be sought.

Annualised job plans are another option, in which staff negotiate a finite number of hours per year, aggregating clinical activity to allow time away. This may suit those who undertake international work requiring repeated short-term commitments. Those wishing to maintain income would need to accept an increased workload while at home, and service pressures may affect their ability to negotiate. In SAO specialties, there is constant pressure to back-fill vacated sessions when colleagues are on leave. Those interested in time away can exploit this pressure by making themselves "super flexible." Employers may agree to such arrangements and compensate with time off in lieu.

A raft of part-time and flexible working options exists in many countries, including part-time or part-year contracts, job sharing, flexitime, annualised contracts, flexible rostering, and voluntary reduced working time. Less-than-full-time clinical contracts have long been paired with academic appointments, and global surgery is one of the fastest expanding areas of surgical research. Taking unpaid annual leave outside a formal career break, or buying or trading additional leave, can sometimes provide time away. Occasionally, study leave may be granted for overseas, humanitarian, or global surgery activities. Equitable solutions and advice are available for working in private practice, including guidance on designing appropriate agreements.[4]

Emergency practice pairs well with global surgery work, both in terms of the conditions encountered and the temporal nature of service delivery. Some hospitals require clinicians to undertake blocks of emergency cover, with periods of compensatory leave afterwards, which could be used abroad.

Lack of time can be a genuine barrier, but people often assume this before having fully explored the options. Time is money, so in many situations it is likely you can negotiate a satisfactory arrangement if you are able to make financial compromises.

ALONE OR IN A GROUP

Are you planning to go alone, as a couple, or is a group option available?

A group is often easier for a first trip. If going alone, seek out and speak with anyone you can who has experience of the place before travel, learning everything possible about the country in advance. How does the healthcare system operate? Who else works at the facility? What is the referral and transport system like? What is the attitude to women?

When going alone, don't underestimate the personal difficulties and actively seek out support.

MONEY MATTERS

Although some organisations pay developed-world salaries in LMICs, these are the exception. Many positions are unpaid or remunerated at local rates. Can you currently afford an expensive hobby? Can you manage with no income, or a nominal one, for a year abroad? Do you need to start saving now to afford this in the future, perhaps through some lucrative locum work?

LANGUAGE

Language is a key consideration and critically important for teaching and training. Our colonial heritage means English is the official language in some LMICs, and the lingua franca in others. Fluency in other languages, especially French, Spanish, and Arabic, can be very helpful.

> **"She is talking deep British and I could not understand it."**
>
> **—Liberian trainee giving the author feedback**

Accents can be challenging. Respect for the "white trainer" is such that local trainees may sit politely through many hours of training, without understanding any of it. I was saddened, for example, when one trainee let me teach a full session, only to state on his feedback form that he could not understand me.

Learning local languages takes time but reaps rewards. Even learning a little can bring significant benefits, at least in building rapport. If you are training local faculty, listening to them teach in their own language gives valuable insight.

CARBON EMISSIONS

Travel and the environmental footprint of overseas work are an important consideration. Does the benefit to healthcare justify the carbon emissions generated by the trip? Is it justified to fly across the world to give just a few days of classroom teaching?

Offsetting should be the basic expectation, but avoiding non-essential travel is better. Face-to-face contact remains necessary for much of what we do, but always consider whether your activity could be conducted, or at least partly conducted, remotely. Better still, could you empower local faculty to deliver the training if the money for this was provided?

EXPLORE FURTHER

1. Hardy, Mark A., and Beth R. Hochman, eds. *Global Surgery: How to Work and Teach in Low- and Middle-Income Countries.* Springer, 2023.
2. Royal Australasian College of Surgeons. *Global Health Deployment Guidebook.* 2021. https://www.surgeons.org/-/media/Project/RACS/surgeons-org/files/global-health/Global-Health-Deployment-Guidebook.pdf.
3. Gana, Tabitha, Simon A. Boyes, and Lesley M. Hunt. "Innovative Job Planning to Facilitate UK Surgeon Engagement with International Development." *British Journal of Healthcare Management* (2022). https://doi.org/10.12968/bjhc.2022.0045.

CHAPTER 19
CHOOSING YOUR FIRST PROGRAMME

STARTING out in global surgery can feel overwhelming. There are many thousands of organisations; how do you choose wisely?

First ventures can be "off the mark." Do not lose heart if your initial efforts do not achieve everything you hoped for. These experiences will inform your future work, and remember that most experienced hands feel it takes around three months in a country before you become productive.

FINDING OPPORTUNITIES

PERSONAL CONNECTIONS AND NETWORKING

Many people begin their path into global surgery, and particularly volunteering, through word of mouth. Colleagues have links, and this sparks interest among others. Increase the chance of making useful personal contacts by joining global surgery groups, attending interest meetings, and taking relevant courses.

ONLINE RESEARCH

Start by visiting websites to get a feel for the work going on. Table 12 in Appendix A (see page 291) lists organisations ranging from major international bodies to small charities. But be sure to do your own searches, particularly if your specialty is niche.

DUE DILIGENCE

Even if you are following a recommendation, you should examine the organisation and the proposed mission carefully before getting too involved. Not all organisations are equally well managed or share the same ethos. Ask yourself: What exactly does the organisation do, and where do your skills fit in? You will be giving your time and often your money, so adopt a "buyer beware" approach.

Read everything you can find. If they have an up-to-date website and published annual reports, this is encouraging. Many organisations also post blogs, stories, and other personal experiences on their websites, but also seek these out independently for unbiased perspective. Request contact details for previous employees, LMIC partners, and volunteers, and speak to them personally. Most organisations require end-of-mission reports, so ask if the non-confidential sections are available to read. If the organisation collates educational materials, also ask to view these.

Sustainability

Consider the life expectancy of the project. What are the long-term goals? Where do they expect to be in five years? Is this something you could be part of for many years, or a one-off initiative? What is their handover and exit strategy? Do they collaborate with others of interest to you?

Financial considerations

Read the organisation's annual reports, which should include financial information and outputs. By exploring reports from other similar organisations, you can develop a rough picture of whether this one appears efficient. It is entirely legitimate to ask these types of questions. If an organisation is offended by you asking about their finances, this is telling.

ORGANISATION-SPECIFIC CONSIDERATIONS

There are specific things to consider for each type of organisation and project. The first few options presented here are not global surgery but may be of interest to readers looking for adventure or personal development, and can act as first steps towards future involvement.

. . .

Voluntourism

Organisations combining volunteering with tourism are popular. It is a rapidly expanding sector, worth billions of dollars globally. They may be, but are not always, operated by not-for-profit groups, allowing individuals to travel to low-resource settings while contributing to local communities. Environmental, health, and social projects are popular. Participants are usually young (15–25 years), and trips often contain an adventure-travel element.

Voluntourism has undergone some recent scrutiny. Some providers are thought to have commodified volunteering, encouraged white saviourism, or even exposed vulnerable groups to harm. Some trips are said to have damaged local environments, strained communities by increasing water and electricity usage, and even encouraged institutionalisation of children to meet the need for volunteer orphanage placements. Additionally, trips can be culturally insensitive and ignore local customs or disrupt traditional social structures.[1,2]

On the other hand, tourism is an important source of income in many LMICs, bringing much-needed foreign exchange and economic benefits. For students with limited time available, carefully selected trips can raise awareness and be a positive introduction to global health.

***Check**: Are the project's environmental credentials sound? Who benefits financially — local communities or tour operators? Is the intervention appropriate and locally led? Are costs transparent and justified? Is your personal safety assured?*

Adventure organisations

Adventure organisations often require doctors to support young people on adventure holidays. Such trips are widely perceived to build resilience, leadership, and organisational skills. Payment, expenses, responsibilities, and indemnity vary between tour operators and should be carefully considered. There are stories of doctors being quite out of their depth, so don't big up your CV to get the post. The Medical Defence Union has advice on preparing for adventure and expedition medicine.[i]

---

[i] Fryar, Caroline. "Dreaming of Far-Flung Places." *MDU Journal*, Summer 2022. https://mdujournal.themdu.com/issue-archive/summer-2022/dreaming-of-far-flung-places.

Check: *Are safety and rescue protocols robust? What is the medical indemnity arrangement? Are responsibilities clearly defined?*

Wilderness

Doctors are required to support exploration and extreme travel. Wilderness medicine has become a niche subspecialty with specific training, texts, and courses available. These combine healthcare delivery training with personal safety and the safety of others in extreme conditions.

Check: *Do you have the necessary wilderness medicine qualifications? Are safety and rescue arrangements possible? What is the medical indemnity arrangement?*

Niche healthcare abroad

Some multinational companies employ agencies to ensure high-level medical care for their workers abroad. Roles include attending sick people during repatriation flights. These are paid posts that may build independent decision-making and understanding of risk management.

Check: *Is medical indemnity explicit? What salary and terms of employment apply? Is personal safety assured? Might there be periods of inactivity?*

Generic health projects or non-SAO provider role in a surgical project

As we develop skills useful in LMICs, life throws up barriers to travel such as relationships, children, and the career ladder. Trainees face a dilemma; they are free to travel while young, but do not yet have the SAO skill set. Non-surgical, and particularly community health projects, may fill this gap, give the satisfaction of contributing, and develop cultural competence, without the pressure of having to perform as an SAO provider or trainer.

Some surgical camps need resident or junior doctor support, allowing volunteers to see surgery in a low-resource setting within a protected framework. Partnerships often involve wide-ranging support to partner hospitals, throwing up opportunities for volunteering in a surgical team, without the necessity to be fully trained. Common themes include capacity measurement, infrastructure support and assessing local requirements.

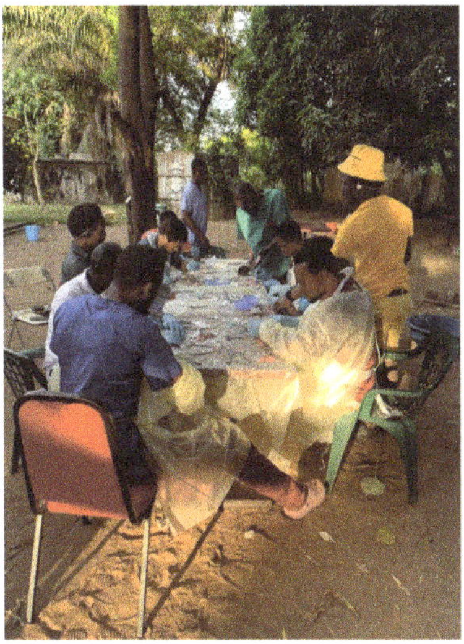

Figure 53. Wet lab, Sierra Leone. Anthony Abbot Kamara, Ishiaka Konneh, and Hassan Sheriff teaching. Photo: author's own.

In UK surgeon Jen Watt's account of camp life (see chapter 17, page 184), she explains how the local team could not access training in theatre as they were too busy with the patients. This could indicate opportunities to shoulder some of the workload of local teams, allowing them to benefit from training in theatre.

Check: *Do you have the appropriate skill set? Could this lead to SAO volunteering later? Is your role clearly defined within a protected environment, or is there risk of mission creep?*

Teaching and training projects

One of the best ways to make sustained change in a LMIC is to train and mentor local teams. Training SAO providers requires SAO providers and, in many LMICs, there are not enough of them to do this within an acceptable timeframe.

For example, in 2016, Sierra Leone had 2.7 SAO providers per 100,000 population.[3] If the existing providers were to train others, the number would organically grow, but to reach a workforce density of 20 providers per 100,000 population would take more than a century. Therefore, if people in LMICs are to get access to surgery, international help is clearly needed.

High-quality teaching requires long-term commitment, familiarity with a country's unique challenges, enduring relationships, and mentorship. Preparing teaching materials takes more time than delivery, and operative teaching is often slow and stressful where resources and backup are limited. Simulation is valuable to shorten the operative learning curve but cannot replace it.

Good teaching programs are undoubtedly laborious, and not for those seeking excitement and adventure. However, a long-term training commitment where you see the patient outcomes achieved by those you trained can be the most rewarding form of volunteering.

"We received intensive, hands-on training from highly skilled and passionate professionals. The curriculum included basic surgical skills, bedside teaching, case presentations, wet lab procedures, and real-time mentorship. These experiences helped build my confidence and competence."

—Ibrahim M. Sesay, surgical officer (Sierra Leone)

However, with high reward often reflecting high risk, teaching projects also present major opportunities to do harm. Great respect is often afforded to expatriate trainers, and naïve audiences may not discriminate the quality of the education. Visiting trainers have been known to teach outside their field of expertise, and training quality is not always monitored. Yet as the challenges faced in LMICs are greater, training quality needs to be at least as good as, if not better than, that in HICs.

In countries where SAO providers are few, the first people trained serve as the seed corn who will set standards and train future generations. This also means that poor or even dangerous practice can become entrenched.

For example, despite poor patient outcomes, we have seen dangerous practices passed along after unusual teaching was delivered a decade earlier. Teaching without follow-up can cause years of harm, of which long gone trainers remain blissfully unaware.

Tokenistic training, such as very short "fly-in fly-out" courses with no follow-up, is also sadly quite common. Some organisations also allow volunteers to teach whatever they fancy, implying that recipients should just be grateful for anything we choose to give them — the educational equivalent of "Junk for Jesus."

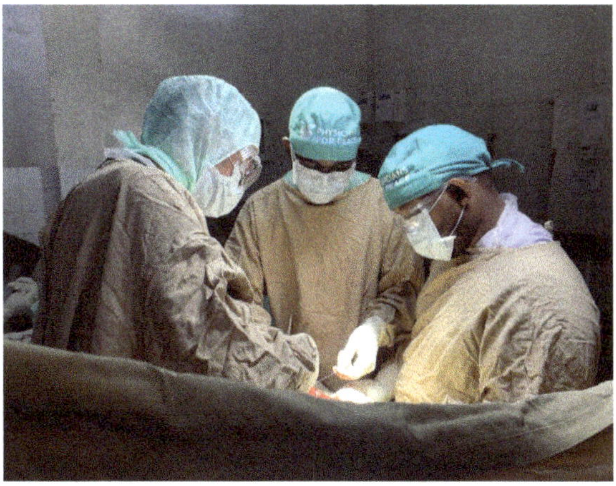

Figure 54. Darwin Nyirenda completing a bowel anastomosis under the supervision of Dominik von Malsen, Blantyre Malawi. Physicians for Peace funded a dedicated weekly list for this training. Photo: Dominik von Malsen.

Residents interested in teaching should consider approaching organisations about shadowing opportunities. This may be welcome, particularly among smaller organisations seeking to attract future trainers. Getting involved early in your career allows you to observe, access training materials and direct your personal study and development to that country's specific needs. You could also help with clerical matters, websites, fundraising, and assisting local trainees.

Some organisations will not accept applications from individuals without prior LMIC experience. Early shadowing helps develop cultural competence and shows long-term commitment, improving your chances of success.

***Check**: Are you responsible for teaching this subject at home? Is this training part of a sustainable programme, or a one-off course? How does the organisation measure effectiveness (i.e. the Kirkpatrick level)?[4] Have you been able to prepare yourself to the standard expected for teaching this subject in a HIC? How do we know training matches local need?*

Working abroad

An alternative to volunteering is to apply for a job abroad. Some mission and LMIC government hospitals, for example, use international doctors to provide day-to-day clinical care, including considerable amounts of obstetrics and sometimes surgery.

The Netherlands International Health and Tropical Medicine (IHTM) programme trains people to become Medical Doctor-Global Health (MD-GH) graduates for these positions. Their course provides a year of obstetrics and gynaecology (O&G) training combined with either a year of paediatrics or surgery and a tropical medicine course. Similar training can be assembled elsewhere, combining clinical placements with tropical medicine diplomas and additional short courses.

These positions typically involve substantial clinical responsibility in low-resource settings, and training is designed to equip doctors with a broad skillset suitable for LMIC hospital work. However, whether this training is sufficient to practise surgery has been questioned. Indeed, some local providers have raised concerns that a minority of individuals have abused these positions to practise surgery before commencing surgical or O&G training in their own countries.

A recent qualitative study found that MD-GH graduates felt they had deficiencies in exposure, particularly in certain surgical competencies, and some reported feeling frustrated when the training profile did not match their needs or equip them to function as independent doctors.[5] The paper states, "Most MD-GHs noted that the global health residency offered the opportunity to further refine their surgical and O&G skills," adding to concerns that vulnerable populations could be exploited or that training opportunities could be taken away from LMIC trainees.

However, other MD-GH graduates reported they did feel adequately prepared, and many graduates of the programme are unsung heroes, demonstrating exemplary professionalism while providing essential care to some of the world's most underserved communities.

Living and working abroad is demanding. People are placed under enormous stress, often charged at a very early stage of their careers, not only with unsupervised clinical duties, but also administrative, managerial and even supervisory roles all happening in an alien culture. Relationships amongst MD-GH providers at the same facility can cause significant angst, due to professional disagreements, differences in clinical judgment,

"I am going back now, and I want to become a GP, simply because I want to be good at what I do. And currently that is not the case. Not at all. I am failing people because of my poor skills."[5]

—MD-GH survey respondent

Tiggelaar et al. BMC Med Educ. 2025 ;25:663.

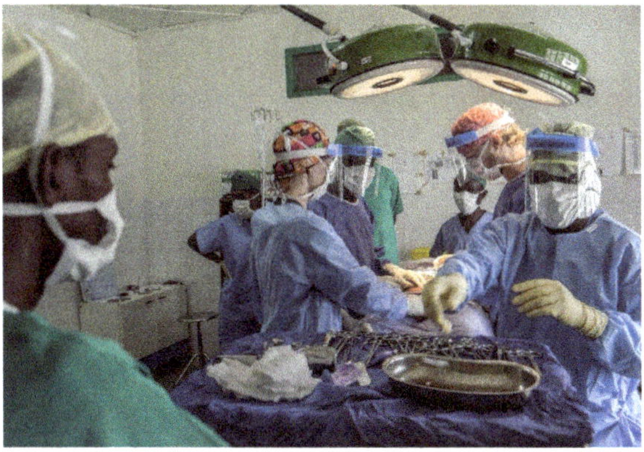

Figure 55. Unsung heroes: Martelien Grootjans and Daniel van Leerdam graduates of the Netherlands MD-GH programme devote their professional lives to providing care for underserved populations. Photo: Magnus Endal.

cultural misunderstandings and power dynamics. The personal stress should not be underestimated.

In larger hospitals, specialist SAO appointments are possible through organisations such as Partners in Health, the World Bank, academic institutions, and local ministries of health and other institutions. Most require board certification (USA) or Certificate of Completion of Training (CCT, UK), although in some places fellowship of a surgical college may suffice.

***Check**: What support will you have? What resources are available on site? Are there additional responsibilities, such as teaching or supervising? What training do you have for any additional roles?*

Disaster relief organisations

A lot of disaster relief work is directly clinical, and surgeons and teams may need to cover obstetrics, war surgery, general surgery, burns and orthopaedics all in the same day. These organisations are often well-resourced compared to surrounding hospitals in the same country, but the environments in which they work can be some of the toughest in the world.

Missions also take place in less challenging settings and are used to train both local and expatriate personnel. 90% of Médecins Sans Frontières' (MSF) 69,000 employees are locally hired. The remaining 10% are internationally mobile staff, specialists or senior managers.

***Check**: Do you have experience across all relevant specialties? Are you prepared for dangerous or unstable conditions, and the personal restrictions and stress this will place on you? Are you available at short notice?*

Medical student electives

The value of electives in LMICs in terms of personal development is well known. Medical schools have established connections and resources. Some LMIC facilities have become familiar with the financial and other advantages of hosting elective students and may therefore accept large numbers. While this can be welcome for social and tourism reasons, students may have an unpleasant reality check when they realise it was their money, rather than themselves, that was wanted.

There are media stories of medical students in small LMIC facilities "doing everything," but I have never witnessed this. I have observed many British, American, European and Scandinavian students in Africa, and never seen bad behaviour on their part. They have behaved in an exemplary way, despite less-than-ideal behaviour from some of their supervisors.

The British Medical Association provides an ethics toolkit for students that addresses several key challenges: the potential pressure to exceed one's competence, language barriers, and cultural differences. [ii] It reminds students they remain under obligation to the General Medical Council, and must decline requests to act beyond their competence, maintain professional ethical standards, minimise the burden they impose, and always put the needs of local trainees ahead of their own.

***Check**: Do you have existing contacts through your medical school? Are there elective opportunities via partnership organisations? Have you sought personal advice and spoken to students with prior experience? Have you explored sponsorship and bursary options?*

ORGANISATION AND PROJECT CHECKLIST

See **Table 10** for suggestions of key criteria for evaluating global health organisations and projects.

[ii] BMA Ethics Toolkit for Medical Students: Medical Students and Electives in Resource-Poor Settings: https://www.bma.org.uk/advice-and-support/ethics/medical-students/ethics-toolkit-for-medical-students/medical-electives-in-resource-poor-settings

EXPLORE FURTHER

1. Fryar, Caroline. "Dreaming of Far-Flung Places." *MDU Journal*, Summer 2022. https://mdujournal.themdu.com/issue-archive/summer-2022/dreaming-of-far-flung-places.
2. UK Government. "Volunteering and Adventure Travel Advice: Safer Adventure Travel and Volunteering Overseas." https://www.gov.uk/guidance/safer-adventure-travel-and-volunteering-overseas.
3. Royal College of Surgeons of Edinburgh. "Introduction to Humanitarian Healthcare Online Course." https://services.rcsed.ac.uk/events-courses/introduction-to-humanitarian-healthcare-online-course.

Organisation and Project Checklist			
Criteria	**Reassuring**	**Non-reassuring**	**Red Flag**
Website	Up to date, informative, clear contact information	Out-of-date, inaccurate	Poor quality, years out of date, contacts expired
Response	Quick, professional	Slow (though remember it may be a temporary issue)	None
References	Required, followed up and, for trainees, supervisor stipulated	Not contacted or slow to contact	For trainees: failure to require supervisor's reference
Previous Volunteers	Enthusiastic yet realistic	Muted or "damned with faint praise," gushing but vague	Open (evidence-based) criticism
Local Team	Prominent; contactable and enthusiastic; local contacts spontaneously offered	Local team not prominent; had to specifically ask for a contact	No local team; local team critical of program
Finances	Available, clear, and careful with resources	Unclear; value difficult to understand	Evidently wasteful or very expensive mode of delivery
Board	Appropriate with financial and clinical governance representation	Unclear	Nepotistic or lacking clinical governance representation
Resources (teaching and reference materials, pre-deployment course, etc.)	Bespoke, up-to-date, evidence-based and setting-specific	Poor quality or inadequate but organisation open to review; or using generic materials, e.g. WHO slides, etc.	Dangerous or out-of-date materials and unwilling to update

Table 10. Key criteria for assessing the quality and reliability of organisations and projects in global surgery.

Criteria	Reassuring	Non-reassuring	Red Flag
Line Management	Clear and appropriate	Unclear	Supervision by inappropriate people
Research Publications (where applicable)	High quality; prominence given to LMIC authors	Tokenistic placement of LMIC authors on papers	Demonstrate risk of exploitation
Your Role	Clear, appropriate and manageable in the time frame	Vague; imprecise match to your skills	Does not match your level or skills; hopelessly unrealistic; unethical
Productivity	Evidenced previous achievement	Lack of evidence about productivity	Long-standing programme unable to show outcomes; reports or evidence of poor outcomes
Climate Change	Active steps to minimise travel; promoting sustainable technology	Aware but could do more	Profligate with CO_2; multiple short trips
Life Expectancy	Clear exit plan with handover process	Unclear	Appears intent on self-perpetuation or blocking local development
Logistics	Clear arrangements for housing, feeding, in-country travel, medical registration etc	Unclear arrangement or housing at far distance	A mess or shows no concern for medical registration
Cost	Clear and reasonable or expenses covered	Unclear; open ended; previous volunteers concerned about costs	Pays for volunteers to stay in expensive hotels etc

Table 10. (cont.)

Criteria	**Reassuring**	**Non-reassuring**	**Red Flag**
Safeguarding Checks	Asked to provide criminal records checks in line with your own country's requirements	Does not require safeguarding information	Does not require safeguarding information, despite working with children or vulnerable groups
Qualifications	Requires verified evidence of all relevant qualifications	Does not require verified evidence of qualifications	Reports of fraudulent people involved in care or teaching
Meet	Opportunity to talk frankly with local team, previous volunteers and board representatives	Opportunity to speak to some but not all	No-one willing to talk or previous volunteers or local partners openly critical
Supervision (as appropriate)	Asked to provide evidence of personal competency and clear supervision arrangements in place for trainees	Vague or danger of making assumptions about competency	Not asked about personal competency; previous post holders working beyond level

Table 10. (cont.)

CHAPTER 20
SELF-IMPROVEMENT

BESIDES BEING good at your day job and finding where those skills are most needed, there are pragmatic clinical and cultural preparations that can help you become more effective, avoid common faux pas, and make you think more deeply about what you are doing.

PROBLEMATIC AREAS FOR DOCTORS IN TRAINING

High-volume surgical care providers tend to get better patient outcomes, leading to specialisation and sub-specialisation in HICs. The combination of this and shorter training hours in the UK and Europe has resulted in tightly focused training programs, because it is usually quicker to train a specialist than a generalist. In countries where SAO providers deal with a wider range of practice, it can be challenging for those with narrow expertise.

> **"I thought I was mentally prepared for death and dying when I came to work here. Nothing could have prepared me for the grief and injustice I felt when I held a peer as he died from a disease that would have had treatment and extended his life expectancy to normal, had he been born where I was born. He could have been a doctor, and I could have been him."**
>
> **—Ong Pei Jean, anesthesia resident and President of GASOC**

We rely heavily on IT, with instant access to information. Connectivity has been a problem in rural and remote locations, but coverage is improving rapidly, enabling better access to information and reference resources.

The IT workload of resident doctors has taken them away from the bedside, eroding clinical skills and confidence. We are heavily dependent on diagnostic adjuncts, such as X-rays, CT scans and blood tests. Working in low-resource settings usually requires a return to old fashioned clinical skills. But making decisions, such as going to theatre or chest drain insertion, solely on the basis of examination can be hard, if you are not used to it.

Challenges for HIC Trainees in LMICs:

Broad clinical responsibilities

Limited IT and diagnostic support

Relying on core clinical skills instead of investigations

Performing open procedures when more familiar with laparoscopic

Independent decision making in high-pressure settings

Adapting to longer, less structured working

A common complaint from surgical trainees in HICs is lack of experience with open surgery, because of the focus on acquiring minimally invasive skills. For instance, performing an appendicectomy via a right iliac fossa incision is tough for those who have never seen it. Lack of both muscle-relaxation anaesthesia and infrastructure in some LICs means laparoscopic surgery is queuing behind developments in anaesthesia.

Transitioning from a decision-light to a decision-heavy role can be difficult. Junior resident doctors in the UK complain they prepare the information necessary for clinical decisions, but their senior makes the actual decision. It can be tough for people to find it's suddenly all on them.

Adapting to a new working pattern can also be difficult. Those accustomed to the European Working Time Directive may struggle with the long hours colleagues endure abroad.

EXTENDING YOUR REPERTOIRE

There are cases of people rapidly trying to master new elective skills because they think they may get the opportunity to perform those

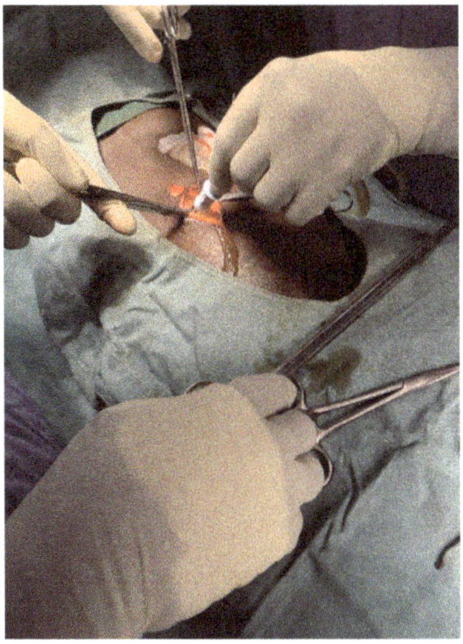

Figure 56. The incision of indecision: a tiny laparotomy to ascertain the colour of the fluid is performed before opening the abdomen where pre-operative imaging is absent Photo: author's own.

procedures during surgical camps or short visits to LMICs. Indeed, the poor outcomes of some camps are thought to be related to practitioners attempting operations outside of their normal practice, and it is rarely necessary to learn elective skills outside of your speciality. However, if you expect to be the sole provider in a remote area, it does make sense to see if there are additional emergency skills you could develop before travelling.

But, before expanding your repertoire, ensure you are fully competent in the skills you should already have. For example, if you have never inserted a chest drain, or if best practice might have changed since you last did it, then update your skills prior to travel. Courses such as Hostile Environment Surgical Training (see Table 13 in Appendix B, page 310) are ideal for this.

Caesarean section

For remote work, the quickest way to maximise your impact is to do obstetrics. Caesarean section and instrumental delivery may be part and parcel of a surgeon's daily work in hard-to-reach areas, and a year of obstetric training at the beginning of your global surgery career could pay dividends for those intending that type of work.

Competency with caesarean section is a requirement for most humanitarian surgery teams, even for non-obstetric surgeons. If you already have surgical skills, attending caesarean lists with an obstetrician or shadowing them on call can be useful.

Ultrasound scanning

In many LICs and parts of MICs, ultrasound scanning (USS) is a bedside adjunct to physical examination, making scanning a useful skill for surgical teams. A two-week course can give you a degree of proficiency which can then be built on by regular use or attending sessions with sonographers and radiologists. The absence of endemic obesity in LICs generally makes scanning easier than in HICs. Digital simulation training and practice modules are also available.

Where findings are unusual or unclear, USS also works well as a "WhatsApp investigation." The local provider performs the scan, while a remote radiologist familiar with the conditions seen in that country views the images live. We have used this approach in Sierra Leone multiple times.

Altering training rotations

Trainees should speak to their educational supervisor and training programme director early on in their thought process, to explore possible adaptations, such as proactively seeking rotations and hospitals providing broad experience. Early-years trainees can also select "taster weeks" to assess interest and future training opportunities.

CULTIVATE CONTACTS

Once you are known in a country, you will find that patients appear whenever you arrive, sometimes with conditions outside your field of expertise. This is one of many reasons it's helpful to nurture contacts in-country, as there may be people around better placed to deal with the problem. The skills available locally are often overlooked by visitors and getting to know who is good at what is very useful. Similarly, knowing the skills of travelling teams is also useful. For instance, when presented with elective head and neck or reconstructive problems, getting the patient on the list for Mercy Ships admission would be a good option. Individual specialists also support programs and travel intermittently, and the patient could be put in touch with them.

Colleagues at home are also an excellent source of information. They can help you avoid walking into something more complicated than you had envisaged and equally reassure you when it is safe to proceed with something straightforward. Video calling with the patient and any available imaging is a huge boon.

It is also nice to know who *cannot* do things. This information takes longer to filter through, as it requires a lot of trust for local teams to share negative information, especially about expatriates. Informal networks may develop, where teams discreetly move patients away from unsafe providers. If you are new to a country, this information is missing to you, but a trusted colleague who has been there before may be able to help.

> **"We are trying to change protocol. We have observed that most, if not all, go back to theatre multiple times, prolonging the hospital stay and end up with stoma."**
>
> **—Darwin Nyirenda, surgical resident talking about ileal typhoid perforations (Malawi)**

UNFAMILIAR DISEASE

You will come across surgical manifestations of unfamiliar, often communicable diseases. Pre-travel preparation includes reading up on these, studying the literature (often scanty), and speaking to those more familiar with the conditions.

The same disease can also vary significantly between regions. For example, I was familiar with the operative decision tree for typhoid perforation in Sierra Leone, but needed to learn a more aggressive strategy to deal with drug-resistant typhoid and difficulties with antibiotic compliance in Malawi.

> **"It's a whole lot harder for various reasons you didn't expect. Even if you have ostensibly appropriate medical experience, you're faced with situations you've not dealt with before. There's no hiding behind anything."**
>
> **—Marianne Stephen, obstetrician, (Plymouth, UK), talking about working for MSF in Pakistan**

FAMILIAR, BUT DIFFERENT

Many of the surgical conditions in LMICs are the same as in HICs. Except they tend to be worse. Hernias are huge, peritonitis well-established, and the foetal head resolutely stuck in the pelvis. This means that things you are just competent at in a HIC may come as an unpleasant surprise in a LIC.

There is a kernel of truth in the story that African surgeons subdivide inguinal hernias into "above knee" and "below knee." These cases are challenging no matter who is operating, especially when they incarcerate, which is also common. A trainee who has only done ten hernia repairs is going to need support from the local surgeons, who will likely have done hundreds of these difficult ones. Surgical trainees could consider preparing themselves by actively seeking out additional hernia training in their programs at home.

> **"A patient with low platelets? In the UK, you'd think ITP or perhaps alcohol-related disease. Here, the likely culprit is malaria. Haemoglobins of 8 g/dL are common and delaying surgery until a "safe" Hb of 12 or 13 g/dL is achieved simply means many patients would never receive surgery."**
>
> **—Jonathon Dean, consultant anaesthetist (UK), talking about working in Malawi**

Ketamine anaesthesia and the lack of laparoscopic infrastructure and equipment mean that operations like appendicectomy are often performed by open surgery in LICs and areas of MICs. Combine this with late presentations, and something you are competent to do in your own setting needs a rethink. Therefore, plan ahead and seek training. Preparatory courses are available (see Table 13 in Appendix B, page 310), but for things like open appendicectomy, also consider approaching the faculty of cadaver courses arranged for other conditions. It may be possible to arrange some bespoke training as an add-on.

AMENDING TEACHING MATERIALS

If you are taking out teaching resources, classroom and simulation training materials will usually need modifying or even rewriting before a trip, so speak to people already familiar, who may have access to setting-specific material. Some things will be minor, such as adding in safe practice for multi-use vials to existing content. For other familiar conditions, HIC evidence-based teaching materials and algorithms may be rendered useless, or even dangerous (**Table 11**). This, of course, is all hard to know when new to a place, so for patient safety, it's important to shadow teaching before working independently and to use country-specific materials.

Key Learning Point	UK	Sierra Leone
Population affected	Frail, elderly, comorbid	Healthy young men
Time from volvulus to presentation	Hours	Days
Assessment of infarction	Clinical, WCC, blood lactate, CT scanning	Clinical
Non-operative devolvulation	Recommended urgently in 95% cases	Contraindicated due to high risk of sudden death from untwisting infarcted colon
Equipment for sigmoidoscopy	Immediately available	Not available +/- unfamiliar
Presence of ileo-sigmoid knotting	Incredibly rare	Common and involved ileum also commonly ischaemic
Timing of surgery	Urgent scheduled daytime	Immediately after resuscitation
Non-operative definitive treatment	PEC	Not available

Table 11. Example showing the entirely different management of sigmoid volvulus in the UK versus Sierra Leone. WCC, white blood cell count. PEC, percutaneous endoscopic colostomy.

My first trip to Sierra Leone, for example, was less productive than I would have liked because I did not understand the training need and had not prepared suitable materials in advance.

LACK OF EQUIPMENT

Surgeons in low-resource settings often use poor quality, broken equipment, and less-than-ideal sutures, without access to surgical staplers, energy devices or even diathermy. Over time, you acquire a set of tricks (usually taught to you by your local colleagues) for getting around situations, such as lack of bowel clamps and shortage of sutures. Help shortcut this process by thoroughly quizzing somebody who is already familiar with the place and polish your basic skills to the highest level. An example of high-skill improvisation is described in the text box:

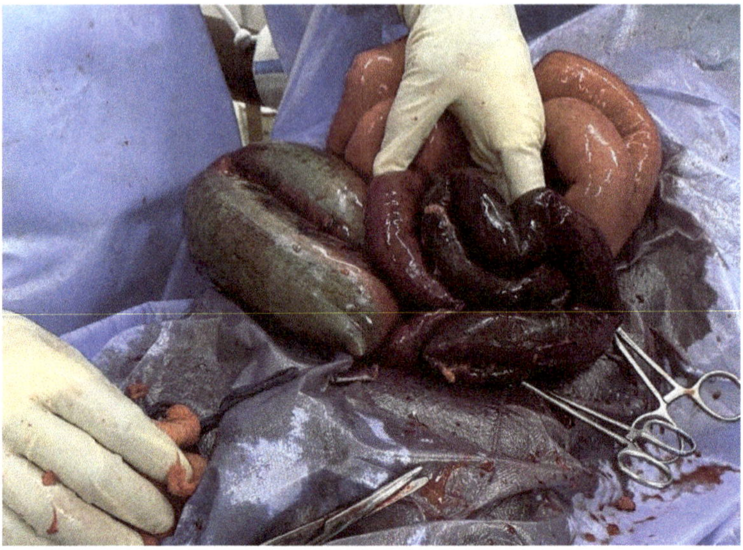

Figure 57. Typical volvulus in Sierra Leone. Ileo-sigmoid knotting with infarction of both ileum and sigmoid. Photo: author's own.

performing an anastomosis with a cutting needle is not recommended, and was only possible here because of exquisite suture technique.

CULTURAL COMPETENCY

> **"From necessity, I once did bowel anastomosis with a reverse cutting 3/0 silk. Each pass of the needle created what felt like a massive hole! ....they recovered very well. So, remember how much you can do with knowledge, some accomplished basic skills and access to only limited basic equipment."**
>
> **—Mark Szymankiewicz, consultant surgeon and founder of SWIFTSS**

We are all encouraged to learn cultural competency before travelling, but in practice this is hard to do. I was stunned, for example, the first time I saw a night-duty scrub nurse set up a corner of the equipment trolley so she could lay down her head and go to sleep during the operation. Her rate of pay was so low, she worked two jobs, and if I was going to spend two hours teaching the local resident, she needed to get some sleep. Cultural competency means developing knowledge, attitudes, and skills to help us understand and appreciate the reasons behind quite profound — or what may initially seem to be profound — differences in values and behaviour.

To become useful contributors in other cultures, we need to actively learn and understand why patients may present late, sometimes abscond, or require significant support to access care. Is the child's mother being lazy or conserving energy as she is reserving the food for him?

Clinicians operating in new contexts without sufficient preparation risk well-meaning interventions causing harm or wasted effort. This can be quite significant, for instance, choosing to build student accommodation when the local population rely heavily on renting rooms to students for their income. Or it may be more casual assumptions of white-man culture, such as painting fairy tale characters on the walls of paediatric wards instead of images recognisable to local children.

Seek out and read everything you can about the country. Do not rely solely on Global North sources, read local news (use a translation as needed), NGO reports, and regional publications. Actively seek perspectives from local healthcare workers, community leaders, and experienced volunteers. Get their insights on the daily realities, challenges, and sensitivities.

Try to understand the context in which history, politics, and inequality shape healthcare access and attitudes, including attitudes to outsiders. Search the news to stay aware of current events; think about how your programme fits into all of these contexts; actively resolve to be open and curious and make friends.

Always think and ask, "why?"

RESOURCES TO INFORM AND PREPARE

Courses

Courses fall roughly into two categories: (1) those focused on the overarching thesis of global surgery such as the unmet need and strategies for improving access, and (2) practical courses providing useful skills and insights for LMICs or austere settings.

Both are likely to be very useful. Courses have the added advantage of meeting like-minded individuals and hearing other people's experiences, valuable in deciding the direction you wish to pursue.

The examples in Appendix B (see Table 13 on page 310) are well known, widely advertised, and either continually available or regularly repeated. However, there are lots more ad hoc courses available to both staff and students, so check your university, hospital and college resources regularly. Medical students will find global health modules and additional elements added to many undergraduate programs. Join global surgery organisations and subscribe to mailing lists, for course notifications.

Strategies to help us learn cultural competence are actively taught. Formal education about poverty, health inequality, systems strengthening and research methodology is widely available, and often paired with learning about ethics and intercultural skills allowing those trained to avoid some of the common pitfalls.

Global health training is still in its infancy in the UK, but many US educational institutions offer courses and online learning.[1] This is a real growth area, and new courses appear regularly, so actively seek out opportunities.

WRITTEN MATERIALS

> *A volunteer who is well-prepared and properly trained is a valuable asset to an aid organisation, whereas well-meaning but poorly prepared volunteers can be a liability, both to themselves and to those they are trying to help.*[2]
>
> —MSF

Many organisations publish useful material on their websites. The list in Appendix C offers representative examples. Bespoke pre-deployment information should also be provided by individual organisations.

One piece of advice: read this info! We have met more than one person who simply turned up saying they did not have time to read the information or could not access the organisation's file storage system. If all of this feels like too much effort, or you are simply too busy, perhaps question whether now is the right moment to volunteer.

CHAPTER 21
PRACTICAL MATTERS

THIS CHAPTER DISCUSSES some of the less familiar, everyday realities of working in low-resource settings. We cover some serious issues and some smaller practical matters. These may seem trivial compared to learning the clinical knowledge and skills, but a few tips and tricks can really make life easier.

STAYING SAFE

BEING OUT OF YOUR DEPTH

Never feel guilty or inadequate if you find yourself in over your head. If you have been honest, either the organisation you are with carries responsibility, or an entirely unexpected misfortune has caused this. Either way, it's not your fault.

> **"...[You) have to have a bit of bravery but also have to be very careful to be transparent and examine your own practice."**
>
> **—Marianne Stephen, obstetrician (Plymouth, UK)**

Immediately contact your line manager and programme organiser, explain what has happened, and ask for help. Speak to the local surgical teams as there may be friendly hospitals around that can support, advise and take patients. One difficulty is knowing who to trust — your organisation's links should be able to help with this.

Being out of your depth in a teaching programme may feel less immediately scary, but the danger here is actually *greater*. Trainees may not recognise misguided instruction or critical omissions. In HICs, one poor teacher rarely derails training, but in countries with few checks and balances, teaching incorrectly can have lasting impact: those you train may not only continue the mistake indefinitely, but also pass it on to others.

Avoid getting into this position by reading everything before the course and highlighting areas you are not qualified to teach. This might include things you do at home but have no experience with in low-resources settings. For example, you may be able to do an appendicectomy at home but have never done it under ketamine anaesthesia. Talk everything through with somebody who has been to the country before.

What if you find yourself unexpectedly in this position? For example, the lead trainer you are shadowing falls sick the day before the obstetric complications course and you have never actually made a Rusch balloon from a condom or done the B-Lynch suture.

Firstly, remember this is not your fault. Secondly, do not compound the situation by trying to teach things you are not familiar with. This could endanger patients. Instead, determine which elements of the course can still go ahead and which need rescheduling. Whatever you do, don't try to bluff your way through. Be completely honest in your report about what has and has not been covered. This ensures that those trainees — and their future patients — are not permanently disadvantaged.

Maintaining your own educational supervision

Continue maintaining your logbook, albeit perhaps in a modified format. Trainees should document cases and learning experiences in their portfolios and discuss them with their training supervisor upon return. Trained staff should ensure the work abroad is covered in their appraisal mechanisms. Reflecting on cases is important to protect learning.

Avoiding professional isolation

This particularly affects those in LMICs for extended periods. Discuss difficult cases with colleagues back home, exactly as you normally would. They may not know the constraints of the environment, but they can offer a different perspective and can stop you developing tunnel vision. Late presentation and delay reaching adequate care means cases can go badly and this is very stressful. Again, talk to colleagues, both locally and at home. Keep up to date with the literature and developments in HICs and attend courses and meetings whenever possible. Work as collaboratively as possible with local colleagues and set up groups such as journal clubs. Join online activities. Investigate the possibility of online clinical multidisciplinary team (MDT) or morbidity and mortality (M&M) meetings to discuss difficult cases, perhaps via a partner organisation or personal contacts.

PERSONAL SAFETY AND LOCAL LAW

SAFETY

Before travel, always check and heed the Foreign Office, or Bureau of Consular Affairs, travel advice or equivalent in other countries. Adhere to host country rules. Different situations require different precautions. Obviously, if you're working in a war zone there will be very tight arrangements. In other places, read everything from your organisation and listen to local advice — if they say it's not safe to walk around at night, don't do it.

VISAS

Check visa requirements and plan ahead. Since the COVID-19 pandemic, many more countries offer online visas. Very importantly, if your destination requires you to renew or confirm your visa while in the country, do not miss this as it can be a very expensive error. This may apply even when online information indicates the visa remains valid.

DRIVING

Ninety percent of the world's road traffic deaths occur in LMICs, despite there being fewer vehicles than in HICs. Conditions vary between countries, but driving can be challenging. Pedestrians and other road users are not as marshalled as they are in HICs. Some countries, like Tanzania, have numerous trucks transporting goods inland and roads are often poorly lit and lack safety features.

Check and follow local licensing requirements. Many countries permit driving for a period (often three months) before you need to get a local or international licence. Always carry your license. Expect to be stopped at roadblocks and pulled over quite often, even without apparent

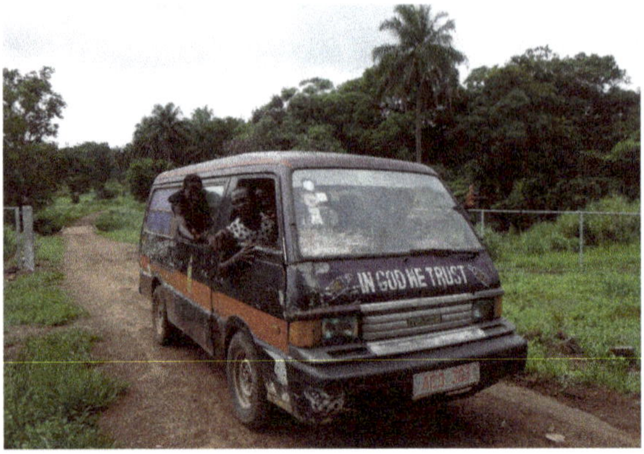

Figure 58. Vehicles in LICs are often old and adapted to carry more passengers than they were designed for. Photo: author's own.

violations. Cash fines are common. Remain polite and accept that you will usually just have to pay up. When expatriates argue their case, the fine is often inflated.

Poor road conditions and congestion mean journeys invariably take longer than you expect. Street lighting is often absent or inadequate, and in some places, potholes make driving at night unsafe. If you are involved in any sort of accident, phone a local friend immediately, as these things are often handled very differently.

If you are white, you are likely to be required to pay for vehicle repairs and hospital costs, for everyone involved, even if the accident was not your fault.

In some countries, women should only travel in female-driven taxis. In others, public transport is rammed, and the vehicles may not be up to standard. Motorbike taxis (*okadas, boda-bodas, velotaxis*) are common and are regulated in many countries, but are an inherently riskier form of transport than closed vehicles and best avoided if possible.

Minibuses (*matatus, danfos, collectivos*) are also common. Roadworthiness varies and they are usually crowded. Be mindful of your luggage, which may well be on the roof. Groups can sometimes negotiate exclusive vehicle use in some regions.

Most NGOs have their own vehicles and will collect you and return you to the airport in comfort. Ask if you can use the organisation's vehicles for your own work and leisure use, and the cost of hiring drivers. Alternatively, ask local partners to help you arrange in-country transport.

Arrest / ID

Understand and follow local laws. However, you may get stopped by the police seemingly without reason, or because of a misunderstanding. Advice on how to proceed will vary from country to country. Phone a local friend immediately and let your line manager know. Corruption can sometimes be a motive for police intervention, but also be well aware of local rules. For instance, plastic bags are illegal in Tanzania and cannot be brought into the country.[i] Always carry ID. In many countries, you are required to carry your passport and visa whenever you are away from your base.

HEALTH

Communicable disease

Hepatitis is endemic across Sub-Saharan Africa, Asia, and South America, and two-thirds of people with HIV live in Sub-Saharan Africa. Even in impoverished areas, hospitals routinely screen patients for both, but lab accuracy varies and system failures, like poor labelling, occur more frequently than in HICs. Always follow universal precautions.

CD4 count testing is becoming more widely available, especially in Southern Africa. Hepatitis viral load measurement is done in some places for monitoring and research but is not usually possible. The clinical picture is usually what you must go on. Take needlestick injuries seriously, especially in areas of high prevalence and where treatment may be suboptimal.

Higher operative workload, higher prevalence, and less adequate treatment increase the risk of occupational HIV transmission.

During the 1990s, the lifetime risk to Zambian surgeons was calculated as 1.5% compared to 0.1% in HICs. Post-exposure prophylaxis (PEP) is readily available, but some organisations and individuals also carry their own. Whether to take it or not is an individual choice. Most healthcare workers we have spoken to say they would take it (or have

---

[i] Part of Tanzania's broader effort to reduce plastic pollution and protect the environment.

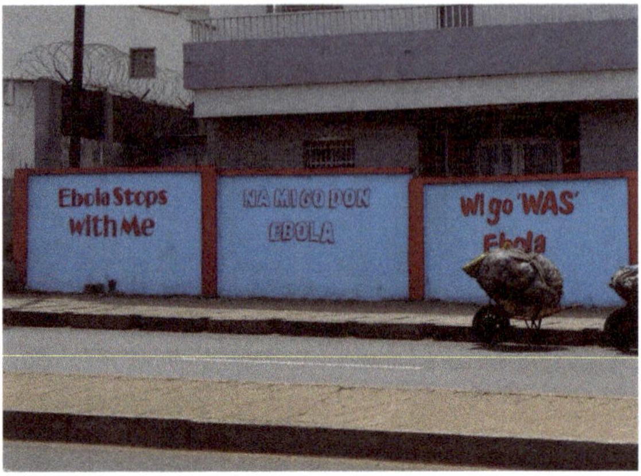
Ebola Stops with Me
NA MI GO DON EBOLA
Wi go 'WAS' Ebola

Figure 59. Freetown, Sierra Leone 2015 During the 2014–15 West African Ebola epidemic, many health workers died, and healthcare delivery was devastated. It is estimated that four times as many deaths resulted from other untreated conditions as from Ebola itself. Photo: author's own.

already taken it), however, the literature suggests compliance with the full course is low.

Viral haemorrhagic fever is endemic in parts of Africa, and Lassa fever and Ebola have killed many health workers. Vigilance is the watchword, with a high index of suspicion for unexplained bleeding or fever. The 2014/15 Ebola epidemic devastated surgical delivery in West Africa, and many healthcare workers lost their lives.

Malaria is endemic in many LMICs. Some expatriates eschew prophylaxis hoping to build resistance, but they usually get sick. Even if you make a good recovery, getting sick usually obviates the purpose of your travel, or at least reduces your effectiveness.

Sleep under a net or, if there is power at night, in front of a fan. Take micropore tape to mend holes in nets. Mosquito nets can be difficult to buy in some countries, because they are provided free of charge by NGOs and there is little commercial market locally. When they appear in markets, it is usually in batches and sometimes illicit business.

Gastrointestinal infections are common. Expatriates are particularly vulnerable, and usual precautions should be taken.

Helminthic infections are also common. If you feel tired or unwell, check your stool. Cutaneous larva migrans is also common and acquired through contact with animals or when skin is exposed to contaminated soil or sand. Anthelmintic treatment is usually readily available.

Vaccinations

Yellow Fever vaccination is mandatory in endemic countries, with certification required for entry or visa issuance. Some temperate countries require you to show your Yellow Fever certificate if you've previously visited endemic areas, so keep it with your passport for all travel. Boosters are no longer required, and travel clinics will upgrade an existing certificate to a lifetime one for a small fee.

Other vaccinations range from highly recommended to optional. Begin planning at least three months ahead as some require booster doses. All bona fide travel clinics follow the same online recommendations, so shop around and maintain clear personal records. It is easy to forget what you had when.

Cholera vaccination lasts only two years and is easily forgotten. During typhoid and cholera outbreaks, vaccination is usually available in-country, but doses are limited, and you may be taking it from somebody at higher risk. Better to get it before travel.

Bugs and snakes and crawling things

Beware of every crawling thing until you have asked local friends about them. Some are deadly and others give nasty stings. Avoid shortcuts through uncleared areas and scan the ground before stepping out of vehicles at night. Ironing shirts after they have been on the washing line is not only important to look good, but it also kills fly larvae.

> "I was bitten by a snake inside the hospital (compound) one Sunday evening and I developed some serious complication that threaten my life. I was admitted to the hospital. But the Doctors with Africa (CUAMM) surgeon was not an obstetrician and could not assess who required C-section. I was carried to the labour ward to examine the patients."
>
> —Hassan Ahmad Sherriff, surgical officer (Sierra Leone)

Heat stroke

We may underestimate the conditions and risk getting heat stroke, dehydration and sunburn. Walk slowly, and be alert to fatigue, headache, dizziness and either cool, clammy or inappropriately dry skin. Immediately seek help and attend to active cooling and hydration.

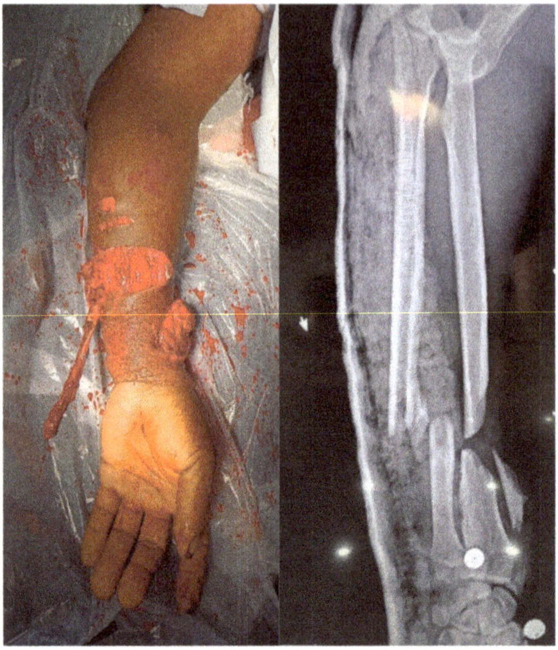

Figure 60. Crocodile bite, Malawi. Photos: Jonathon Dean.

Drugs

It is handy to take a small supply of common drugs, such as analgesia, loperamide, oral rehydration salts and certain antibiotics, plus all regular medication, contraceptives and country-appropriate malaria prophylaxis. Counterfeit drugs are an issue in some countries. Don't forget sunblock and mosquito repellent.

Contact and insurance

Ensure friends and family can easily contact you. Most organisations require you to provide an emergency contact and share your travel insurance details. Insurance is generally available, although in extreme places and during crises and epidemics it can be expensive.

> "It's not unusual to have a crocodile bite on the trauma list or a snake bite in intensive care — and these are only the patients who make it to hospital."
>
> —Jonathon Dean, consultant anaesthetist (UK), talking about Malawi

Insurance is not always as good as you would like in an emergency. In case of illness or injury, a lot of policies fund emergency transportation to the nearest "safe centre," which is likely to be another hospital in the region, when you would rather get home. Make sure you have somebody to find you a flight and get you home if that is what you want.

DAILY LIVING

Clothes

Check climate and season and pack accordingly. Follow local dress codes, which may include specific coverage for women. Remember a sun hat. Expatriates have a reputation for being scruffy, and this can come across as disrespectful. Err on the side of dressing smartly for work and remember a travel iron — you don't want to look like you're on a beach holiday. There may be local customs which are nice to join in with, such as dressing African on Fridays. At dawn and dusk, try to stay covered and socks are nice. Take a strong umbrella in rainy season or the monsoon, and if walking in the sun.

For meetings, conferences, medical registration interviews, etc. dress as you would for the same event at home, with adjustment for local weather conditions. Except if your country has a very relaxed dress code, in which case smarten up a bit for these events in LMICs.

In many places, you will need to take your own scrubs, theatre footwear, hats and sometimes gloves. Surgeons with smaller hands be aware some hospitals in LMICs only stock larger sizes. Also watch out for powdered gloves which are quite common and must be rinsed off before use.

Laundry is often done by hand and can be rough on delicate items. In the rainy season, it can be difficult to get clothes dry, and they may stink a bit even when they do, so for short trips consider taking additional clothes.

Food

You may be lucky enough to volunteer somewhere with fabulous food, but often the quality and variety is not as you are used to. In cities and some centres, there is easy access to supermarkets and restaurants, but in remote and rural areas, the availability of food can be a problem for expatriates used to instant gratification.

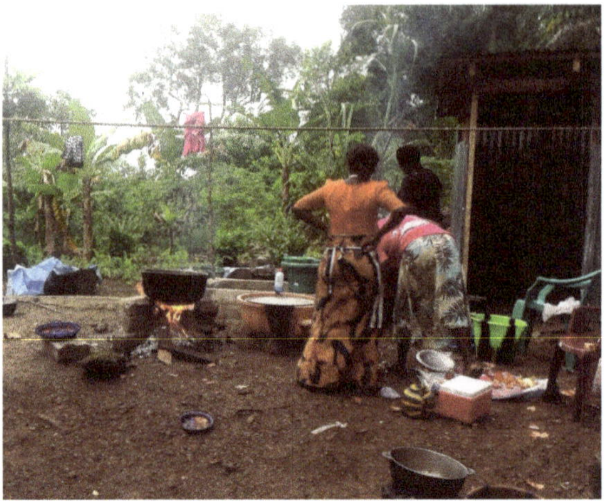

Figure 61. Cooking on open fires. Burns, especially childhood burns, are a disease associated with poverty. Photo: Magnus Endal.

Many NGOs employ cooks, and making dinner may start with killing a chicken.

Depending on where you are going, consider having a small supply of instant nutrition, such as cereal bars, in case you arrive at night and nothing is available, and a few sneaky treats from duty free are nice. Regarding street food — it often smells delicious but can have hidden surprises, so the advice is don't risk it. In most low-resource areas all water should be either bottled, in packets, boiled for two minutes, or passed through a microbiological purification filter.

Luggage

Checked bags don't always get through, and delayed bags are not reliably delivered to you in some countries. It may be wise to collect the late bag personally at the airport, which is especially inconvenient when there are few flights. Carry 24–48 hours' worth of clothes, all drugs and essential work items in your hand luggage. But be aware that airlines tend to use older planes on routes to LICs, and hand luggage space is usually limited.

Trolley cases can be taken from you, so have a zipped non-woven polypropylene (NWPP) or similar bag to decant everything into, as we heard stories of hand baggage never being seen again. You will see long

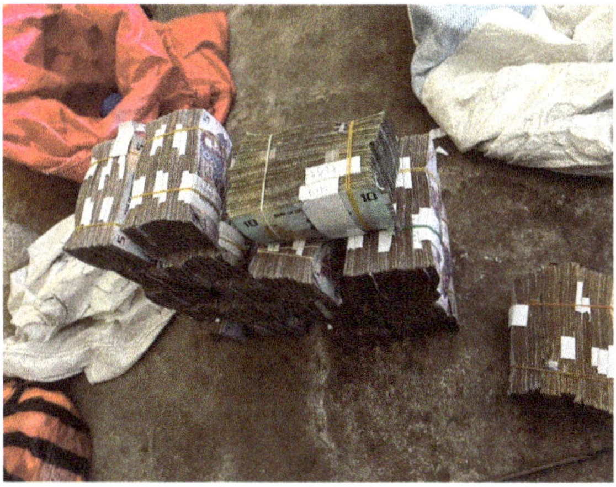

Figure 62. Large stack of Leones: inflation means cash gets bulky in many countries where notes lose value fast. Photo: author's own.

queues form early to board flights to LICs, as people want to get on while there is still luggage space available.

Money

In LIC cities, cash machines (ATMs) are as available as they are in the less well-endowed parts of British cities, however they do not always dispense. In rural areas, and as backup, cash is better. US dollars are almost universal, and Sterling and Euros are fairly easy to exchange in most places. Check the best currency for your destination.

You usually get a better exchange rate for large denomination notes. Small dollars should be avoided as they give poor value. Electronic means of payment are increasing, and a lot of people use mobile phone-based services such as Orange Money. Western Union and Ria are widely present if you need to send or receive cash.

Walking wallet

It is common in LMICs to be viewed as a "walking wallet" by casual acquaintances. You will likely receive more requests for help, sponsorship, and new phones than you can support. Your organisation may have gift-giving policies, and there may also be formal sponsorship programs in place that you can contribute to and put people forward for. Weigh up which contributions will make a sustainable difference.

It is unwise and rude to "flash the cash." Expensive equipment like MacBooks and certain phones cost more than the annual salary of the majority of people around you. Laptops are pretty much essential when working abroad, but don't be casual about them, and make sure all your materials are backed up in case of loss.

Differential pricing exists whereby most traders will charge "white guy prices." You might willingly accept this as the reality of the situation, but if you want to avoid it, get a friend to make the purchase for you. Approaching traders in a vehicle rather than on foot also ups the price.

Toiletries

For a short trip, take your own products and sanitary supplies. Global North items are available in most places, but quickly "nipping" to the shops is not always easy. Toilet paper is available in supermarkets but is an HIC concept and may not be provided, especially in workplace toilets.

Post and parcels

Postal services vary enormously and may be liable to interference, but increasingly international parcel delivery services can and do work well even in impoverished areas.

WELLBEING AND ADAPTATION

Loneliness

Isolation can be physical but can also be cultural. Local communities are usually very welcoming and friendly, but relationships inevitably take time. You will likely be treated very respectfully, and people do not want to intrude. You may also be put on a pedestal, which can be a lonely place. Find somebody you can kick back with. Expatriates do tend to group together for socialising and touristic experiences, and it does help to discuss things.

Don't accept loneliness. It is surprising how quickly people can get down, especially if the work side of life is not going well — or not going well *yet*. Voluntary Service Overseas (VSO) often deploy volunteers to unfamiliar environments for two years and include strategies for dealing with loneliness in their pre-deployment training.[ii]

Talk to as many people as possible ahead of your visit and actively seek out friends and other expatriates, if you need them. Don't stay quiet; although there may be others around who are settled and not looking for new friends, they may know people in the same position as you and can connect you.

Talking to family and friends at home can be difficult as they may encourage you to come home, even if you're not at that point. Spend whatever it takes on data to keep in touch, make regular contact and share concerns, but explain why you are planning to stay.

There are also some practical steps you can take before you go. Download a few TV series and movies on a hard drive and load up an e-reader. Determine to use any alone time productively. Write those papers, or that book you've been planning but never had the time for.

Your efforts to learn the local language will be greatly welcomed by the majority and serve as a good ice breaker. It allows you to engage more directly and the language teacher may run groups or be able to put you in touch with other expatriates. LMIC hospitals tend to employ a lot of security staff, many of whom are often quite bored. Recruit the guys on the gate as additional language teachers. Every evening you learn a new phrase and then get tested the next morning.

PRIVACY AND NOISE

The equal and opposite problem can occur, and some people complain of a lack of privacy. Shared facilities, noise and no escape from work can be stressful. In the UK, loud music late at night is considered a public nuisance; in parts of West Africa, it is considered a public service. A good night's sleep is invaluable if you're feeling down. Consider taking your own pillow and ear plugs and take a weekend off someplace nice every now and then.

SEX

Some organisations, particularly humanitarian ones, have codes of conduct about sexual behaviour. Relationships between expatriate colleagues can become problematic, especially in confined, unsafe envi-

---

ii https://www.vsointernational.org/volunteering/professional/how-volunteering-works/before-you-start

ronments. If relationships sour, this can affect the working of the entire team.[1]

Relationships outside the expatriate community present additional challenges. In some countries, sex outside marriage is frowned upon, and local partners and organisations can suffer backlash. Same-sex relationships are illegal in some countries, and some aid workers therefore hide their sexuality.

> **"Making decisions on the best way for staff to visit brothels is a familiar dilemma for some humanitarian logistics managers."**
>
> **—Pauline Oosterhoff, *The Guardian*, July 10, 2014**

Transactional sex is fraught with extreme moral difficulty in situations where wealth inequality is extreme or where individuals may be selling sex because of the desperate circumstances they have been thrown into.

Female humanitarian workers are warned of the "George Clooney Effect." After three months on a lonely mission, every man looks like George Clooney. Unsafe sex is reported by one-third of returning aid workers.[2]

Alcohol and drugs

Witnessing suffering is hard. Poor mental health and distress is common amongst humanitarian workers, especially young women and those with previous mental health problems. Risk-taking behaviours, such as substance abuse and unsafe sex, tend to increase when there is a high effort-reward imbalance, with hazardous drinking being especially common.[3,4]

CULTURAL AND PROFESSIONAL CHALLENGES

Respect and disrespect

Most people gain respect at work according to their knowledge, skills, and behaviour. Being treated with either too much or too little respect is unusual, and it jars when it happens. However, when people from HICs suddenly drop into LMICs, these mechanisms can go awry. Discussions with colleagues at all levels indicate that the most common issue is "over-respect."

Unearned privilege is common. Even at junior level, you may be treated as an expert and quickly get out of your depth. Most people adapt, being ultra-careful not to express opinions casually and pointing out where they do not have expertise. However, if forays abroad coincide with the overconfident stage of early careers or declining competency after retirement, excessive respect can lead to exaggerated self-belief.

Rarely, lack of respect can also be an issue, especially if local staff feel you have been parachuted in. This is also a serious problem, as it can lead to underutilisation of your skills and lost opportunities to help. In rolling programs, you may get respect (or lack thereof), based on your predecessor's behaviour.

UNDERUTILISATION

The apocryphal scenario is you arrive at a bush hospital to find the incumbent has just left, as she's not had a day off in six months. Things are going to be very tough for the first few weeks.

However, there are worse situations than being too busy. A few years ago, a major European donor offered funding to hospitals in LICs if they had a resident doctor. Organisations placing volunteers were asked to send people in the hope of securing this funding, and some found themselves at facilities where they could not establish a role. Similarly, some partnerships are important to LMIC institutions because they provide sponsorship and funding for various things, but the volunteers the organisations send as part of the package may not be valued, or have clear roles, especially if specialities vary with each posting.

Such underutilisation ranks among the worst expatriate experiences. Having given up a lot to volunteer, one wants to do something worthwhile. Finding yourself underutilised or tasked with unproductive work can be soul destroying, especially if useful skills are being wasted.

Don't become too discouraged too quickly — take a few weeks to see where your skill set can help. You may end up doing something useful, albeit not what you originally planned. Even worse than feeling useless is feeling that you are a burden, perhaps by continually asking for translation. This is particularly a risk for medical students.

Learn as much as possible about your specific role before departure. It will likely change, perhaps dramatically, but at least it indicates someone has considered your skillset in relation to the needs of the organisation.

. . .

Indifference to patients

Most SAO providers in LMIC countries are doing all they can to help patients. However, there are places where there is systemic indifference to patient suffering and easily avoidable death. It may be eminently possible to improve outcomes within existing resources, but where local individuals are not motivated to help patients this process will be painfully slow.

All you can do is demonstrate how easy it is to make a difference and wait for caring individuals to rise through the ranks. This is a very difficult scenario to cope with emotionally.

Cutting a trip short

Remember, if it is really not working — for whatever reason — you can always leave. You may need to pay the NGO back, but this is better than being stuck where you cannot achieve anything and are wasting both money and time, or in a situation so overwhelming it is going to destroy you. Having the knowledge that you can leave, empowers you stay. Look at flights but promise yourself you will give it "two more weeks."

> - Me: "I've got to come home...."
> - My mother: "Well, come home then'
> - Me: "I can't."
> - My mother: "Well, don't then...."
>
> —Marianne Stephen, obstetrician (Plymouth, UK) talking about her first humanitarian mission

Most people we have talked to found that after three to four weeks, those inundated with work had developed coping mechanisms, and those underutilised were able to establish enough local contact to become productive. It is quite common to hear repeat visitors to a place describe that they had a rough time initially. They got past it, and some even fell in love with the place.

The morning meeting

In many hospitals, and departments of larger hospitals, the day begins with the morning meeting, aka the morning report, where the patients admitted during the last 24 hours are presented. Effective morning meetings improve communication and situational awareness, as everybody is fully informed of the sick patients and the day can be planned efficiently. They can also be used as an educational opportunity.

The reality can be a bit harder to take. For example, they are not infrequently used as an opportunity to exercise ritual humiliation on trainees. You may witness behaviour that would result in suspension and dismissal if it happened in a HIC. Trainees in LICs say they hate it, but also partly defend the system, saying that surgery is hard, and getting through this stress "toughens them up."

It may be that all you can do to counter this is to use the opportunity to publicly heap praise on those who have done a good job. The respect in which expatriates are held means your public approval of somebody may carry weight.

Another challenging aspect is the tendency to decide patient management at a distance during these meetings, rather than senior doctors conducting post-take ward rounds.

Formal introductions

The high degree of respect afforded to expatriates means you may be formally introduced and welcomed by senior hospital staff, such as the general manager and medical superintendent. Factor in the time for this type of process into your proposed timetable. There may also be a grand send off at the end of your trip.

Frustration, slowness and inertia

We travel with all our lifelong behavioural practices and biases neatly packed. Frustration at the slowness of some things can be very challenging when working in LMICs. *Imagine how much we could do if the system was running well?* This emotion is, of course, completely illogical because if it was, why would you even be there? We travel in the hope of contributing to useful change, but the nature and pace of change must be directed by the host team. Bulls can contribute to a lot of change in china shops.

Cultural differences in care and training

The nursing system in LICs and some parts of MICs is different. Nursing tasks are often limited to taking observations, administering drugs and doing dressings. Patients are required to bring their own caretakers for feeding, hygiene and mobilisation, with presence of a caretaker often an absolute requirement for admission. Caretakers are often very motivated, and some can be trained up to provide niche care, such as stoma or fistula care, and enteral feeding.

Informed consent practice can be very different from that in HICs, and patients have been known to run away from lifesaving surgery as "too much information was provided." Consent, rather than informed consent, is normal in many places and makes patients vulnerable to rogue providers.

Husbands or even family elders may be required to give consent for the surgery of women. This is alien in societies where women are more equal, but confronting this head on is not usually the answer. Nearly all development agencies have empowerment of women as high-level aims.

> **"I found if I took a male member of staff with me, and my head was covered, it was possible to explain that the mother or the baby's life was in danger and nine out of ten people responded to that...."**
>
> **—Marianne Stephen, obstetrician (Plymouth, UK), on talking to male family members who made decisions on behalf of women**

Bringing relatives into the operating theatre was something that came as shock to me. Surgical teams fear being criticised for not saving an unsalvageable situation, so call the relatives in to show them things like infarction of the entire gut.

It is essential to understand local culture. We were once conducting an oral examination, for example, where there was a question about a retained gauze. All the candidates expressed dismay at the thought of telling the patient what had happened during the previous surgery, and felt it was preferable to keep this information secret.

Brain drain

Countries such as the UK systematically fail to train enough doctors and rely on migration from poorer countries. In 2019, a third of UK doctors were trained abroad, mainly on the Indian subcontinent. Brain drain can be cited by some as a reason not to bother — why train them if they are likely to leave anyway? However, training opportunities and career progression are cited as the main drivers of migration. Improving career structures and local job satisfaction is essential.[5]

GOVERNANCE AND MEDICOLEGAL

CLINICAL GOVERNANCE

Aid organisations and those working within them are sometimes criticised and at times, rightly so. Always adhere to the standards mandated by both your licensing body at home and the host country. Medical registration requirements vary: most countries require full registration, but some will grant a letter of authorisation based on good standing in your home country, after an interview and presentation of your documentation.

International guidelines exist for some fields of expertise, e.g. anaesthesia have international clinical standards and best practice guidelines exist for emergency responses.[iii] In certain situations, legal accountability can be difficult, and it is therefore imperative to always adhere to the highest standards of ethical behaviour and good practice.

Licensing, regulation and continuing professional development may be underdeveloped. There can also be an excessive focus on paper qualifications and a failure to respond to poor clinical outcomes, so residents who are getting terrible results may eschew practical training and concentrate on exam study, since passing exams is all they need to progress.

MEDICAL INDEMNITY

Find out the arrangements for indemnity in the country you are visiting. Maintain your existing Good Samaritan indemnity if you can possibly afford to do so. Advisors from these organisations have been helpful in managing ethical issues, although whether advice is given may be at the discretion of the individual advisor. We know of colleagues, for example, who faced difficulty after they helped a very sick colleague in a LIC.

Although clinicians in HICs complain about litigation, it is far worse to be in an environment where it does not exist. In most impoverished countries, the medicolegal system is not at all established, allowing

---

[iii] Alan F. Merry et al., "International Standards for a Safe Practice of Anesthesia 2010," *Canadian Journal of Anesthesia* 57, no. 11 (2010), https://pmc.ncbi.nlm.nih.gov/articles/PMC2957572/; World Health Organization, *Classification and Minimum Standards for Emergency Medical Teams* (Geneva: World Health Organization, 2021), https://www.who.int/publications/i/item/9789240029330.

rogue operators to function without challenge. Occasionally, after egregious cases resulting in death, relatives may approach the police.

Weirdos and misfits

The overwhelming majority of expatriates are kind, committed and appropriately trained. In fact, many are truly extraordinary in helping the world's poorest. However, given it is hardly "normal" to volunteer in LMICs (in that most people don't do it), we must all be weirdos and misfits to some extent.

However, some expatriates are not there for the right reasons, with white privilege protecting them from the scrutiny they would be subject to in their own countries. These people can be harmless freeloaders or dangerous liabilities. We have come across alcoholics moving from organisation to organisation, protected by their itinerant lifestyle, as well as people who have fraudulently misrepresented themselves.

Photographs

In some countries, patients actively solicit you to take their photograph, want pictures with the team, and will chase you down to take them. But this is not the case everywhere. Patient confidentiality needs to be maintained, and permission given for all photographs. There have even been cases where people have fallen foul of local law enforcement by inappropriate sharing of clinical images.

> "Sometimes, it feels like they just come for tourism. They take pictures, post online, say they are helping. Then they go. But we are still here, doing the hard work every day."
>
> —Sayoh Kanneh, emergency surgical officer (Sierra Leone)

Record keeping

The system of patient notes is often problematic in LMICs, and the default situation in some places is that notes will not be available for follow-up admissions. Some countries, such as Malawi, provide individual patients with their own Patient Passport, which is a précis of interactions. Others are moving early to electronic records. When preparing for a re-operation, such as stoma closure, it can be hard to find the first operation note. However, given the small size of the surgical community, it is often possible to speak to the original operator, who may have kept their own record, knowing further surgery will be needed.

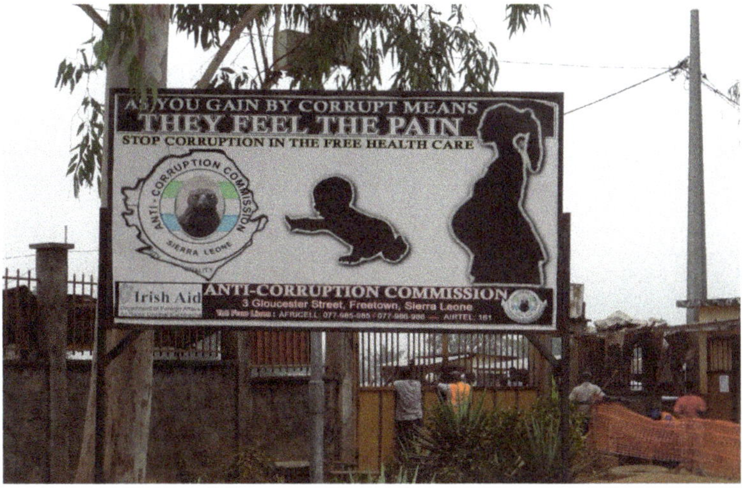
YOU GAIN BY CORRUPT MEANS
THEY FEEL THE PAIN
STOP CORRUPTION IN THE FREE HEALTH CARE
ANTI-CORRUPTION COMMISSION
SIERRA LEONE
Irish Aid
ANTI-CORRUPTION COMMISSION
3 Gloucester Street, Freetown, Sierra Leone

Figure 63. Makeni Government Hospital Sierra Leone. Patients may be pressurised to make payments for free healthcare. Photo: author's own.

Keeping your own record of certain operations can work, if data protection and patient confidentiality is adhered to. Any patient details can only be stored with the patient's consent and in a robust password protected system.

CORRUPTION

Corruption is widespread in healthcare, and rich countries are not immune, where priorities may favour certain groups and educated patients can work the system. In LMICs, patients may pay bribes to access care which should be free, and political corruption may lead to a lack of focus on those most in need.

There can even be deliberate hindering of beneficial change, such as blocking an increase in the number of medical school places. India, Georgia and Rwanda have systematically tackled corruption in healthcare, through community organisations, transparency and aggressive prosecution of corrupt individuals.

Corruption can also be present in healthcare training, and some graduates of some institutions may have been helped through the system, leading to variability in the quality of output from medical schools and other training institutions. Those entering further training may be

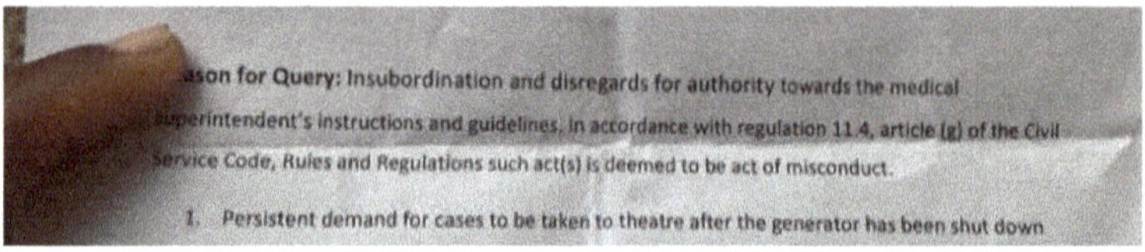

ason for Query: Insubordination and disregards for authority towards the medical uperintendent's instructions and guidelines, in accordance with regulation 11.4, article (g) of the Civil ervice Code, Rules and Regulations such act(s) is deemed to be act of misconduct.

1. Persistent demand for cases to be taken to theatre after the generator has been shut down

Figure 64. Running the generator at night solely to power the operating theatre is expensive. Teams face the challenge of balancing optimal care for individual patients with the costs of care delivery. Shown: snippet from a letter to an individual disciplined for trying to get emergency patients to theatre at night. Photo: Anon.

inconsistent in knowledge and ability. Licensing and regulation of SAO providers can also be lacking.

TECHNOLOGY

Equipment quality and spares

Laptops, cables, and USB sticks in LICs are often poor quality. African colleagues report difficulty obtaining durable goods even when they can afford them. Take spares of essential items. Tropical climates are unforgiving, and equipment malfunctions due to humidity and temperature extremes. Magnetic laptop charging is particularly problematic, so bring an additional charging option.

Electricity supply and power management

Electricity supply and voltage is unreliable in many LMICs. Some places have power 24/7 and generators in case of interruption, but remote hospitals may only have intermittent power. Take and regularly charge power banks for phones and headtorches.

Some mobile phones react badly to heat and if not optimally charged, so plugging them into a power bank overnight is useful. Tropical storms are a threat to electrical devices, with devices getting fried by lightning strikes, so unplug things during electrical storms. Random power surges also happen, and voltage regulating adapters are useful. Finding stuff in the dark, or half-light is challenging, so be organised and know where you put things.

Headtorches

You will sometimes have to assess and operate on patients by headtorch. Get the best rechargeable one you can, commensurate with comfort. It's unlikely you will be able to take it home; somebody will beg it off you.

Mobile connectivity

Coverage can be patchy. Consider having two phones or a dual SIM phone to connect to two networks. Local SIM cards are available at airports and from roadside vendors. Countries vary in their adherence to SIM card registration, especially where national ID numbers are not universal, but many do require passport identification for SIM registration. Data purchased on a local SIM can be hot spotted to your other SIM or devices. WhatsApp is the dominant communication platform in many places.

Preparing and sharing teaching materials

If you know the content, prepare teaching materials before travel, as you may have little downtime once there. Share content with local partners for feedback in advance. While materials can be amended on arrival, downloading images and fact checking is difficult with limited bandwidth.

Prepare a hard drive with teaching materials, reference material, and books you might need. Take an anatomy atlas (digital or physical). For video presentations, compress files for easier sharing, except those showing operative detail. If you will be sharing materials with a lot of people, preload things onto USB sticks to avoid numerous devices connecting to your laptop. If you are travelling with both your laptop and hard drive, create a backup and leave it at home.

Verify projection facility availability with local partners or bring a portable projector and quality screen for projecting operative images. Remember most people in LMICs use Android.

Clinical WhatsApp groups

Consultation and clinical discussion groups are common, but ensuring advice is safe is difficult. The loudest voice may not be giving the best advice. Do not give your opinion unless everybody using the forum knows your qualifications and experience. If you do, be clear whether you are giving opinion, advice, direct instruction, or just putting an idea out there.

Ideally, groups should have rules of engagement making it mandatory to supply all relevant fields before requesting advice. But in practice, requests are often incomplete regarding both patient information and the local capabilities. It is often better to have a direct conversation with the requester and perhaps the patient and let the group know the outcome in due course. There is a clear role for a HIC trainee here — policing and organising requests and summarising interactions for group education.

On a one-to-one basis, WhatsApp is invaluable for mentoring colleagues and trainees abroad. It allows you to virtually pop into theatre and look at operative findings, advise on difficult cases, talk to patients and put colleagues in touch with others who can help when you are asked things outside your remit.

RESOURCES AND SUPPLIES

Where to get stuff

Taking stuff is often necessary, and once you've been to a place you get to know what is needed. Ask staff at home to save out-of-date items. Don't be too specific, ask them to save everything and then filter out what is useful, because occasionally you get unexpected wins like suprapubic or emergency tracheostomy kits.

A lot of things are available to buy online. Some HIC organisations, specialise in equipment for LMICs. However, also look at purely commercial sites which might be better value. Companies such as GB Medical offer reconditioned operating theatre equipment at reasonable prices. eBay is also useful, and if there are specific things needed set alerts. New, but good-value items can be bought from online shopping sites.

Transportation

Your luggage is likely to be crammed with sutures, mesh and various bits of tubing. When taking large items such as diathermy machines, expect to get stopped at customs. Have the paperwork available, if possible, along with a letter from your organisation stating that the item is a donation of expired equipment. You may need to pay to get items through, and there may be a

> "Pack the equipment in the middle and pack your underwear over the top. A few panties seem to reduce enthusiasm for the search."
>
> —Carolyn Ramwell, nurse educator (Washington DC and Malawi)

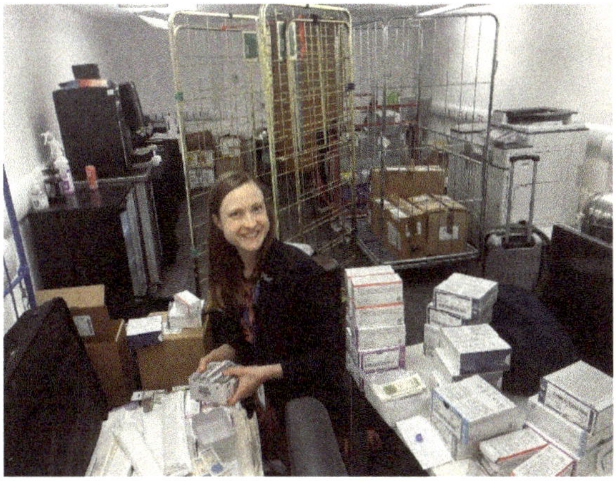

Figure 65. Helen Please sorting sutures donated by Medtronic plc. Photo: Jen Watt.

different price depending on whether a receipt is issued or not. Luggage may be searched.

People like to help

Make friends with your bioengineering department. Staff in Sheffield have supported LMICs by checking and servicing donated equipment in their own time. Our procurement manager and supplies team also obtain near-expiry items for LICs, through relationships with commercial partners. Commercial representatives will often source and blag specific items for you. Resuscitation officers can be good friends. When the trolleys are refreshed you can pick up unused i-gels, airways and ET tubes very easily.

Some US hospitals have a section in supplies devoted to expired and unwanted equipment for volunteers to pick through. Also liaise with volunteers in other specialities. I get offered various radiological items, which can be passed on to colleagues. Follow your employer's policy, declaring all donations, even if they do not have commercial value.

If it's broken, or so niche nobody used it in your home country, it will remain broken and so niche nobody uses it in an LMIC.

Remember not everything is useful. Follow the WHO donation guideline and checklist. Shipping containers work well for larger items, but the luxury of space creates the temptation to include junk. Recipients usually pay local taxes, and sometimes unofficial payments, to release containers from the docks, so it is important everything is actively wanted.

Expired or near expired drugs

Government bodies in HIC issue the expected warnings that using expired drugs can be harmful to health. However, there is also pragmatism about the issue, with the US FDA stating that drugs can remain durable after expiry and accepting that, for some patients, the choice is between expired medication or no medication. Theoretically, most drugs on the WHO Essential Medications list maintain potency for up to ten years, with more detailed information and signposting available.[6]

> **"Low-quality and out-of-date sutures tend to separate from the needle swage, so I advise drawing sutures by the thread, not the needle."**
>
> **—Raymond Nyirenda, consultant surgeon (Malawi)**

The International Dispensary Association (IDA) Foundation in Amsterdam is a not-for-profit supplier of essential medicines and supplies to LMICs.

Absorbable sutures

The desperate shortage of suture material in LICs appears to be getting worse rather than better. Colleagues in West Africa report that there are simply no sutures available to buy, even where patients have the money for them. Most surgeons in LICs use expired sutures, as the alternative is nothing. After several years, absorbable sutures can lose strength, so stress the suture hard to check it before use.

MISCELLANEOUS

Per diems

Per diems are payments given for expenses and to compensate lost time and income from attendance at meetings and education. There were introduced in the 1970s when aid workers wanted to ensure their work was effective, and address inequity between expatriate researchers and less well-paid African colleagues.

They are often essential, allowing those who cannot otherwise afford to travel to attend meetings and courses. But they can have negative consequences, such as creating a handout culture where disinterested individuals attend solely for the payment. Some healthcare workers regard them as a right, and hierarchies have developed with people of differing ranks getting different payments for the same travel and expenses. Organised corruption, multiple signings, attending multiple workshops unrelated to the field of practice, and signing for non-attending colleagues have all happened.

This became known as "acute perdiemitis" and prompted legislation in some countries.[7] Expatriates are not immune, occasionally accepting, not only per diems, but stipends, free accommodation, and every allowance going, while delivering minimal work.

Charitable boards and governance

Charitable boards are run by trustees. Governments provide both law and guidance on this, to ensure that charities carry out their purposes for public benefit and comply with their governing document and the law. Trustees must always act in their charity's best interests, manage its resources responsibly, act with care and skill and make sure the charity is accountable.

Festivals and holidays

Important religious occasions, fasting periods, festivals, public holidays, and other significant events require consideration when planning schedules.

Leaving

Short visits tend to have little impact on the emotions but longer stays can make leaving more emotional. Cultures vary from not really acknowledging you are going to a big send-off party and gift-giving, with the latter being more common. The things people say in these moments can have a profound effect on you and be the reason for returning. Leaving is usually easier if you know you are coming back. Perhaps one reason the pragmatic solidarity approach to capacity building works well is because it is mutually satisfactory.

End of mission reports

These are needed to share information and reflect on what happened. Like everything else, they tend to be biased to Global North perspectives, the format often paying more attention to the traveller's experience than the needs of the hosts. They may also be generic and not generated by an expert in the subject area.

Therefore, you are likely to add in additional information as well as the requested reflections, particularly for training programs, where knowledge, behaviour and competency assessments are vital to maintain continuity, and allow subsequent training to focus on who needs what.

The report is a drag at the end of trip. Tricks are to keep on top of it during the trip, by detailing each day's outcomes, and to try and finish a first draft on the journey home. Then leave it a few days to reflect before checking and submitting it promptly.

> **"It's very important when you come back to realise this is a completely different context. It's a different life and you can't go through comparing both situations. It's not possible and if you did, you'd end up not being able to come back at all."**
>
> **—Marianne Stephen, obstetrician (Plymouth, UK)**

> **Re-entry Syndrome Tactics:**
>
> - Maintain contact, plan the next trip, build pragmatic solidarity
> - Meet up with expatriates with similar experiences
> - Give presentations, write and reflect on the work
> - Manage profligacy in HIC healthcare by treating discarded useful items as opportunities ("Can I have that?")
> - Take a few days off or dive back into the day job — both approaches can work!
> - Set immediate and longer-term goals

Re-entry syndrome

Most return invigorated and motivated to advocate for the colleagues and patients left behind. But "reverse culture (or repatriation) shock" is a thing, particularly for those working in very challenging situations or away for extended periods. Family and friends may have moved on or seem to inhabit different worlds with different values. Others may miss the excitement or face the loss of immediate goals.

Sixty percent of humanitarian workers report negative emotions upon returning home to HICs, typically initial euphoria followed by feelings of loss, guilt, and relationship difficulties. Missions with relentless or hopeless workloads can lead to emotional burnout and even PTSD, either directly or vicariously after witnessing terrible things happen to others. If organisations or colleagues behave badly, this can cause anger, betrayal, and moral distress that tend to cause pessimism.

EXPLORE FURTHER

1. World Health Organization. *Guidelines for Medicine Donations.* 3rd ed. World Health Organization, 2011. https://www.who.int/teams/health-product-and-policy-standards/medicines-selection-ip-and-affordability/donations.
2. Storti, Craig. *The Art of Crossing Cultures*. John Murray Business, 2015.
3. Storti, Craig. *The Art of Coming Home*. John Murray Business, 2016.

CHAPTER 22
POOR BEHAVIOUR — PRIMUM NON NOCERE

SADLY, expatriates working and volunteering in LMICs sometimes behave badly. If this is simply due to lack of knowledge or naivety, it can be avoided with a little more information. Other problems are more challenging and can be destructive. We outline some common issues, and the contexts in which they arise; a heads up about what you might see, and how others have responded.

LACK OF COMPETENCY

HIC TRAINEES

> "You aren't allowed to be amateurish if you are in the game of saving lives. The one human right that the poor and the vulnerable should have at the very least is to be protected from incompetence."
>
> —Jan Egeland, UN Undersecretary-General for Humanitarian Affairs and Emergency Relief (2003–2007), speaking to the *New York Times*, 2004

Stories abound among African surgeons of expatriate doctors ostensibly coming to help, but in practice performing unlicensed surgery. Some genuinely seem to believe "anything is better than nothing," or what they have to offer is the best available. No matter how poor or underdeveloped a country, there is no place for self-taught surgery or anaesthesia. You will almost certainly do more harm than good. It is also fraudulent and happening in countries where people face catastrophic expenditure from surgery.

To put a generous slant on this, trainees may genuinely believe they are more competent than they are. It is hard to recognise how much the trainer is helping by organising the retraction or intervening just before an error. Play safe: if you are not doing a procedure unsupervised at home, do not feel tempted to do so in a LIC.

Colleagues in LICs say there are also a small minority of HIC trainees actively exploiting the situation to do things they've never seen. There are extreme examples — the young European faced with a perforated ulcer, who cuts off a square of omentum, leaving the local health officer holding the retractors to explain this is not a free flap procedure, or the trainee who had never seen hernia mesh inserted yet felt confident to teach it to LIC trainees.

In explaining, or even forgiving this behaviour, we must note very junior people are being exposed to situations they cannot fully appreciate, and the blame does not rest entirely with the individual. This behaviour is effectively condoned by the Global North organisations who facilitate it and reflects bigger issues of systemic inequality and power imbalance in global health. *Global Surgery: How to Work and Teach in Low- and Middle-Income Countries* (2023) by Hardy and Hochman offers useful insight into these issues.[1]

Employer of last resort

SAO providers unable to get, or remain in employment back home, either because of poor outcomes or poor behaviour, may find employment in LICs, where governance and regulation are less mature (see chapter 8, page 81).

Taking opportunities from local trainees

If your planned trip abroad suggests a training opportunity for you, do due diligence to make sure the opportunity is not being taken from a local trainee. Practising surgery abroad should not be used to compensate for deficiencies in the training programs of developed countries. It is challenging to obtain certain competencies and suggestions for addressing this are made in chapter 19.

The Lancet Commission's paper "Global Surgery 2030: A Roadmap for High-Income Country Actors" explicitly addresses "surgical colonialism," highlighting the risks it poses to both trainees and patients in

LMICs.[2] It also provides recommendations for HIC trainees on how to avoid this.

White saviour syndrome

It is not a huge step from the above to full-blown white saviour syndrome, where expatriates (of any race) act as if they know best how to save the poor locals. This is highlighted by cases such as Renee Bach, the unqualified missionary who was accused of behaving as a doctor in a Ugandan mission where children died.[i]

Some think white saviours are motivated by a desire to get glory or narcissism; however, the complex can be associated with deeply held religious conviction. "God does not call the qualified, he qualifies the called," can, and has, led people into the belief they do not need to be trained for a post.

Respecting local expertise

Some expatriates resist advice or feedback, particularly from health officer SAO providers, even when the latter are more skilled, knowledgeable, and experienced. However, it can be genuinely difficult to know who to trust when you are new to town. The friendly person may be spouting nonsense while the knowledgeable one respectfully hangs back.

(White) Saviour Syndrome: when someone from a more privileged background tries to "rescue" less privileged people without listening to their needs or perspectives, reinforcing stereotypes and ignoring local agency, expertise and solutions.

POOR BEHAVIOUR BY ORGANISATIONS

Nepotism

Small MONGOs (My Own NGO; see chapter 16, page 162) do not have to follow employment rules. They may appoint unqualified friends or relatives, without the accountability that would apply in regulated industries. Decisions about who to appoint to various roles may go directly against the wishes of LMIC partners.

In small organisations, there is not necessarily much that can be done,

---

[i] Jesko, Jackie, director. *Savior Complex.* HBO Documentary Films, Latchkey Films, and One Story Up Productions, 2023. 3 episodes.

other than to keep in mind that the good ones outnumber the bad. However, larger organisations, and those taking donor aid, cannot behave with impunity. Where nepotism causes harm, you should report it. Abuse of the power imbalance between HIC and LMIC partners is well recognised and will concern donors.

> **"It's important not to fall into the trap of the 'white saviour'. You still see it. And often, unfortunately. A sense of 'better-ness'."**
>
> **—Mark Szymankiewicz, UK surgeon and founder of SWIFTSS**

Institutionalised bullying

In HICs, the destructive effect of bullying on the development of organisations is known. However, in some LMICs, an attitude persists that, once you get to the top, you bully those below. You may therefore see formulaic humiliation of trainees go unchallenged.

You may also be bullied yourself. We are aware of volunteers who shouldered large parts of the workload of paid expatriate colleagues and then found themselves humiliated and verbally abused by those same colleagues. The unearned privilege and deference afforded to expatriates can also lead them to bully and abuse local staff and trainees, and this can be extreme, even resulting in dismissal of the victim.

Where systems are immature, bullying can be difficult to deal with. Being very careful about your own behaviour and setting a good example is likely to be helpful. Talk to someone to maintain perspective and prevent becoming inured to it. Report concerns to your organisation.

The Oxfam scandal of 2011

In all walks of life, there are those who use power to exploit the most vulnerable. Roland van Hauwermeiren (RVH) and colleagues were sexual predators who used senior positions in aid organisations to exploit survivors of humanitarian disasters.

But what shocked the world most was the aid sector's (lack of) response, and the ease with which predators simply moved from NGO to NGO after serious allegations. There was evidence that Oxfam ignored or covered up initial accusations, and a confidential Oxfam report later referred to a culture of impunity among aid workers in Haiti.[3]

Whistleblowers described this case as the tip of the iceberg, with no proper regulation in place and organisations covering things up to protect their reputations. Whistleblowers have had to resort to going to the press after the organisations responsible failed to act.

On a lesser scale, those working on the ground in LMICs will see abuse of power and white privilege playing out. The simple test is "would this behaviour be acceptable at home?" If not, don't do it. This might be carrying out procedures that you are not trained to do, bullying other staff, abusing hospital and NGO vehicles and property, or inappropriate actions within the local community. Be mindful and speak to your organisation if you have any concerns. Written reports are also of value. Remember: although the truth often does come out in the end, someone must bring it to light.

Liberia: in the Wake of the Civil War

"The behaviour at that time in Monrovia was insane, I think Merlin were a bit worse, but plenty of UN types [were] doing the same."

—Amira Malik Miller, Swedish whistleblower describing sexual misconduct amongst INGO staff in 2002

Poor outcomes

Late and extreme presentations mean complications and mortality are unavoidable. However, geographically or systemically isolated hospitals, and perhaps a saviour mentality in some cases, can result in mortality being higher in certain facilities where expatriates operate than local surgeons would expect, or than those local surgeons themselves achieve with fewer resources. Audit and clinical governance are not well developed in some places and working in isolation can lead to loss of perspective.

RESEARCH

Poor research practice and unethical behaviour in research is discussed in chapter 12 (see page 117).

POOR TEACHING

Poor teaching from expatriates is disappointingly common in LMICs. The desire to help sometimes leads to inappropriate or unqualified people delivering teaching — and "delivering" is often the operative word. Some provide training abroad when they are not involved with it at home. Lacking the skills to evaluate whether what they are doing has any real value, they may take "happy sheets" and multiple-choice questionnaires as evidence of satisfactory training. Expatriates may also teach outside their speciality and beyond their expertise. Camps wishing to create the appearance of sustainability sometimes add tokenistic teaching onto pre-planned activity.

> **"It was clear she didn't know much about surgery. From the start, you could tell something was not right. When foreigners come, they don't listen to us. They listen to each other. They later told me she would help plan how the program should run. That shocked me."**
>
> **—Sayoh Kanneh, emergency surgical officer (Sierra Leone)**

The Essential Surgery Package may be disregarded in favour of a trainer's preferred subject matter, or evidence-based practice may be ignored altogether. In the best case, this results in a small benefit achieved at the cost of time, money, and carbon emissions. In the worst-case scenario, poor teaching produces poor practice, which then goes unchallenged and is passed down to others.

Occasionally, there are extreme cases. An expatriate trainer, for example, was reported to have supplied trainees with a wet-lab model and told them to teach themselves. If only it was that easy, the shortage of SAO providers in LMICs would have been solved long ago. A facility with a high anastomotic leak rate had been trying to follow a highly unorthodox mixture of bowel anastomosis techniques, taught to them a decade earlier.

Failings also occur at an organisational level, with trainee numbers exceeding training capacity, lack of proper competency assessments, and radical departures from standard training practices, without formal risk assessment. Expatriates sometimes fail to listen to concerns raised by local partners, even where these involve patient safety.

The multiplier effect associated with teaching and training means the potential benefit is great. However, when teaching is misguided or substandard, the potential for harm is equally great.

POOR PRACTICE FROM LOCAL SURGEONS

This can be a very difficult situation to be faced with. At the straightforward end of the spectrum, it may be a simple understanding or a skills gap, which handled with tact and diplomacy can be addressed to great satisfaction by both parties. But it can also be a difficult balancing act. What if somebody is doing a certain procedure tolerably well? Do you leave them to continue as is, or show them how to do it with a bit more finesse? One option is to offer to show them one procedure "in the UK/US/HIC style" and see their reaction.

"In my role as Head of Education for the Students and Graduates Union, I formally raised concerns about the program's quality. This came when the quality of training started to decline, and many supervisors started complaining about the low level of students on rotation."

—Hassan Sheriff, emergency surgical officer (Sierra Leone)

Another challenge is when the most senior person has been expounding false beliefs for a long time and correcting them would humiliate them in front of their subordinates.

Most people who have spent time on the ground have endured the agony of watching something done badly and weighing up the damage to future working relationships of speaking out, when loss of that relationship could in turn harm many future patients. This will always be very challenging. Do nothing rash. Talk the problem through with a trusted colleague and the clinical governance lead of your organisation.

SEEING (AND KNOWING) IT ALL IN THE FIRST COUPLE OF WEEKS

As discussed in chapter 16, it takes a few weeks on the ground to start to understand local systems, people and culture. However, there is a tendency ("rapid appraisal bias") for us all to feel we have crystal-clear insight into everything after about two weeks. To counter this bias, it's best to stay quiet at first and observe. Even the most well-intentioned international partnerships have undermined existing systems through rash decisions made without seeing the full picture. The person who befriended you in the first week, for example, may be using you to push their personal agenda.

Make friends, practice cultural humility, interact with respect and openness, listen more than you speak, and be prepared to adapt your views. Alternatively, it could be that you, as the outsider, have stumbled on a valuable insight, in which case you can raise it in due course.

Innovation and new ideas are needed. But it is risky to disregard standard practice or throw out things that have been working well.

JEALOUSY

Jealousy is a normal human emotion, and this type of work is no exception. Small NGOs can sometimes be blighted by it. People can feel threatened by much-needed help and even sabotage development if it jeopardises their personal position.

THEFT

Theft does not always mean of movable things. Time and infrastructure can also be stolen. Turning up for work only to sleep through a shift or renting out parts of the hospital complex as a guesthouse are not uncommon. Poor systems breed corruption and bad behaviour, even in decent people. If you have not been paid for several months, it is understandable you look for ways to make ends meet. However, there are also expatriates who eke out a livelihood living for free courtesy of NGOs without actually delivering on any of their agenda.

ETHICS

One recently qualified volunteer doctor reported challenging the legitimacy of a research project in a LIC, only to be told "ethics are a luxury in this country." Attitudes like this show how deeply cultural prejudice and exploitation can be embedded. Suffice to say, the worse the local conditions, the greater the duty to uphold ethical standards.

There are excellent reviews of ethical matters in global surgery in several of the textbooks cited in Appendix C (see page 317).

PROBITY

Imagine a scenario, where a trainee from your own country states in a meeting they recently performed numerous self-taught laparotomies in South Africa. This may be a naïve brag from someone who thinks the audience will be impressed. However, it could also be a lie, made with the nefarious intent of gaining access to operative cases for personal development. Then, of course, there is the possibility it is actually true, and the individual represents a material risk to the population of any country he/she is in.

What would you do about this? Do you report him/her to the Health Professional Council of South Africa, or the medical council at home? Do you contact his/her educational supervisors and ask them to deal with this as a likely probity issue? Do you pretend you never heard it?

The most sensible first step is to consult your professional indemnity provider for advice. They are experts in guiding people through this type of minefield. Your indemnity provider will likely help you prepare a written statement, reporting this upwards, with a view to the NGO's governance structures managing the situation. The NGO may conclude the claim is false, help the trainee reflect on the importance of probity, and arrange an increase in direct supervision. If they conclude there is veracity in the claim, they must report this to the South African authorities.

Ignoring this is no more possible abroad than it is at home; the professional responsibility to protect patients knows no geographical boundaries. Unacceptable practice is unacceptable practice wherever you are in the world.

However, it is possible your indemnity provider will not be able to help, as this type of advice is at the discretion of the medical advisor. In which case you can seek advice from another trusted colleague, such as your department clinical governance lead, medical council responsible officer, or the clinical governance lead of the NGO concerned.

DON'T LET IT GET YOU DOWN

This is a depressing chapter, and the negative behaviour of others can be draining and deflect attention away from the real issues. It is likely you will run into some difficult people, and some well-intentioned but ill-prepared ones. Otherwise, decent people can also react badly under stress abroad.

Don't let this bring you down. The overwhelming majority of people you will encounter are genuine, doing meaningful work under difficult circumstances and doing so with great grace. You will meet some of the most wonderful people in the world.

So, join them.

EXPLORE FURTHER

1. Ng-Kamstra, Joshua S., Sarah L. M. Greenberg, Fizan Abdullah et al. "Global Surgery 2030: A Roadmap for High-Income Country Actors." *BMJ Global Health* 1, no. 1 (2016): e000011. https://doi.org/10.1136/bmjgh-2015-000011.
2. Hardy, Mark A., and Beth R. Hochman, eds. 2023. *Global Surgery: How to Work and Teach in Low- and Middle-Income Countries*. Springer. ISBN 978-3-031-28126-6. —*The ethics chapter in this textbook is excellent.*
3. Jesko, Jackie, director. *Savior Complex.* HBO Documentary Films, Latchkey Films, and One Story Up Productions, 2023. 3 episodes.

AFTERWORD

The benefits of meaningful work in LMICs are felt by both the volunteer/worker and local partners.

Much is said about work-life balance, as if work and life are somehow separate entities. Working in areas of great need offers the chance for work-life integration, where this meaningful work becomes an essential part of who you are.

> **"In all my twenty-plus years of working in the NHS, without a shadow of doubt the most professionally rewarding time I have spent in my life has been in Africa."**
>
> **—Mark Szymankiewicz, surgeon (Salisbury, UK)**

Take inspiration from the remarkable individuals described and featured throughout this book, and above all, from the local surgical, anaesthetic, and obstetric providers and trainers who persevere every day to make surgery accessible and safe for their communities.

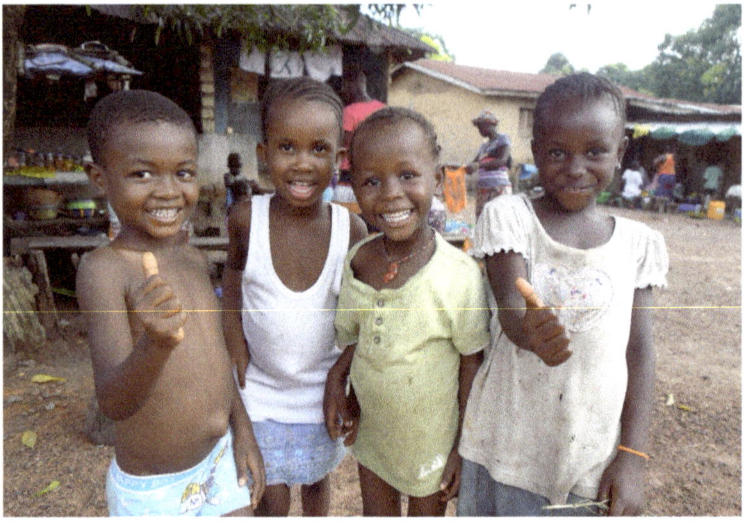

Figure 66. Children in Masanga, Sierra Leone. Photo: author's own.

GLOSSARY

BCA: Benefit–Cost Analysis; estimates net economic benefit, allowing comparisons across diverse interventions.

Capacity building: Process of developing skills, knowledge, and resources to scale interventions.

CEA: Cost-Effectiveness Analysis.

CIGH: Center for Innovation in Global Health at Stanford University.

Clusters: Humanitarian groups coordinating actions in technical sectors (for example, health clusters) during crises.

DALY: Disability-Adjusted Life-Years; a key metric that can be used to measure the effect of untreated surgical conditions, measuring years of healthy life lost.

DCP3: *Disease Control Priorities*, 3rd Edition; World Bank publication containing a separate volume dedicated to Essential Surgery. Published in 2015.

Dunning-Kruger effect: Cognitive bias where low-skill individuals overestimate their ability, while experts tend to underestimate theirs.

EESA: Emergency and Essential Surgery and Anaesthesia.

EESC: World Health Organization training resources for Emergency and Essential Surgical Care.

EMTs: Emergency Medical Teams; groups of healthcare professionals providing emergency surgical and medical care during crises.

FIGO: International Federation of Gynecology and Obstetrics.

FRP: Financial Risk Protection data; measures how well financial exposure to health costs is mitigated.

GASOC: Global Anaesthesia Surgery and Obstetric Collaboration.

GBD: Global Burden of Disease; measures health loss from diseases or injuries at the population level.

GDP: Gross Domestic Product; total economic output of a country.

GIEESC: World Health Organization Global Initiative for Emergency and Essential Surgical Care; promotes international policy collaboration to improve surgical care access.

GSPU: Global Surgery Policy Unit at London School of Economics and RCS England.

HIC: High-Income Country.

HIPC: Heavily Indebted Poor Country.

HIS: Humanitarian Surgery Initiative; developing surgical education and training for crisis situations.

ICRC: International Committee of the Red Cross.

IFRC: International Federation of Red Cross and Red Crescent Societies; the world's largest humanitarian network.

IMEESC toolkit: World Health Organization's 2009 Integrated Management tool for surgical care policymakers.

IMF: International Monetary Fund; United Nations specialised agency for monetary cooperation.

ISOFS: International Society of Obstetric Fistula Surgeons.

Kirkpatrick evaluation: Model used to assess the impact of healthcare training beyond trainee reactions, including behavioural changes and patient outcomes.

LCoGS: Lancet Commission on Global Surgery.

LIC: Low-Income Country.

LMIC: Low- and Middle-Income Country.

Maternal mortality: deaths from any cause related to, or aggravated by, pregnancy and childbirth, and within 42 days of the end of pregnancy.

Maternal Mortality Rate: number of maternal deaths divided by the number of women of reproductive age

MDGs: United Nations Millennium Development Goals, established in 2000 and targeting extreme poverty, gender equality and health

MDR: Multi-Drug-Resistant pathogens.

MIC: Middle-Income Country.

MMR: Maternal Mortality Ratio; number of maternal deaths per 100,000 live births.

MONGO: Informal term meaning "My Own NGO," referring to small, unregulated charities operating with minimal oversight.

NGO: Non-Governmental Organisation.

NHPSP: National Health Policies, Strategies, and Plans; country-wide frameworks guiding health system development.

NOTSS: Non-Technical Skills for Surgeons.

NSOAP: National Surgical Obstetric and Anaesthesia Plan.

NSOANP: National Surgical Obstetric Anaesthesia and Nursing Plan.

OGB: Operation Giving Back; American College of Surgeons volunteer programme for surgical education in underserved regions.

OOP: Out-of-Pocket patient healthcare payments.

PEP: Post-Exposure Prophylaxis; treatment to prevent infection after potential exposure to disease such as HIV.

PGSSC: Program in Global Surgery and Social Change; a collaboration between Harvard University and Partners in Health.

PIH: Partners in Health; NGO strengthening health systems in LMICs.

RCT: randomised controlled trial.

RVF: Rectovaginal Fistula.

SAO workforce: Surgeons, Anaesthetists, and Obstetrician providers, of all cadres.

SAOD: Surgical, Anaesthetic, and Obstetric Density; number of specialists per 100,000 population.

SAT: Situational Analysis Tool; quantifies surgical activity in LMICs. Can also (confusingly) stand for Surgical Assessment Tool, which evaluates hospital surgical capacity.

SDGs: United Nations Sustainable Development Goals, adopted in 2015 to promote global development.

STG: Strategic Development Goal.

STMM: Short-Term Medical Mission.

Surgical care: Operative and non-operative management of treatable conditions, including perioperative stages, as defined in Disease Control Priorities, 3rd Edition.

Surgical disability: Physical deficits resulting from surgical complications or sequelae as outlined in Disease Control Priorities, 3rd Edition.

Surgical procedure: Tissue manipulation requiring anaesthesia, categorised in Disease Control Priorities, 3rd Edition.

Surgical provider: Trained individual qualified to perform surgical procedures.

Surgical sequelae: Complications resulting from untreated conditions or adverse surgical events, as defined in Disease Control Priorities, 3rd Edition.

Surgically treatable condition: Medical condition amenable to improvement through surgical care, according to Disease Control Priorities, 3rd Edition.

UCES: Universal Coverage of Essential Surgery.

UHC: Universal Health Coverage; World Health Organization-defined access to quality health services without financial hardship.

UNFPA: United Nations Population Fund; sexual and reproductive health agency.

UNICEF: United Nations Children's Fund.

VVF: Vesicovaginal Fistula.

WFSA: World Federation of Societies of Anaesthesiologists.

WHA: World Health Assembly; decision-making body of the World Health Organization.

WHO: World Health Organization.

WHO-CHOICE: World Health Organization Choosing Interventions that are Cost-Effective; a standardized NGO reporting system for intervention cost-effectiveness.

APPENDIX A: EXAMPLE ORGANISATIONS IN GLOBAL SURGERY

Thousands of organisations work in global surgery. The list in **Table 12** was compiled by starting with well-known groups and those encountered through our work, then expanded using internet searches such as "global surgery and training." Inclusion or omission may reflect online visibility rather than actual quality or impact. As this field continually evolves, organisations listed in other books are often unavailable, and the same may happen here. The intention is to offer a window onto the world of volunteering.

Exploring these websites should prompt critical thinking about your own situation. Updated searches will then allow you to see what has appeared and changed since we compiled this list. The organisations listed here are biased towards English or have an English-language online presence. If you speak other languages, you should also search online in those languages.

We have been deliberately inclusive with these listings, including opportunities for doctors to support adventure holidays, voluntourism with a humanitarian element, right through to long-term commitments within teaching programs. As you browse through websites and materials, begin to consider what you can contribute.

We make no endorsements or attest for the veracity of what organisations have posted about themselves online. Finally, do get in touch if you wish us to consider adding your organisation in future editions.[i]

[i] gasocdirectors@gmail.com

Organisation	Description & Website
American College of Surgeons Health Outreach Program for Equity in Global Surgery (ACS HOPE)	Platform for surgeons to explore and engage in volunteer opportunities. Update of Operation Giving Back with emphasis on equal partnership. Resources, education, advocacy and useful list of volunteering opportunities.
	https://www.facs.org/for-medical-professionals/membership-community/acs-hope/
Adventure Medic	Free online magazine for healthcare professionals and students interested in wilderness, expedition and humanitarian medicine. Inspirational stories, links to courses (with feedback from previous participants), vacancy board and links to organisations with overlapping interests.
	https://www.theadventuremedic.com
African Health Placements	A recruitment agency initially formed to recruit qualified doctors in rural South Africa.
	https://www.ahp.org.za
African Mission and Healthcare	Supporting African mission hospitals with infrastructure, equipment, supporting education and training programs and grants.
	https://africanmissionhealthcare.org/
Agape Volunteers	Affordable medical volunteering in Tanzania, Ghana and Kenya which include the opportunities for adventure breaks as part of the package. Costs from £675.
	https://www.agape-volunteers.com/programmes/
Alliance for Global Clinical Training	AGCT links clinical educators and residents with clinical departments in educational institutions in LMICs. Currently looking for surgical educators and residents for a programme of attachments in Tanzania.
	http://www.agct.info
Americares	US NGO working to guide short-term missions on best practice and help local services.
	https://www.americares.org

Table 12. Selected organisations involved in global surgery.

Organisation	Description & Website
AO Alliance	Education, training and guidelines in fracture management for LMICs.
	https://ao-alliance.org/
Backpacker Medics	Provides and trains local teams to provide prehospital paramedic care after disasters and in isolated communities.
	https://www.backpackermedics.org
Better Lives Foundations	Started by an altruistic family group, the BLF provide medical and surgical camps and programs which empower local communities in health, education and social development. Projects in India and Africa.
	https://www.betterlivesfoundation.org/
Blavatnik Institute Global Health and Social Medicine: Program in Global Surgery and Social Change	Surgical Systems Strengthening through Research, Advocacy/Policy, Capacity Building, and Implementation Science. Resources, projects and fellowships and opportunities for students.
	https://www.pgssc.org/
Blue Ventures	Offer reduced rates for medics on their marine conservation-based expeditions.
	https://www.blueventures.org
British Exploring Society	Adventures for those 16 to 25 years in many countries including the UK. Looking for medical expedition leaders with full GMC registration.
	https://www.britishexploring.org/wp-content/uploads/2019/12/bes-medicalleaderinfo.pdf
British Foundation for International Reconstructive Surgery and Training	Trains local surgeons/teams to independence in re-constructive plastic surgery. Hands-on F2F in-country training and fellowships and provision of instru-mentation. Needs surgeons, nursesallied specialists.
	https://bfirst.org.uk/default.aspx
British Medical Association	Provides advice and pointers for doctors and medical students volunteering abroad and publishes guides covering benefits to you and host countries. Has resources to aid decision making and advice on the impact of volunteering on your career and finances.
	https://www.bma.org.uk/advice-and-support/career-progression/volunteering/volunteering-abroad-as-a-doctor

Table 12. (cont.)

Organisation	Description & Website
British Medical Association *(con.)*	Advice about medical student electives: https://www.bma.org.uk/advice-and-support/ethics/medical-students/ethics-toolkit-for-medical-students/medical-electives-in-poor-countries
British Society for Surgery of the Hand	Partnerships in 10 LMICs.
	https://www.bssh.ac.uk/overseas.aspx
Building Anaesthesia Training in the ECSA Region	Irish Aid funded partnership supporting College of Anaesthesiologists of East Central and Southern Africa (CANECSA) to build training capacity, curricula, training materials and quality assessments.
	https://www.rcsi.com/surgery/global-surgery/our-projects/building-anaesthesia-training
CapaCare	Projects in Liberia and Sierra Leone.
	https://www.capacare.org
Cardiostart International	Aims to educate and assist local medical teams in providing heart surgery and cardiac care in LMICs. Require cardiac surgical teams, cardiologists, technicians and coordinators.
	https://cardiostart.org/
Centre for Health Equity in Surgery and Anesthesia (CHESA) University of California	Wide range of projects and activity. Website has abundant resources and information. Opportunities for trainees and fellowships open to international applicants.
	https://globalsurgery.org/
Charity Challenge	Provide adventure trips for groups raising money for charity. Looking for doctors to support these adventures. Costs and indemnity cover provided.
	https://www.charitychallenge.com
Cinterandes Foundation	Using a mobile operating theatre on a truck, this organisation performs surgery in Honduras and Ecuador. Junior doctors and students are invited to apply for programs involving surgical assisting and pre- and postoperative care.
	https://www.cinterandes.org

Table 12. (cont.)

Organisation	Description & Website
Critical Care International	Sophisticated healthcare in remote environments. Focus on staffing, consultancy and training. Recruit doctors three years post qualification with ALS and ATLS/PHTLs and experience of remote environments.
	https://www.critcareint.com
CTSNet	A not-for-profit organisation connecting cardiothoracic surgeons globally. Volunteering opportunities and scholarships for surgical residents and newly qualified surgeons.
	https://www.ctsnet.org/
DDRC Healthcare	Deliver 24/7 emergency diving and hyperbaric medical emergency service. Numerous training courses and few paid positions.
	https://www.ddrc.org
Doctors of the World	More than 400 programs in 80 countries, ranging from HIV work to surgical camps. Also known as Médecins Du Monde.
	https://www.doctorsoftheworld.org.uk/our-work/international/
Doctors with Africa (CUAMM)	Design and implement long-term healthcare cooperation projects to create or strengthen health systems in Africa. Primarily focused on maternal health but looking for suitably trained surgeons, paediatricians and junior doctors. CUAMM: Collegio Universitario Aspiranti Medici Missionari and Colleges Universtaires Aspirants et Médecins Missionaires.
	https://doctorswithafrica.org/en/who-we-are/
Doc Tours	Tour company specialising in medical electives and volunteering for students and doctors.
	https://www.doctours.com.au
European Global Surgery Network	Organising conferences, meetings and workshops.
	https://www.linkedin.com/company/european-global-surgery-network-egsn
Exile Medics	Provide medical support for expeditions and consultancy services. Opportunities to learn expedition medicine with supervised roles and range of courses provided.

Table 12. (cont.)

Organisation	Description & Website
Exile Medics *(con.)*	https://www.exile-medics.com
Facing Africa Noma	Short missions to Ethiopia treating Noma, facial tumours and the aftermath of trauma. Require consultant plastic, maxillo-facial and craniofacial surgeons for two-week surgical camps and junior doctors for patient preparation. 8-week missions.
	http://www.facingafrica.org/get-involved/medical-volunteers/
FIGO (International Federation of Gynaecology and Obstetrics)	Women's and maternal health advocacy; fistula surgery training program, competency and standard-setting
	https://www.figo.org/
The G 4 Alliance — Global Alliance for Surgical, Obstetric, Trauma and Anesthesia Care	Coalition of associations increasing access to surgery, obstetric care and anaesthesia, via education, partnership projects, research and advocacy. Require experienced surgeons and obstetricians (including recently retired) to help train local surgeons in accredited hospitals in 17 countries.
	https://www.theg4alliance.org
Gap Force	As well as gap year opportunities they run courses (online and in-country) in expedition leadership.
	https://gapforce.org/gb/gap-year-programs/program/expedition-leader-training-work
Global Adventure Challenges	Create challenges and adventures for groups and individuals who wish to raise funds for charity. Looking for GPs or doctors with A&E experience to work as volunteers with expenses covered.
	https://www.globaladventurechallanges.com
Global Anaesthesia, Surgery and Obstetric Collaboration (GASOC)	UK based trainee organisation, sharing knowledge and experience to improve surgical outcomes in LMICs. Journal clubs, skills teaching, summer school, annual conference, innovation and bursaries.
	https://www.gasocuk.co.uk/about
Global Emergency Care Collaborative (GECCo)	Emergency Care teams involved in and advocating for global health issues.
	https://geccouk.com/

Table 12 (cont.)

Organisation	Description & Website
Global ENT Outreach	Bone labs, teaching fellowships, pro bono surgery in LMICs.
	https://www.geoutreach.org/
Global Surgery Amsterdam	Organisation aiming to initiate, facilitate and collaborate by research and educational projects. Provides summer schools (in English) for students and surgical trainees.
	https://www.globalsurgeryamsterdam.com
Gezondheidszorg en Tropengeneeskunde	The Netherlands Tropical Doctor Training Scheme (Arts Internationale Gezondheidszorg en Tropengeneeskunde, the AIGT). Responsible for organising the training of doctors in Global Health and Tropical Medicine.
	https://www.oigt.nl/?home
Global Initiative for Children's surgery	Collaborations, advocacy, partnerships, competitions and research to raise profile and capacity build in paediatric surgery. Website merging old GICS website with the Global Paediatric Surgery Network.
	https://www.globalchildrenssurgery.org/
Global Surgery Germany	German speaking surgical teams working in multiple countries.
	https://globalsurgery-germany.de/
The Global Surgical and Medical Support Group	Provide surgery including complex operations in Northern Iraq. Seeking surgeons to work in secure facilities for 1-4 weeks.
	http://www.GSMSG.org
Global Surgery Student Alliance	Aims to educate, inspire, and unite students through engagement and mentorship in global surgery, anaesthesia and O&G. Resources, inspiration, conference and support.
	https://www.globalsurgerystudents.org/
Health Education England *(now merged into NHS England which itself is being merged into Department of Health)*	Works with LMICs to seek new bilateral relationships to strengthen workforce development in the UK and overseas. Global Learners and International Postgraduate Medical Training Schemes and an International Volunteering Program, supporting volunteering opportunities.

Table 12. (cont.)

Organisation	Description & Website
Health Education England *(con.)*	https://www.hee.nhs.uk/our-work/global-engagement
	Guidance for trainees planning to volunteer: https://www.hee.nhs.uk/sites/default/files/documents/HEE%20Guidance%20for%20Trainees%20planning%20to%20volunteer%20or%20work%20overseas%20v2%20%28Low%20resolution%29.pdf
Health Volunteers Overseas Transforming Lives Through Education	Short missions delivering clinical training, education and operative training for local surgeons. Hand surgery projects in Ghana and Honduras; orthopaedic projects in Africa, Asia, South America and the Caribbean. Require fully trained surgeons but for some projects will accept final year residents paired with a consultant.
	https://hvousa.org
	Hand surgery: https://hvousa.org/get-involved/programs/hand-surgery/
	Orthopaedics: https://hvousa.org/get-involved/programs/orthopaedics/
Hernia International	Surgery, anaesthesia capacity building and training for hernia in 23 countries.
	https://www.herniainternational.org.uk/
InciSioN	Student and junior doctor-led group promoting access to safe surgery. Groups in several countries.
	https://www.incisionetwork.org/
Innovations in Global Surgery	A platform bringing together innovations for safe affordable surgery. Runs conferences and workshops and brings together expertise.
	https://www.surgicalinnovations.org/
International College of Surgeons	Projects in Nigeria and Paraguay.
	https://icsglobal.org/
International Healthcare Volunteers	Missions to Ghana with large expatriate teams for women's health and surgical care. Opportunities for trained providers, residents and medical student electives.
	https://www.ihcv.org/volunteering

Table 12. (cont.)

Organisation	Description & Website
International Medical Core (IMC) UK	Maintains a worldwide roster of experts, including surgical teams able to deploy to humanitarian emergencies when needed. May require volunteers to deploy rapidly for missions of 2 to 8 weeks.
	https://www.internationalmedicalcorps.org.uk/volunteer
International Society of Obstetric Fistula Surgeons (ISOFS)	African organisation promoting the highest standards of obstetric fistula care in cooperation with national and international providers.
	https://isofs-global.org/
International Volunteers in Urology (IVU)	Travelling urology mentors and team. Providing education, training and service in urology in LMICs. Fellowships for residents travelling with mentors.
	https://www.ivumed.org/
Inter Surgeon Global Surgical Partnerships	An interactive website designed to bring individuals and organisations together to improve surgical care. A dating agency for volunteers to match with organisations who can best use their skills.
	https://intersurgeon.org
Islamic Medical Association of North America	Funds and medical teams for disaster relief and other aid and support.
	https://www.imana.org/
KidsOR	Provide education and training, equipment, campaigning and research for paediatric surgery in LMICs.
	https://kidsor.org
King's Centre for Global Health and Health Partnerships	Paid and voluntary positions with stipend in many areas of healthcare including surgery. Working in Somaliland, Sierra Leone, DCR and Zambia. Opportunities for medical student electives and doctors including via MedicineAfrica platform.
	https://www.kcl.ac.uk/lsm/research/divisions/global-health

Table 12. (cont.)

Organisation	Description & Website
Lifebox: Saving lives through safer surgery	Improving safety: anaesthesia, teamwork, surgical safety. Provides education and essential equipment such as oximeters and headlights. Opportunities for all including residents and students.
	https://www.lifebox.org/
Médecins Sans Frontières (MSF)	Humanitarian Medical aid for people affected by disasters, conflict and poverty. Short-term placements in war zones and longer term and first mission placements. Requires anaesthetists, O&G, nurses and experienced surgeons competent at emergency and trauma surgery and willing to learn obstetric surgery.
	https://msf.org.uk
	Volunteering booklet: https://www.msf.org.uk/sites/uk/files/Surgeon_bookletweb_201111173714.pdf
Medical Ministry International	Christian organisation providing short missions and capacity building in surgical, speciality and dental care.
	http://www.mmi.org/
MedicineAfrica	Platform supporting organisations provide low-cost online education training and mentoring.
	https://medicineafrica.com
Mending kids	Cardiac, ENT and other surgical missions and individual patient transfers.
	https://www.mendingkids.org/
Mercy Ships	Well-resourced hospital ships travelling to LMICs to provide complex surgery not otherwise available in the countries visited. Training of local staff and specific courses. Recruits surgeons and other doctors with specific skills as required.
	https://www.mercyships.es/about-us-mercy-ships/
Mission to Heal	Medical missions including training the trainers.
	http://missiontoheal.org
National Health Service (UK)	The NHS website has a limited number of volunteering opportunities suitable for surgeons-in-training.
	https://www.healthcareers.nhs.uk/explore-roles/doctors/career-opportunities-doctors/medical-experience-abroad/volunteering-abroad-doctors

Table 12. (cont.)

Organisation	Description & Website
NGO Jobs In Africa	Large African job site focusing on Non-Governmental Organisations.
	https://ngojobsinafrica.com/job/general-surgeon/
NIHR Global Health Research Unit on Global Surgery	Funding links to ongoing projects and research outputs. Fellowships, information gathering and building research capacity in LMICs.
	https://www.globalsurgeryunit.org/
Oana Namibia	Variety of expeditions with emphasis on nature and the environment. Looking for post FY2 doctors with emergency experience, ALS and ATLS or equivalent as volunteer medics to oversee gap year students.
	https://www.theconservationnetwork.org
One World Surgery	Surgical missions and capacity building in Honduras and the Dominican Republic. Opportunities for paying accompanying persons.
	https://oneworldsurgery.org/
Operation Giving Back	See ACS HOPE above
Operation Hernia	Long established NGO providing surgical camps and increasingly training local surgeons. Pioneers of low-cost mesh. Opportunities for consultants and surgical registrars/residents.
	https://www.operationhernia.org.uk
Operation International	Surgical camps and additional educational activities. Support for disadvantaged individuals.
	https://www.operationinternational.org/
	UK team: https://www.operationinternational.org/teams/uk
Operation Smile	Providing cleft lip surgery, paediatrics and support services. Recruits international volunteers for 10–12-week missions at low cost to volunteer. Also offers resident leadership fellowships.
	https://www.operationsmile.org
	https://www.healthcareers.nhs.uk/explore-roles/doctors/career-opportunities-doctors/medical-experience-abroad/volunteering-abroad-doctors

Table 12. (cont.)

Organisation	Description & Website
Orbis	Flying eye hospital, partnerships and long-term programs and training. Looking for all types of ophthalmology specialist, surgical teams, biomedical engineers and ophthalmic technicians.
	https://gbr.orbis.org/en
Oxford University Global Surgery Group	International partnerships supporting teaching and clinical work including paediatric surgery, clubfoot, O&G, and trauma care.
	https://www.globalsurgery.ox.ac.uk/
OxPal Medlink	Connects doctors and medical students in UK with counterparts in Palestinian Territories to deliver online teaching.
	http://www.oxpal.org/
Palestinian Children's Relief Fund	Humanitarian Aid and Children's Healthcare.
	https://www.pcrf.net/
Pan-African Academy of Christian Surgeons	Require surgeons with an active Christian faith to train local surgeons in rural African settings.
	https://paacs.net
Partners In Health (PIH)	Works long-term with local sister organisations to strengthen systems building and train in Africa, America and Kazakhstan. Employment and volunteering opportunities for surgical care providers.
	https://www.pih.org
Physicians for Peace	Providing hands on surgical and anaesthesia training in Malawi. Require experienced practising or recently retired general surgeons and anaesthetists for three months or more. Expenses and stipend paid.
	Recently merged into ReSurge (see below)
	https://www.physciansforpeace.org/
PRIME Partnerships in Medical Education	Associated with Christian Medical Fellowship. GP group promoting care worldwide. Offer opportunities to junior doctors and medical students.
	https://www.cmf.org.uk

Table 12. (cont.)

Organisation	Description & Website
Raleigh International	Require expedition doctors (two years' experience) to support young volunteers in Tanzania, Costa Rica and Nepal. Leadership on treks and office-based work in-country.
	https://raleighinternational.org/medics/
Recruit.net	Agency advertising positions for surgeons in South Africa.
	https://za.recruit.net/search-surgeon-jobs
Resident Global Surgery Collaborative (RGSC)	Canadian plastic surgery residents' group for collaboration and learning.
	http://www.rgscollab.com/
ReSurge International	Volunteer surgeons doing plastic and reconstructive surgery and training the local surgical workforce; also supporting other surgical fields
	https://resurge.org/about-us/ https://resurgeafrica.org
Royal College of Anaesthetists	Global partnerships; opportunities for anaesthetists in LMICs; SAFE project
	https://www.rcoa.ac.uk/about-us/global-partnerships
Royal Australasian College of Surgeons	Active Global surgery program, focus on capacity building and monitoring. Scholarships, grants and aid programs. Pacific Islands Program strengthens specialised clinical services, clinical governance, education, training, and workforce development.
	https://www.surgeons.org/about-racs/global-health
Royal College of Obstetricians and Gynaecologists	Advocacy, volunteering opportunities and position statements
	https://www.rcog.org.uk/site-search?ss360Query=global+surgery
Royal College of Surgeons of Edinburgh	Global CARE. Grants and travel bursaries, and scholarships. Ad hoc events. Developing education and targeting training.
	https://www.rcsed.ac.uk/

Table 12. (cont.)

Organisation	Description & Website
Royal College of Surgeons of Edinburgh *(con.)*	Has a Faculty of Remote Rural and Humanitarian Healthcare and free courses: https://www.rcsed.ac.uk/faculties/faculty-of-remote-rural-and-humanitarian-healthcare
Royal College of Surgeons of England	Sign posting to a number of organisations. Some grants and travel bursaries.
	https://www.rcseng.ac.uk/information
RCS England-LSE Global Surgery Policy Unit	A collaboration between RCSE and London School of Economics, aiming to translate research into policy, advocate for access to surgery and develop leaders.
	https://www.lse.ac.uk/lse-health/research/GSPU/GSPU
Royal College of Surgeons of Ireland	The most active of all the Royal Colleges in global surgery with education, partnerships, projects and funding.
	https://www.rcsi.com/surgery/
Royal College of Surgeons of Ireland Institute of Global Surgery	Extensive portfolio of global surgery education, courses at undergraduate, postgraduate masters level, PhD supervision and continuing professional development (CPD) courses. Facilitates short-term clinical exchanges at ST5–8, medical student electives in Sub-Saharan Africa and global surgery internships.
	https://www.rcsi.com/surgery/global-surgery
Royal College of Surgeons of Glasgow	RCPSG International Postgraduate Diploma in Expedition and Wilderness Medicine considered a must for those participating in or leading expeditions in extreme and challenging environments.
	https://rcpsg.ac.uk/travel-medicine/qualifications-in-travel-medicine/rcpsg-international-postgraduate-diploma-in-expedition-and-wilderness-medicine
Royal Flying Doctor Service	Comprehensive aeromedical organisation providing primary healthcare and emergency services to people in remote parts of Australia. Posts advertised on website and journals. Has student placements.
	https://www.flyingdoctor.org.au

Table 12. (cont.)

Organisation	Description & Website
Safer Anaesthesia from Education (SAFE)	Joint project Association of Anaesthetists and WFSA training; equipping anaesthesia providers. Trained > 6500 clinicians in 48 countries. Volunteering and funding opportunities.
	https://anaesthetists.org/Home/International/Our-international-work/safer-anaesthesia-from-education-safe
Skyline Events	Organise charity fund raisers in UK and abroad. Looking for post FY2 doctors with cycling or trekking experience and training in expedition medicine to support overseas challenges.
	https://www.skylineevents.co.uk
Smile Train	Capacity building to empower local teams to do cleft surgery including innovative digital training.
	https://www.smiletrain.org/
Solidarity Bridge	Works alongside Bolivian healthcare professional to provide and train in advanced surgical care.
	https://www.solidaritybridge.org
SURG-Africa	Collaboration between RCSI, COSECSA and Surgical organisations and European Universities for education, training, monitoring and research.
	https://www.surgafrica.eu/
Surgeons for Cambodia	Clinics and surgical camps, medical student and some surgical teaching. Require trained surgeons and trainees (US resident years R3–R5). Accepts junior trainees with supervisor.
	http://www.surgeonsforcambodia.org
Surgeons OverSeas	Direct interventions, missions, advocacy and research. A forum for surgeons and trainees in HICs to connect with colleagues in LMICs.
	https://www.surgeonsoverseas.org/
Surgical Education Learners Forum (SELF)	Sponsored by Intuitive SELF supports development and evaluation of training modules for LMICs allowing learners to work independently. All SELF models are free and publicly available. Development grants and supportive expertise.
	https://www.self.surgery

Table 12. (cont.)

Organisation	Description & Website
SELF *(con.)*	Developed from the Global Surgery Training Challenge: https://globalsurgicaltraining.challenges.org/
Surgical teams Working in aFrica Together for Safer Surgery (SWIFTSS)	Capacity building across surgical care. Paradigm shift in mesh hernia; training local teams to prepare and use mesh. Supporting safe surgery and data collection. African mesh hernia registry.
	https://swiftss.org/
Surgical Volunteers International	Short surgical missions in many countries (North Africa, Far East and South America) addressing specific conditions. Involved with training local staff.
	https://www.surgicalvolunteers.org/
Surgeons of Hope	Missions and educational initiatives supporting paediatric heart surgery in Nicaragua.
	https://www.surgeonsofhope.org
SURG-hub	UN global surgery learning hub with multiple online courses and education.
	https://www.surghub.org/
UK-Med	Emergency response teams, expertise, training of local staff, and applied research in response to disasters, outbreaks and conflict. Register of trained staff and pre-deployment training. Specialist roles available to support surge and emergency response.
	https://www.uk-med.org
United Surgeons for Children (La Chaîne de l'Espoir International)	Working in 30 countries in Africa, Asia, Middle East and South America providing surgical treatment, infrastructure and training. Require surgeons and other doctors working with children.
	https://usfc.org
University of Global Health Equity	Providing high-level university education for the underserved. Calendar of events and recorded educational materials of interest to all surgical teams. Global Surgery Advocacy Certificate Program for LMIC surgical teams.
	https://ughe.org/

Table 12. (cont.)

Organisation	Description & Website
Urolink	Supports links with organisations in LMICs and facilitates professional visits to build capacity in urological surgery. Inspirational Urolink website.
	https://www.baus.org.uk/professionals/urolink/urolink_home.aspx
The Vine Trust	Medical care in Tanzania and Peru using medical ships. Volunteers and full-time staff in activities including minor surgery. Trainees in A&E, paediatrics or GP and senior doctors.
	https://www.vinetrust.org
The Virtual Doctors	Remote telemedical advice for Zambia and Malawi. Volunteers with CCT or board accreditation in vascular, maxillofacial, plastic, burns, general, paediatric, urological, orthopaedic and trauma surgery. Accepts experienced residents on a case-by-case basis.
	https://www.virtualdoctors.org/become-a-volunteer-doctor
Voluntary Service Overseas (VSO)	Particularly interested in maternal, neonatal and child health but other opportunities arise. Will accept junior doctors and has links to some Royal Colleges.
	https://www.vsointernational.org
Volunteer Forever	Wide-ranging volunteering and internship projects, including for resident doctors and medical students, in Argentina, Bali, Costa Rica, Ghana, Guatemala, India, Nepal, Peru, Sri Lanka, Tanzania, Uganda, Vietnam. Affordable costs.
	https://www.volunteerforever.com/volunteer-abroad/
Wilderness Medical Training	Courses for medics and students in mountain and expedition skills.
	https://www.wildernessmedicaltraining.co.uk
World Federation of Societies of Anaesthesiologists	Global surgery advocacy and SAFE global educational initiative for safer anaesthesia
	https://wfsahq.org/?s=global+surgery

Table 12. (cont.)

Organisation	Description & Website
World Medical Mission / Samaritan's Purse	Rolling programme of activities for Christian surgeons.
	http://www.smaritanspurse.org/what-we-do/world-medical-mission-2/

Table 12. (cont.)

APPENDIX B: COURSES IN GLOBAL HEALTH AND SURGERY

Organisation	Description & Website
ASiT Courses	Ad hoc courses relevant to global surgery topics from time to time.
	https://asit.org/conference/programme-2025/friday-7th-march-courses/pre-conference-courses/global-surgery-challenges-innovations-and-collaborations-sunday-10th-march
Blavatnik Institute Global Health and Social Medicine: Program in Global Surgery and Social Change	Online research seminars, educational opportunities, repository of materials.
	https://www.pgssc.org/
Faculty of Remote Rural and Humanitarian Healthcare RCSEd	Webinar series and library on subjects relevant to global surgery.
	https://services.rcsed.ac.uk/faculties/faculty-of-remote-rural-and-humanitarian-healthcare/202526-webinar-series
FutureLearn	Online courses on multiple subjects including global health and an excellent Train the Healthcare Trainer Course — many free to UK NHS staff and low cost to others.
	https://www.futurelearn.com
Global Frugal Innovations Course	Online course covering range of innovation and research skills.
	https://www.gasocuk.co.uk/innovation-course
Global Surgery Foundation	Champions in Global Surgery programme (learning internships).
	https://www.globalsurgeryfoundation.org/champions
Global Surgery Amsterdam	Interest group providing clinical courses and ad hoc events.
	https://courses.basicsofglobalsurgery.org/

Table 13. Courses in global health and surgery.

Organisation	Description & Website
Hostile Environment Surgical Training, United Kingdom (HEST-UK)	Hands-on course to ready consultants and senior residents for humanitarian crisis situations. Also, very useful to those working in other austere environments. Expensive but very high value.
	https://services.rcsed.ac.uk/events-courses/hostile-environment-surgical-training-united-kingdom-hest-uk
Introduction to Humanitarian Healthcare Online Course	Developed in partnership with Faculty Remote, Rural and Humanitarian Healthcare of RCSEd and UK-Med. A comprehensive overview helping potential volunteers make informed decisions. Free to faculty members.
	Introduction to Humanitarian Healthcare Online Course RCSEdhttps://services.rcsed.ac.uk/events-courses/introduction-to-humanitarian-healthcare-online-course
King's Global Health Institute	Undergraduate and postgraduate courses, events and speakers on global health topics.
	https://www.kcl.ac.uk/kghi/study-with-us
Liverpool School of Tropical Medicine	Programme of MSc, PgD and PgC courses in global health and allied subjects; MSc in Tropical and Infectious disease; 13-week Diploma course in Tropical Medicine and Hygiene; various short courses and ad hoc opportunities.
	https://www.lstmed.ac.uk/
London School of Hygiene and Tropical Medicine	Programme of MSc, PgD and PcC courses in global health and allied subjects; Professional Diploma in Tropical Medicine and Hygiene; short courses and occasional study options.
	https://www.lshtm.ac.uk/study
Médecins San Frontieres	Part-time online global health & humanitarian medicine course: medical knowledge and skills required to work in low-resource settings and humanitarian crisis contexts.
	https://msf.org.uk/global-health-and-humanitarian-medicine-course
NIHR Global Health Research Unit on Global Surgery	Range of free online courses on global surgery and general research topics.
	https://www.globalsurgeryunit.org/research_capacity_strengthening/global-surgery-education-training-faculty/
	https://education.globalsurgeryunit.org/courses

Table 13. (continued)

Organisation	Description & Website
International Postgraduate Diploma in Expedition and Wilderness Medicine, Royal College of Surgeons and Physicians of Glasgow	Considered a must for those seeking to participate in or lead expeditions in extreme and challenging environments.
	https://rcpsg.ac.uk/travel-medicine/qualifications-in-travel-medicine/rcpsg-international-postgraduate-diploma-in-expedition-and-wilderness-medicine
McGill University Faculty of Medicine and Health Sciences Montreal	Master of Science (M.Sc.) Surgical and Interventional Sciences (Thesis): Global Surgery.
	https://www.mcgill.ca/study/2024-2025/faculties/medicine/graduate/programs/master-science-msc-surgical-and-interventional-sciences-thesis-global-surgery
Royal College of Surgeons of Ireland Global Surgery Courses	Undergraduate and postgraduate global surgery courses, trainee exchanges, medical student electives and internships, extensive learning opportunities.
	https://www.rcsi.com/surgery/global-surgery/education
Stanford Centre for Innovation in Global Health	Global Health courses and residency.
	https://globalhealth.stanford.edu/
Stanford University Center for Global Health and the Johns Hopkins University Berman Institute of Bioethics	Insightful online learning about ethical issues related to global health and volunteering abroad. Ethical Challenges in Short-Term Global Health Training.
	https://www.ethicsandglobalhealth.org
SURGhub UN Global Surgery Learning Hub	Online learning on wide variety of anaesthesia, O&G, surgery and non-technical subjects.
	https://www.surghub.org/courses

Table 13. (continued)

Organisation	Description & Website
University of British Columbia	Master of Global Surgical Care online course.
	https://www.grad.ubc.ca/prospective-students/graduate-degree-programs/master-global-surgical-care
University of British Columbia, Branch for Global Surgical Care (BGSC)	Graduate level programs in global surgery and focused topics, F2F and online courses and Global Surgery Lab forum, undergraduate options in development.
	https://globalsurgery.med.ubc.ca/
University of Central Lancashire	Several short postgraduate courses leading to MSC/PGDIP/PGCert of interest to those involved in global surgery such as Rural Medicine / Urgent Care, Disaster Medicine and Point of Care Ultrasound.
	https://www.uclan.ac.uk/schools/medicine/courses.php#medicinePG
University of Colorado	Global surgery fellowship and humanitarian surgical skills workshop.
	https://medschool.cuanschutz.edu/surgery/education/global-surgery-program/education
University of Manchester Humanitarian and Conflict Response Institute	Undergraduate and postgraduate courses, research opportunities and projects.
	https://www.hcri.manchester.ac.uk/
University of Oxford Global Surgery Anaesthesia and Obstetrics	Range of courses, summer schools, research degrees and fellowships, undergraduate education and global surgery elective information.
	https://www.globalsurgery.ox.ac.uk/about
The Utrecht Summer School (Utrecht University, the Netherlands)	Global surgery and O&G short courses mixing academic and clinical topics.
	https://utrechtsummerschool.nl/courses/healthcare/global-surgery-obgyn

Table 13. (continued)

Organisation	Description & Website
Wilderness Medical Training	Courses for medics and students in mountain and expedition skills.
	https://www.wildernessmedicaltraining.co.uk
The World Bank Academy	Internships and online learning courses on development including health.
	https://olc.worldbank.org/wbg-academy

Table 13. (continued)

APPENDIX C: WRITTEN RESOURCES

ONLINE RESOURCES AND GUIDANCE DOCUMENTS

American College of Surgeons — Operation Giving Back
Resources and opportunities for surgeons volunteering internationally.
https://www.facs.org/for-medical-professionals/membership-community/operation-giving-back/.

Association of Anaesthetists — Quick Reference Handbook
https://anaesthetists.org/Home/Resources-publications/Safety-alerts/Anaesthesia-emergencies/Quick-Reference-Handbook.

Association of Surgeons of Great Britain and Ireland — How to Work as a Surgeon Overseas: Practical advice for humanitarian surgeons and teams. Booklet.
https://www.asgbi.org.uk/userfiles/file/ipp/_iipp-how-to-work-as-a-surgeon-overseas-as-gone-to-press.pdf.

Australian Medical Association — Guide to Working Abroad for Australian Medical Students and Junior Doctors.
https://ama.com.au/sites/default/files/Guide_to_Working_Abroad.pdf.

British Association of Urological Surgeons — UK Urologists Working Abroad

Information for urologists and others working in LMICs.
https://www.baus.org.uk/professionals/urolink/uk_urologists_working_abroad.aspx.

British Medical Association — Broadening Your Horizons: A Guide to Taking Time Out to Work and Train in Developing Countries.
Booklet (no longer posted on BMA website; available via BAUS).
https://www.baus.org.uk/_userfiles/pages/files/urolink/Bma%20guidance%20on%20working%20abroad.pdf.

Consortium of Universities for Global Health — Global Health Competencies Toolkit, 3rd edition, 2025.
Covers health and planetary issues of relevance to global health teams.
https://www.cugh.org/wp-content/uploads/sites/95/2025/03/Global-Health-Competencies-Tool-Kit-3rd-Ed-Updated-3_4.pdf.

International Committee of the Red Cross — Anaesthesia Handbook shop.icrc.org/anaesthesia-handbook-print-en.html.

Médecins Sans Frontières — Working in the Field: FAQ
Practical information for those considering work with MSF.
https://www.msf-me.org/media-centre/story/working-field-faq.

Médecins Sans Frontières UK — Reports and Publications
Resources documenting humanitarian work and challenges.
https://msf.org.uk/reports-and-publications.

NGO Explorer — NGOs in Africa
Activities and income of over 9,000 NGOs worldwide.
https://ngoexplorer.org/region/continent/africa.

Royal Australasian College of Surgeons — Pre-deployment Handbook
Comprehensive guide for surgeons planning international work.
https://www.surgeons.org/-media/Project/RACS/surgeons-org/files/global-health/Global-Health-Deployment-Guidebook.pdf?rev=2ca356373f264441a412e6d8f3409dfa.

Royal College of Anaesthetists — Green Theatre Checklist, Version 2.0.
Compendium of advice for teams addressing global issues.

https://rcoa.ac.uk/news/green-theatre-checklist-version-20.

Tropical Health and Education Trust — Volunteer Toolkit, 2021
Practical guidance for healthcare volunteers.
https://www.thet.org/wp-content/uploads/2021/09/Volunteer-Toolkit_THET.pdf.

World Health Organization — Online Toolkits and Training Module in Surgery & Anaesthesia Care
Official WHO resources for surgical and anaesthesia care.
https://www.who.int/teams/integrated-health-services/clinical-services-and-systems/surgical-care.

JOURNAL ARTICLES AND GUIDELINES

Crump, Jonathan A., Jeremy Sugarman, and Working Group for Ethics Guidelines on Global Health Training (WEIGHT). "**Ethics and Best Practice Guidelines for Training Experiences in Global Health**." *American Journal of Tropical Medicine and Hygiene* 83, no. 6 (2010): 1178–82. https://doi.org/10.4269/ajtmh.2010.10-0527. — *Important ethical guidelines for global health training experiences.*

Leow, Justin J., Robert S. Groen, Thomas P. Kingham et al. "**Preparation Guide for Surgical Resident and Student Rotations to Underserved Regions**." *Surgery* 151, no. 6 (2012): 770–8. https://doi.org/10.1016/j.surg.2012.03.002. — *Practical preparation guidance for trainees in underserved areas.*

TEXTBOOKS AND ACADEMIC REFERENCES

There are few books on global surgery, as it is a new field. Clinical and operative texts tailored for those working in LMICs remain limited. Material is typically created for HICs, then trickles down to LMICs.

Mukherjee, Joia. ***An Introduction to Global Health Delivery: Practice, Equity, Human Rights***. Oxford University Press, 2017. ISBN 978-0197607251. — *History of the global health movement and the role of advocacy.*

Swaroop, Mamta, and SreyRam Krishnaswami, editors. ***Academic Global Surgery*** *(Success in Academic Surgery)*. Springer, 2015. ISBN

978-3319142975. — *Current knowledge needs and pathways for future leaders in academic global surgery.*

Clinical texts

Ameh, Emmanuel A., Stephen W. Bickler, and Kokila Lakhoo, eds. ***Paediatric Surgery: A Comprehensive Textbook for Africa***. 2 vols. Springer International Publishing, 2020. ISBN 9783030417239. — *A free downloadable copy is available. https://global-help.org/products/paediatric_surgery_a_comprehensive_text_for_africa/#basicprinciples.*

Archampong, Edward Q., Simon B. Naaeder, and Benard Ugwu, editors. ***BAJA's Principles and Practice of Surgery Including Pathology in the Tropics***. 5th ed. University of Ghana Medical School, 2015. ISBN 978-9988222895. — *Considered the text for West African surgery.*

Baillière Tindall. *Surgery in the Tropics (Baillière's **Clinical Tropical Medicine & Communicable Diseases**)*. Baillière Tindall, 1988. ISBN 978-0702013096.

Carter, Louis L., ed. ***Principles of Reconstructive Surgery in Africa***. Pan-African Academy of Christian Surgeons, 2013. — *Free download: https://web.archive.org/web/20161226070514/http://paacs.net/wp-content/uploads/2012/09/PAACS-Principles-of-Reconstructive-Surgery-in-Africa-v.2-072413.pdf.*

Cohen, Ricardo V., Fernando Aun, and Dennis Up, editors. ***Tropical Surgery: Vademecum***. Karger Landes Systems, 1997. ISBN 978-3805564977. — *Concise handbook for doctors less familiar with tropical disease.*

Dallimore, Jon, Sarah R. Anderson, and Chris Imray, editors. ***Oxford Handbook of Expedition and Wilderness Medicine***. 3rd ed. Oxford University Press, 2023. ASIN B01K0SS53A.

Davey, William W. ***Companion to Surgery in Africa***. Harcourt Brace/Churchill Livingstone, 1967. ISBN 978-0443001437. — *Old but useful, includes photographs of tropical conditions.*

Dobson, Michael. ***The Right Stuff: Anaesthetic Equipment and Techniques That Work Best in Low-Resource Countries.*** Lulu.com, 2017.

Giannou, Christos, and Marco Baldan. ***War Surgery: Working with Limited Resources in Armed Conflict and Other Situations of Violence***. International Committee of the Red Cross, 2010. — Available online:

- Vol. 1: https://www.icrc.org/sites/default/files/external/doc/en/assets/files/other/icrc-002-0973.pdf
- Vol. 2: https://www.icrc.org/sites/default/files/external/doc/fr/assets/files/publications/icrc-002-4105.pdf

Kamel, Refaat, and John Lumley. ***Textbook of Tropical Surgery***. Westminster Publishing Ltd, 2004. ISBN 978-0954685508. — *Detailed information about parasitic infections.*

King, Maurice, Peter Bewes, James Cairns, and Jim Thornton, editors. ***Primary Surgery***. Vol. 1: Non-Trauma; Vol. 2: Trauma. Oxford University Press, 1990. Vol. 1 ISBN 978-0192616944; Vol. 2 ISBN 978-0192615985. — *Often considered the bible of tropical surgery. Older but valuable.*

See also:

> Cotton, Michael et al., editors. *Primary Surgery, Vol. 1: Non-Trauma*, 2nd ed. GHO Publications, 2024. https://global-help.org/products/primary-surgery-vol-1/
> Cotton, Michael et al., editors. *Primary Surgery, Vol. 2: Trauma*, 2nd ed. GHO Publications, 2024. https://global-help.org/products/primary-surgery-vol-2-2/

King, Maurice et al. ***Primary Anaesthesia***. Oxford University Press, 1986. ISBN 978-0192615923.

Kravitz, Amy, editor. ***Oxford Handbook of Humanitarian Medicine***. Oxford University Press, 2019. ISBN 978-0199565276.

World Health Organization. ***Surgical Care at the District Hospital — WHO Manual***. WHO, 2003. https://www.who.int/publications/i/item/9241545755.

Combination texts

Hardy, Mark A., and Beth R. Hochman, eds. ***Global Surgery: How to Work and Teach in Low- and Middle-Income Countries***. Springer International Publishing, 2023. https://doi.org/10.1007/978-3-031-28127-3. — *Emphasises established frameworks and standards, with "how to" guides, ethics, and expat insights.*

Meara, John G., Christopher D. McClain, and S. O. Rogers, editors. ***Global Surgery and Anaesthesia Manual: Providing Care in***

Resource-Limited Settings. CRC Press, 2014. ISBN 978-1482247305.

Park, Adrian, and Rachael Price, editors. ***Global Surgery: The Essentials***. Springer, 2017. ISBN 978-3319494807.

PERSPECTIVE AND INSPIRATION

Biddle, Pippa. ***Ours to Explore: Privilege, Power, and the Paradox of Voluntourism***. University of Nebraska Press, 2021. ISBN 978-1640124417.

Hamlin, Catherine. ***The Hospital by the River: A Story of Hope***. Monarch Books, 2004. ISBN 978-1854246738.

Hummerlen, Marlies. ***Into the World: Experiences of Medical Doctors in Global Health and Tropical Medicine***. Edited by Matthijs Bottman. Uitgeverij Boekschap, 2017. ISBN 978-94-90357-21-4 — *Available on Apple Books & Kindle.*

Kidder, Tracy. ***Mountains Beyond Mountains: The Quest of Dr Paul Farmer,*** *a Man Who Would Cure the World*. Profile Books, 2009. ISBN 978-1846684319.

Nott, David. ***War Doctor: Surgery on the Front Line***. Picador, 2020. ISBN 978-1509837045.

Polman, Linda. ***The Crisis Caravan: What's Wrong with Humanitarian Aid***. Picador, 2010. ISBN 978-0312610586.

Polman, Linda. ***War Games: The Story of Aid and War in Modern Times***. Viking, 2010. ISBN 978-0670919772.

NOVELS

Do not overlook the power of novels to offer insight into different cultures. Here is just one example: I was talking to an African college about an honest man who had been accused of embezzlement. He told me if I wanted to understand I should read this novel.

Armah, Ayi Kwei. ***The Beautyful Ones Are Not Yet Born***. Heinemann, 1989.

SOCIAL MEDIA

Many educational opportunities are first advertised on social media. Handles include:

@GlobalSurg, @GSCommission, @HarvardPGSSC, @GlobalNeurosurg, @TheG4Alliance, @GASOC.

PODCASTS

Brown Surgery Podcast: Getting Involved with Global Surgery and Global Surgery Research
https://www.ivoox.com/en/getting-involved-with-global-surgery-and-global-surgery-audios-mp3_rf_87968976_1.html.

Cold Steel podcast: Global Surgery and the Power of Purpose
https://www.globalhealthunfiltered.com/.

EAST Traumacast: Global Surgery
https://www.east.org/education-resources/traumacasts?categoryId=29.

Global Health Unfiltered
https://www.globalhealthunfiltered.com/.

Global Scalpels: A Global Surgery Podcast
https://www.globalscalpels.com/.

Off the Table: A Global Surgery Podcast
https://podtail.com/podcast/off-the-table-a-global-surgery-podcast/.

Magee DJ. Global Surgery: A Tale of Two Colleges. 2024 International Society of Surgery Lecture, 17 Jan 2025.
https://houseofsurgery.podbean.com/e/2024-international-society-of-surgery-lecture-%e2%80%a2-global-surgery-a-tale-of-two-colleges/.

VIDEOS

Global Surgery Student Alliance (video talks): https://www.youtube.com/channel/UCkETsQ6XRaYBZ7lmSv6xtoA

Harvard PGSSC: https://www.youtube.com/@harvardpgssc752

Humanitarian Aid — Nobhojit Roy keynote: https://www.youtube.com/watch?v=h7wP20kdhC8

LCoGS lectures: https://www.youtube.com/@thelancetcommissiononglobal6940/videos

Oxford University Global Surgery lectures: https://www.youtube.com/playlist?list=PLqUC1bDIuY7pG-q73derrsEp4iKLZ-kHv

RCSI Institute of Global Surgery: https://www.youtube.com/channel/UC2tgwC5E0h_6kYygaKATr1w

TED Talks (global surgery): https://www.ted.com/search?q=global%20surgery

BLOGS AND VLOGS

Seek out blogs and vlogs with firsthand accounts of working in LMIC environments or countries of interest. Personal writings provide frank, practical insights.

REFERENCES

1. INTRODUCTION: A CALL TO ARMS — SURGERY AND HEALTH FOR ALL

1. Address by H Mahler Director-General of the World health organisation to the XX11 Biennial World Congress of the International College of Surgeons [cited 2025 June 22]. https://cdn.who.int/media/docs/default-source/integrated-health-services-(ihs)/csy/surgical-care/mahler1980speech.pdf?sfvrsn=18072fa8_11.
2. Meara, John G., Andrew J. M. Leather, Lars Hagander et al. "Global Surgery 2030: Evidence and Solutions for Achieving Health, Welfare, and Economic Development." *The Lancet* 386, no. 9993 (2015): 569–624. https://doi.org/10.1016/S0140-6736(15)60160-X.
3. "Global Surgery 2030: A Roadmap for High-Income Country Actors." *BMJ Global Health* 1, no. 1 (2016): e000011. https://doi.org/10.1136/bmjgh-2015-000011.; Lozano R, Naghavi M, Foreman K et al. Global and regional mortality from 235 causes of death for 20 age groups in 1990 and 2010: a systematic analysis for the Global Burden of Disease Study 2010. Lancet. 2012;380(9859):2095–2128.
4. Bickler, Stephen N., Thomas G. Weiser, Nicholas Kassebaum, Hidetaka Higashi, David C. Chang, Jan J. Barendregt et al. "Global Burden of Surgical Conditions." In *Essential Surgery. Disease Control Priorities*, third edition, volume 1, edited by Haile T. Debas, Peter Donkor, Atul Gawande, Dean T. Jamison, Margaret E. Kruk, and Charles N. Mock, 19–40. World Bank, 2015. doi:10.1596/978-1-4648-0346-8. License: Creative Commons Attribution CC BY 3.0 IGO. http://www.ncbi.nlm.nih.gov/books/NBK333518/.
5. Farmer, Paul E., and Jim Y. Kim. "Surgery and Global Health: A View from Beyond the OR." *World Journal of Surgery* 32, no. 4 (2008): 533–36. https://doi.org/10.1007/s00268-008-9525-9.
6. Copenhagen Consensus Center. "Copenhagen Consensus 2008 – Results." Copenhagen Consensus Center, 2008. http://www.copenhagenconsensus. com/sites/default/fi les/cc08_results_final_0.pdf (accessed 22 June 2025).

2. WHAT IS GLOBAL SURGERY?

1. Alkire, Blake C., Nakul P. Raykar, Mark G. Shrime et al. "Global Access to Surgical Care: A Modelling Study." *The Lancet Global Health* 3, no. 6 (2015): e316–23. https://doi.org/10.1016/S2214-109X(15)70115-4.
2. Rose, John, Thomas G. Weiser, Phil Hider, Leona Wilson, Russell L. Gruen, and Stephen W. Bickler. "Estimated Need for Surgery Worldwide Based on Prevalence of Diseases: A Modelling Strategy for the WHO Global Health Estimate." *The Lancet. Global Health* 3 Suppl 2, no. Suppl 2 (2015): S13-20. https://doi.org/10.1016/S2214-109X(15)70087-2.
3. Murray, C. J., A. D. Lopez, and D. T. Jamison. "The Global Burden of Disease in 1990: Summary Results, Sensitivity Analysis and Future Directions." *Bulletin of the World Health Organization* 72, no. 3 (1994): 495–509.
4. World Health Organization, United Nations Population Fund, United Nations Children's Fund, and Averting Maternal Death and Disability Program. *Monitoring Emergency Obstetric Care: A Handbook*. World Health Organization, 2009. https://www.

unfpa.org/sites/default/files/pub-pdf/obstetric_monitoring.pdf (accessed June 22, 2025).

5. Pearson, L., and R. Shoo. “Availability and Use of Emergency Obstetric Services: Kenya, Rwanda, Southern Sudan, and Uganda.” *International Journal of Gynaecology and Obstetrics* 88, no. 2 (2005): 208–15. https://doi.org/10.1016/j.ijgo.2004.09.027.

3. MATERNAL HEALTH AND SURGICAL CAPACITY IN LOW- AND MIDDLE-INCOME COUNTRIES

1. World Health Organization, United Nations Children’s Fund, United Nations Population Fund, World Bank Group, and United Nations Department of Economic and Social Affairs, Population Division. *Trends in Maternal Mortality: Estimates 2000 to 2023.* World Health Organization, 2025. https://www.unfpa.org/sites/default/files/pub-pdf/9789240108462-eng.pdf.
2. Debas, H. T., P. Donkor, A. Gawande, D. T. Jamison, M. E. Kruk, and C. N. Mock, editors. 2015. *Essential Surgery. Disease Control Priorities*, third edition, volume 1. World Bank. doi:10.1596/978-1-4648-0346-8. License: Creative Commons Attribution CC BY 3.0 IGO.
3. Ibid.
4. Gibbons, Luz, José M. Belizán, Jeremy A. Lauer, Ana P. Betrán, Mario Merialdi, and Fernando Althabe. "Inequities in the Use of Cesarean Section Deliveries in the World." *American Journal of Obstetrics and Gynecology* 206, no. 4 (2012): 331.e1–331.e19. Erratum in *American Journal of Obstetrics and Gynecology* 210 (2014): 162.
5. Bouchard, Megan E., Jeanine Justiniano, Dominique Vervoort, Julian Gore-Booth, Adupa Emmanuel, and Monica Langer. “Cross-Sectional Analysis Tracking Workforce Density in Surgery, Anesthesia, and Obstetrics as an Indicator of Progress toward Improved Global Surgical Access.” *IJS Global Health* 3, no. 6 (2020): e26. https://doi.org/10.1097/GH9.0000000000000026.
6. Holmer, Hampus, Mark G. Shrime, Johanna N. Riesel, Adam Lantz, Teena Kunjumen, Walt Johnson, Andy Leather, John G. Meara, and Lars Hagander. "Towards Closing the Gap of the Global Surgeon, Anaesthesiologist and Obstetrician Workforce: Thresholds and Projections Towards 2030." *The Lancet* 385 (global surgery special issue) (2015): S40.
7. Bouchard, Megan E., Jeanine Justiniano, Dominique Vervoort, Julian Gore-Booth, Adupa Emmanuel, and Monica Langer. “Cross-Sectional Analysis Tracking Workforce Density in Surgery, Anesthesia, and Obstetrics as an Indicator of Progress toward Improved Global Surgical Access.” *IJS Global Health* 3, no. 6 (2020): e26. https://doi.org/10.1097/GH9.0000000000000026.
8. United Nations. "Millennium Development Goals." United Nations, 2000. https://www.un.org/millenniumgoals/maternal.shtml.
9. Ibid.
10. World Health Organization, United Nations Children’s Fund, United Nations Population Fund, World Bank Group, and United Nations Department of Economic and Social Affairs, Population Division. *Trends in Maternal Mortality: Estimates 2000 to 2023.* World Health Organization, 2025. https://www.unfpa.org/sites/default/files/pub-pdf/9789240108462-eng.pdf.
11. Ibid.
12. UNFPA. *Second Meeting of the Working Group for the Prevention and Treatment of Obstetric Fistula, Addis Ababa, 30 October–1 November 2002.* UNFPA, 2003.

4. BARRIERS AND DELAYS

1. Thaddeus, Sereen, and Deborah Maine. "Too Far to Walk: Maternal Mortality in Context." Social *Science & Medicine* 38, no. 8 (1994): 1091–110. https://doi.org/10.1016/0277-9536(94)90226-7.
2. Dare, Anna J., Joshua S. Ng-Kamstra, Jayadeep Patra et al. "Deaths from Acute Abdominal Conditions and Geographical Access to Surgical Care in India: A Nationally Representative Spatial Analysis." *The Lancet. Global Health* 3, no. 10 (2015): e646-653. https://doi.org/10.1016/S2214-109X(15)00079-0.

5. THE BARE NECESSITIES OF ADEQUATE SURGICAL CARE

1. Meara, John G., Andrew J. M. Leather, Lars Hagander et al. "Global Surgery 2030: Evidence and Solutions for Achieving Health, Welfare, and Economic Development." *The Lancet* 386, no. 9993 (2015): 569–624. https://doi.org/10.1016/S0140-6736(15)60160-X.
2. Zadey, Siddhesh, Himanshu Iyer, Anveshi Nayan et al. "Evaluating the Status of the Lancet Commission on Global Surgery Indicators for India." *The Lancet Regional Health.* Southeast Asia 13 (June 2023): 100178. https://doi.org/10.1016/j.lansea.2023.100178.
3. Funk, Luke M., Thomas G. Weiser, William R. Berry et al. "Global Operating Theatre Distribution and Pulse Oximetry Supply: An Estimation from Reported Data." *The Lancet* 376, no. 9746 (2010): 1055–61. https://doi.org/10.1016/S0140-6736(10)60392-3.
4. Copenhagen Consensus Center. "Copenhagen Consensus 2008 – Results." Copenhagen Consensus Center, 2008. https://copenhagenconsensus.com/sites/default/files/cc08_results_final_0.pdf.
5. Meara, John G., Andrew J. M. Leather, Lars Hagander et al. "Global Surgery 2030: Evidence and Solutions for Achieving Health, Welfare, and Economic Development." *The Lancet* 386, no. 9993 (2015): 569–624. https://doi.org/10.1016/S0140-6736(15)60160-X.
6. World Health Organization. *Safe Surgery: Tool and Resources.* World Health Organization. Accessed September 26, 2025. https://www.who.int/teams/integrated-health-services/patient-safety/research/safe-surgery/tool-and-resources.

6. THE WORLD'S BEST OPERATIONS — DEFINING ESSENTIAL SURGERY

1. Botman, Matthijs, Rinse J. Meester, Roeland Voorhoeve et al. "The Amsterdam Declaration on Essential Surgical Care." *World Journal of Surgery* 39, no. 6 (2015): 1335–40. https://doi.org/10.1007/s00268-015-3057-x.
2. Dobson, Michael, Paul Fenton, Richard Fisher et al. *Surgical Care at the District Hospital.* Edited by Michael Dobson and Richard Fisher. World Health Organization, 2003. https://www.who.int/publications/i/item/9241545755.
3. WHO World Health Organization. *WHO Global Initiative for Emergency and Essential Surgical Care.* World Health Organization. Accessed October 23, 2025. https://www.who.int/initiatives/who-global-initiative-for-emergency-and-essential-surgical-care.
4. Debas, H. T., P. Donkor, A. Gawande, D. T. Jamison, M. E. Kruk, and C. N. Mock, editors. 2015. *Essential Surgery. Disease Control Priorities*, third edition, volume 1.

World Bank. doi:10.1596/978-1-4648-0346-8. License: Creative Commons Attribution CC BY 3.0 IGO.

5. Ibid.
6. Botman, Matthijs, Rinse J. Meester, Roeland Voorhoeve et al. "The Amsterdam Declaration on Essential Surgical Care." *World Journal of Surgery* 39, no. 6 (2015): 1335–40. https://doi.org/10.1007/s00268-015-3057-x.
7. Meara, John G., Andrew J. M. Leather, Lars Hagander et al. "Global Surgery 2030: Evidence and Solutions for Achieving Health, Welfare, and Economic Development." *The Lancet* 386, no. 9993 (2015): 569–624. https://doi.org/10.1016/S0140-6736(15)60160-X.
8. Stewart, Barclay T., Gavin Tansley, Adam Gyedu et al. "Mapping Population-Level Spatial Access to Essential Surgical Care in Ghana Using Availability of Bellwether Procedures." *JAMA Surgery* 151, no. 8 (2016): e161239. https://doi.org/10.1001/jamasurg.2016.1239.
9. James, Kennedy, Isaiah Borchem, Rodney Talo et al. "Universal Access to Safe, Affordable, Timely Surgical and Anaesthetic Care in Papua New Guinea: The Six Global Health Indicators." *ANZ Journal of Surgery* 90, no. 10 (2020): 1903–9. https://doi.org/10.1111/ans.16148.
10. Hoh, Su Mei, Mohamed Y. A. Wahab, Abdullah N. Hisham, Glenn D. Guest, and David A. K. Watters. "Mapping Timely Access to Emergency and Essential Surgical Services: The Malaysian Experience." *ANZ Journal of Surgery* 92, nos. 1–2 (2022): 223–27. https://doi.org/10.1111/ans.16986.
11. Kamali, Parisa, Issy Marks, Godfrey Sama, Dominique Vervoort, and Justine Davies. "Measuring Surgical Systems Worldwide: An Update." *World Bank Blogs*, February 12, 2018. https://blogs.worldbank.org/en/opendata/measuring-surgical-systems-worldwide-update.

7. MAJOR INITIATIVES IN GLOBAL SURGERY

1. Jamison, Dean T., W. Henry Mosley, Anthony R. Measham, and José Luis Bobadilla, eds. *Disease Control Priorities in Developing Countries.* Oxford University Press for the World Bank, 1993. https://documents1.worldbank.org/curated/en/705591468320064221/pdf/multi0page.pdf.
2. Jamison, Dean T.; Breman, Joel G.; Measham, Anthony R.; Alleyne, George; Claeson, Mariam; Evans, David B.; Jha, Prabhat; Mills, Ann; Musgrove, Philip. 2006. *Disease Control Priorities in Developing Countries*, Second Edition. © World Bank. http://hdl.handle.net/10986/7242 License: CC BY 3.0 IGO.
3. Debas, H. T., P. Donkor, A. Gawande, D. T. Jamison, M. E. Kruk, and C. N. Mock, editors. 2015. *Essential Surgery. Disease Control Priorities*, third edition, volume 1. World Bank. doi:10.1596/978-1-4648-0346-8. License: Creative Commons Attribution CC BY 3.0 IGO.
4. Ibid.
5. Botman, Matthijs, Rinse J. Meester, Roeland Voorhoeve et al. "The Amsterdam Declaration on Essential Surgical Care." *World Journal of Surgery* 39, no. 6 (2015): 1335–40. https://doi.org/10.1007/s00268-015-3057-x.
6. Ng-Kamstra, Joshua S., Sarah L. M. Greenberg, Fizan Abdullah et al. "Global Surgery 2030: A Roadmap for High Income Country Actors." *BMJ Global Health* 1, no. 1 (2016): e000011. https://doi.org/10.1136/bmjgh-2015-000011.
7. Nepogodiev, Dmitri et al. "Surgical Health Policy 2025-35: Strengthening Essential Services for Tomorrow's Needs." *The Lancet*, Volume 406, Issue 10505,860-880. https:/doi.org/10.1016/S0140-6736(25)00985-7.
8. World Health Organization. *Sixty-eighth World Health Assembly: Resolution WHA68.15, Agenda Item 17.1, 26 May 2015. Strengthening Emergency and Essential*

Surgical Care and Anaesthesia as a Component of Universal Health Coverage. Document A68/31. World Health Organization, 2015. https://apps.who.int/gb/ebwha/pdf_files/wha68/a68_r15-en.pdf.

9. World Health Organization. *Surgical Care Systems Strengthening: Developing National Surgical, Obstetric and Anaesthesia Plans*. World Health Organization, 2017. https://iris.who.int/bitstream/handle/10665/255566/9789241512244-eng.pdf. Licensed under CC BY-NC-SA 3.0 IGO.
10. World Health Organization. *Seventy-sixth World Health Assembly: Resolution WHA76.2, Agenda Item 13.1, 30 May 2023. Integrated Emergency, Critical and Operative Care for Universal Health Coverage and Protection from Health Emergencies.* World Health Organization, 2023. https://apps.who.int/gb/ebwha/pdf_files/WHA76/A76_R2-en.pdf.
11. M'pele, Pierre, Justina O. Seyi-Olajide, Tarcisse Elongo, Jorn Lemvik, Delanyo Dovlo, and Emmanuel A. Ameh. "From Research to a Political Commitment to Strengthen Access to Surgical, Obstetric, and Anesthesia Care in Africa by 2030." *Frontiers in Public Health* 11 (May 2023). https://doi.org/10.3389/fpubh.2023.1168805.
12. United Nations Development Programme. *Sustainable Development Goals*. Accessed August 21, 2025. https://www.undp.org/sustainable-development-goals.
13. World Health Organization. *Millennium Development Goals (MDGs)*. Updated August 2025. World Health Organization. https://www.who.int/news-room/fact-sheets/detail/millennium-development-goals-(mdgs).
14. Bose, Dipan, Sheila Dutta, and Patricio Vicente Marquez. *The High Toll of Traffic Injuries: Unacceptable and Preventable*. Washington, DC: World Bank Group, 2018. https://documents.worldbank.org/curated/en/374881515180592957.
15. World Health Organization, United Nations Children's Fund, United Nations Population Fund, World Bank Group, and United Nations Department of Economic and Social Affairs, Population Division. *Trends in Maternal Mortality: Estimates 2000 to 2023*. World Health Organization, 2025. https://www.unfpa.org/sites/default/files/pub-pdf/9789240108462-eng.pdf.
16. Bose, Dipan, Sheila Dutta, and Patricio Vicente Marquez. *The High Toll of Traffic Injuries: Unacceptable and Preventable*. Washington, DC: World Bank Group. https://documents.worldbank.org/curated/en/374881515180592957.
17. United Nations General Assembly. *Resolution 70/1: Transforming Our World: The 2030 Agenda for Sustainable Development.* Adopted September 25, 2015. A/RES/70/1. https://sdgs.un.org/2030agenda.
18. United Nations. *The Sustainable Development Goals Report 2024*. United Nations, 2024. https://unstats.un.org/sdgs/report/2024/The-Sustainable-Development-Goals-Report-2024.pdf.

8. QUALITY MATTERS

1. Arya, Sumedha, Joshua Ng-Kamstra, John G. Meara, and Ana Langer. "Tracking Perioperative Mortality and Maternal Mortality: Challenges and Opportunities." *The Lancet Global Health* 4, no. 7 (2016): e440–41. https://doi.org/10.1016/S2214-109X(16)30082-1.
2. Abbott, T. E. F., A. J. Fowler, T. D. Dobbs, E. M. Harrison, M. A. Gillies, and R. M. Pearse. "Frequency of Surgical Treatment and Related Hospital Procedures in the UK: A National Ecological Study Using Hospital Episode Statistics." *British Journal of Anaesthesia* 119, no. 2 (2017): 249–57. https://doi.org/10.1093/bja/aex137.
3. National Emergency Laparotomy Audit, "NELA Data Collection Web Tool," accessed 3 December 2025, https://data.nela.org.uk/.
4. Weiser, Thomas G., and Atul Gawande. "Excess Surgical Mortality: Strategies for Improving Quality of Care." In *Essential Surgery. Disease Control Priorities*, third

edition, volume 1, edited by Haile T. Debas, Peter Donkor, Atul Gawande, Dean T. Jamison, Margaret E. Kruk, and Charles N. Mock. World Bank, 2015. https://doi.org/10.1596/978-1-4648-0346-8. License: Creative Commons Attribution CC BY 3.0 IGO.

5. Abbott, T. E. F., A. J. Fowler, T. D. Dobbs, E. M. Harrison, M. A. Gillies, and R. M. Pearse. "Frequency of Surgical Treatment and Related Hospital Procedures in the UK: A National Ecological Study Using Hospital Episode Statistics." *British Journal of Anaesthesia* 119, no. 2 (2017): 249–57. https://doi.org/10.1093/bja/aex137.
6. Lindheim-Minde, Barbro, Andreas Gjøra, Juul M. Bakker et al. "Changes in Surgical Volume, Workforce, and Productivity in Sierra Leone between 2012 and 2017." *Surgery* 170, no. 1 (2021): 126–33. https://doi.org/10.1016/j.surg.2021.02.043.
7. Contini, Sandro. "Typhoid Intestinal Perforation in Developing Countries: Still Unavoidable Deaths?" *World Journal of Gastroenterology* 23, no. 11 (2017): 1925–31. https://doi.org/10.3748/wjg.v23.i11.1925.
8. World Health Organization. "WHO Surgical Safety Checklist." *Safe Surgery: Tool and Resources*. World Health Organization. Accessed October 23, 2025. https://www.who.int/teams/integrated-health-services/patient-safety/research/safe-surgery/tool-and-resources.
9. Haynes, Alex B., Thomas G. Weiser, William R. Berry et al. "A Surgical Safety Checklist to Reduce Morbidity and Mortality in a Global Population." *The New England Journal of Medicine* 360, no. 5 (2009): 491–99. https://doi.org/10.1056/NEJMsa0810119.
10. World Health Organization. *WHO Guidelines for Safe Surgery 2009: Safe Surgery Saves Lives*. World Health Organization, 2009. https://apps.who.int/iris/bitstream/handle/10665/44185/9789241598552_eng.pdf.
11. Jin, James, Salesi 'Akau'ola, Cheng-Har Yip et al. "The Impact of Quality Improvement Interventions in Improving Surgical Infections and Mortality in Low and Middle-Income Countries: A Systematic Review and Meta-Analysis." *World Journal of Surgery* 45, no. 10 (2021): 1. https://doi.org/10.1007/s00268-021-06208-y.
12. Aveling, Emma-Louise, Peter McCulloch, and Mary Dixon-Woods. "A Qualitative Study Comparing Experiences of the Surgical Safety Checklist in Hospitals in High-Income and Low-Income Countries." *BMJ Open* 3, no. 8 (2013): e003039. https://doi.org/10.1136/bmjopen-2013-003039.
13. NIHR Global Health Research Unit on Global Surgery, Sivesh Kathir Kamarajah, and Philip Alexander. "Structures, Processes and Outcomes between First Referral and Referral Hospitals in Low-Income and Middle-Income Countries: A Secondary Preplanned Analysis of the FALCON and ChEETAh Randomised Trials." *BMJ Global Health* 9, no. Suppl 4 (2024): e015599. https://doi.org/10.1136/bmjgh-2024-015599.
14. Ibid.
15. World Health Organization. "Safe Surgery." In *Patient Safety: Research and Resources*, Integrated Health Services Department. World Health Organization, 2025. https://www.who.int/teams/integrated-health-services/patient-safety/research/safe-surgery.
16. World Health Organization. *Guidelines for Trauma Quality Improvement Programmes*. World Health Organization, 2009. Accessed September 19, 2025. https://iris.who.int/handle/10665/44061.
17. Kamali, Parisa, Issy Marks, Godfrey Sama, Dominique Vervoort, and Justine Davies. "Measuring Surgical Systems Worldwide: An Update." *World Bank Blogs*, February 12, 2018. https://blogs.worldbank.org/en/opendata/measuring-surgical-systems-worldwide-update.
18. Klein, Rosemary, and Adrian Park. "Surgical Training in Low-Resource Settings." In *Global Surgery: The Essentials*, edited by Adrian Park and Raymond Price. Springer International Publishing, 2017. https://doi.org/10.1007/978-3-319-49482-1_4.
19. Maki, Joni, Michael Qualls, Barbara White, Scott Kleefield et al. "Health Impact Assessment and Short-Term Medical Missions: A Methods Study to Evaluate Quality of Care." *BMC Health Services Research* 8, no. 121 (2008).

20. Ibid.
21. Ibid.
22. Jones, Andrew. "Medical Equipment Donated to Developing Nations Usually Ends Up on the Junk Heap." *Scientific American*, May 6, 2013. https://www.scientificamerican.com/article/medical-equipment-donated-developing-nations-junk-heap/.
23. Mark, Ian H., Hilary Thomas, Edward Fitzgerald et al. "Medical Equipment Donation in Low-Resource Settings: A Review of the Literature and Guidelines for Surgery and Anaesthesia in Low-Income and Middle-Income Countries." *BMJ Global Health* 4, no. 5 (2019): e001785. https://doi.org/10.1136/bmjgh-2019-001785.

9. ANAESTHESIA AND SAFETY CULTURE

1. Citron, Isabelle, and John G. Meara. "A Global Surgery, Obstetrics and Anaesthesia Metamorphosis: The SAFE-T Summit 2018 Reports." *Update in Anaesthesia* 33 (2019): 6–8. https://resources.wfsahq.org/wp-content/uploads/uia33-A-global-surgery-obstetrics-and-anaesthesia-metamorphosis.pdf.
2. Meara, John G., Andrew J. M. Leather, Lars Hagander et al. "Global Surgery 2030: Evidence and Solutions for Achieving Health, Welfare, and Economic Development." *The Lancet* 386, no. 9993 (2015): 569–624. https://doi.org/10.1016/S0140-6736(15)60160-X.
3. Debas, H. T., P. Donkor, A. Gawande, D. T. Jamison, M. E. Kruk, and C. N. Mock, editors. 2015. *Essential Surgery. Disease Control Priorities*, third edition, volume 1. World Bank. doi:10.1596/978-1-4648-0346-8. License: Creative Commons Attribution CC BY 3.0 IGO.
4. Ouro-Bang'na Maman, A. F., K. Tomta, S. Ahouangbévi, and M. Chobli. "Deaths Associated with Anaesthesia in Togo, West Africa." *Tropical Doctor* 35, no. 4 (2005): 220–22. https://doi.org/10.1258/004947505774938666.
5. Debas, H. T., P. Donkor, A. Gawande, D. T. Jamison, M. E. Kruk, and C. N. Mock, editors. 2015. *Essential Surgery. Disease Control Priorities,* third edition, volume 1. World Bank. doi:10.1596/978-1-4648-0346-8. License: Creative Commons Attribution CC BY 3.0 IGO.
6. O'Neill, Kate, Kaitlin M. Daniels, Shailvi Greenberg, and Niraj Raykar. "Appendix 2.2: Situational Analysis Tool." In J. G. Meara et al., "Global Surgery 2030: Evidence and Solutions for Achieving Health, Welfare, and Economic Development." *The Lancet* 386, no. 9993 (2015): 569–624. Supplementary appendix. https://www.thelancet.com/journals/lancet/article/PIIS0140-6736(15)60160-X/fulltext.
7. Kushner, Adam L., Meena N. Cherian, Luc Noel, David A. Spiegel, Steffen Groth, and Carissa Etienne. "Addressing the Millennium Development Goals from a Surgical Perspective: Essential Surgery and Anesthesia in 8 Low- and Middle-Income Countries." *Archives of Surgery* (Chicago, Ill.: 1960) 145, no. 2 (2010): 154–59. https://doi.org/10.1001/archsurg.2009.263.
8. Funk, Luke M., Thomas G. Weiser, William R. Berry et al. "Global Operating Theatre Distribution and Pulse Oximetry Supply: An Estimation from Reported Data." *The Lancet* 376, no. 9746 (2010): 1055–61. https://doi.org/10.1016/S0140-6736(10)60392-3.
9. World Health Organization. *Zambia Service Availability and Readiness Assessment 2010: Summary Report.* Ministry of Health, Republic of Zambia, and World Health Organization, 2010. https://web.archive.org/web/20220119165218/https://www.who.int/healthinfo/systems/zmb_sara_report_2010_web.pdf.
10. Henry, Jaymie A., Olubayo Windapo, Adam L. Kushner, Reinou S. Groen, and Benedict C. Nwomeh. "A Survey of Surgical Capacity in Rural Southern Nigeria: Opportunities for Change." *World Journal of Surgery* 36, no. 12 (2012): 2811–18. https://doi.org/10.1007/s00268-012-1764-0.

11. Walker, Isabeau A., Apunyo D. Obua, Falan Mouton, Steven Ttendo, and Iain H. Wilson. "Paediatric Surgery and Anaesthesia in South-Western Uganda: A Cross-Sectional Survey." *Bulletin of the World Health Organization* 88, no. 12 (2010): 897–906. https://doi.org/10.2471/BLT.10.076703.
12. Pedersen, Tom, Bente Dyrlund Pedersen, and Ann Merete Møller. "Pulse Oximetry for Perioperative Monitoring." *Cochrane Database of Systematic Reviews*, no. 2 (2003). https://doi.org/10.1002/14651858.CD002013.
13. Albert, V., S. Mndolo, E. M. Harrison, E. O'Sullivan, I. H. Wilson, and I. A. Walker. "Lifebox Pulse Oximeter Implementation in Malawi: Evaluation of Educational Outcomes and Impact on Oxygen Desaturation Episodes during Anaesthesia." *Anaesthesia* 72, no. 6 (2017): 686–93. https://doi.org/10.1111/anae.13838.
14. Oodit, Ravi, Bruce M. Biccard, Eugenio Panieri et al. "Guidelines for Perioperative Care in Elective Abdominal and Pelvic Surgery at Primary and Secondary Hospitals in Low-Middle-Income Countries (LMIC's): Enhanced Recovery After Surgery (ERAS) Society Recommendation." *World Journal of Surgery* 46, no. 8 (2022): 1826–43. https://doi.org/10.1007/s00268-022-06587-w.

10. MONEY, MONEY, MONEY

1. Harvard PGSSC. "Jim Yong Kim – Inaugural Lancet Commission on Global Surgery 2014." Featuring Jim Yong Kim. Recorded January 17, 2014, Boston, MA. Published December 14, 2017. YouTube video, 2:27. https://www.youtube.com/watch?v=61iM4Qjk-q4.
2. Meara, John G., Andrew J. M. Leather, Lars Hagander et al. "Global Surgery 2030: Evidence and Solutions for Achieving Health, Welfare, and Economic Development." *The Lancet* 386, no. 9993 (2015): 569–624. https://doi.org/10.1016/S0140-6736(15)60160-X.
3. Ibid.
4. Kamali, Parisa, Issy Marks, Godfrey Sama, Dominique Vervoort, and Justine Davies. "Measuring Surgical Systems Worldwide: An Update." *World Bank Blogs*, February 12, 2018. https://blogs.worldbank.org/en/opendata/measuring-surgical-systems-worldwide-update.
5. Ibid.
6. Meara, John G., Andrew J. M. Leather, Lars Hagander et al. "Global Surgery 2030: Evidence and Solutions for Achieving Health, Welfare, and Economic Development." *The Lancet* 386, no. 9993 (2015): 569–624. https://doi.org/10.1016/S0140-6736(15)60160-X.
7. Ibid.
8. Ibid.
9. Ibid.
10. Alkire, Blake C., Nakul P. Raykar, Mark G. Shrime et al. "Global Access to Surgical Care: A Modelling Study." *The Lancet Global Health* 3, no. 6 (2015): e316–23. https://doi.org/10.1016/S2214-109X(15)70115-4.
11. Ifeanyichi, Martilord, Jose Luis Mosso Lara, Phyllis Tenkorang et al. "Cost-Effectiveness of Surgical Interventions in Low-Income and Middle-Income Countries: A Systematic Review and Critical Analysis of Recent Evidence." *BMJ Global Health* 9, no. 10 (2024). https://doi.org/10.1136/bmjgh-2024-016439.
12. Alkire, Blake C., Jeffrey R. Vincent, and John G. Meara. "Benefit-Cost Analysis for Selected Surgical Interventions in Low- and Middle-Income Countries." In *Essential Surgery. Disease Control Priorities*, third edition, volume 1, edited by Haile T. Debas, Peter Donkor, Atul Gawande, Dean T. Jamison, Margaret E. Kruk, and Charles N. Mock. World Bank, 2015. https://doi.org/10.1596/978-1-4648-0346-8. License: Creative Commons Attribution CC BY 3.0 IGO.

13. Ibid.
14. Ibid.
15. Ibid.
16. Alkire, Blake C, Mark G Shrime, Anna J Dare, Jeffrey R Vincent, and John G Meara. "Global Economic Consequences of Selected Surgical Diseases: A Modelling Study." *The Lancet Global Health* 3 (April 2015): S21–27. https://doi.org/10.1016/S2214-109X(15)70088-4.
17. Meara, John G., Andrew J. M. Leather, Lars Hagander et al. "Global Surgery 2030: Evidence and Solutions for Achieving Health, Welfare, and Economic Development." *The Lancet* 386, no. 9993 (2015): 569–624. https://doi.org/10.1016/S0140-6736(15)60160-X.
18. Alkire, Blake C, Mark G Shrime, Anna J Dare, Jeffrey R Vincent, and John G Meara. "Global Economic Consequences of Selected Surgical Diseases: A Modelling Study." *The Lancet Global Health* 3 (April 2015): S21–27. https://doi.org/10.1016/S2214-109X(15)70088-4.
19. Nasser, Jacob S., and Kevin C. Chung. "Economic Analyses of Surgical Trips to the Developing World: Current Concepts and Future Strategies." *Hand Clinics* 35, no. 4 (2019): 381–89. https://doi.org/10.1016/j.hcl.2019.06.001.
20. World Health Organization. "New Cost-Effectiveness Updates from WHO-CHOICE." 15 October 2021. https://www.who.int/news-room/feature-stories/detail/new-cost-effectiveness-updates-from-who-choice.
21. Zitzman, Elena, Holly Berkley, and Rahul M. Jindal. "Accountability in Global Surgery Missions." *BMJ Global Health* 3, no. 6 (2018). https://doi.org/10.1136/bmjgh-2018-001025.
22. Hamer, Mirjam, Dennis Alcorn, Raphiou Oumar Diallo et al. "A Comparative Analysis of the Health, Financial, Distributive, and Cost-Effectiveness Impacts of Maxillofacial Surgery in Guinea." *Impact Surgery* 1, no. 4 (2024): 136–44. https://doi.org/10.62463/surgery.79.

11. TASK SHIFTING AND TASK SHARING

1. World Health Organization, PEPFAR, and UNAIDS. *Task Shifting: Rational Redistribution of Tasks among Health Workforce Teams: Global Recommendations and Guidelines.* World Health Organization, 2007. https://iris.who.int/handle/10665/43821.
2. Ryan, Isabel, Keshav V. Shah, Carlos E. Barrero, Tjinjeka Uamunovandu, Andre Ilbawi, and Jordan Swanson. "Task Shifting and Task Sharing to Strengthen the Surgical Workforce in Sub-Saharan Africa: A Systematic Review of the Existing Literature." *World Journal of Surgery* 47, no. 12 (2023): 3070–80. https://doi.org/10.1007/s00268-023-07197-w.
3. Debas, H. T., P. Donkor, A. Gawande, D. T. Jamison, M. E. Kruk, and C. N. Mock, editors. 2015. *Essential Surgery. Disease Control Priorities*, third edition, volume 1. World Bank. doi:10.1596/978-1-4648-0346-8. License: Creative Commons Attribution CC BY 3.0 IGO.
4. World Health Organization. *Sixty-eighth World Health Assembly: Resolution WHA68.15, Agenda Item 17.1, 26 May 2015. Strengthening Emergency and Essential Surgical Care and Anaesthesia as a Component of Universal Health Coverage. Document A68/31.* World Health Organization, 2015. https://apps.who.int/gb/ebwha/pdf_files/wha68/a68_r15-en.pdf.
5. Meara, John G., Andrew J. M. Leather, Lars Hagander et al. "Global Surgery 2030: Evidence and Solutions for Achieving Health, Welfare, and Economic Development." *The Lancet* 386, no. 9993 (2015): 569–624. https://doi.org/10.1016/S0140-6736(15)60160-X.

6. Ryan, Isabel, Keshav V. Shah, Carlos E. Barrero, Tjinjeka Uamunovandu, Andre Ilbawi, and Jordan Swanson. "Task Shifting and Task Sharing to Strengthen the Surgical Workforce in Sub-Saharan Africa: A Systematic Review of the Existing Literature." *World Journal of Surgery* 47, no. 12 (2023): 3070–80. https://doi.org/10.1007/s00268-023-07197-w.
7. Bognini, Maeve S., Christian I. Oko, Meskerem A. Kebede et al. "Assessing the Impact of Anaesthetic and Surgical Task-Shifting Globally: A Systematic Literature Review." *Health Policy and Planning* 38, no. 8 (2023): 960–994. https://doi.org/10.1093/heapol/czad059.
8. van Duinen, A. J., M. M. Kamara, L. Hagander, T. Ashley, A. P. Koroma, A. Leather, M. Elhassein, E. Darj, Ø. Salvesen, A. Wibe, and H. A. Bolkan. "Caesarean Section Performed by Medical Doctors and Associate Clinicians in Sierra Leone." *The British Journal of Surgery* 106, no. 2 (2019): e129–37. https://doi.org/10.1002/bjs.11076.
9. Beard, Jessica H., Lawrence B. Oresanya, Larry Akoko, Ally Mwanga, Charles A. Mkony, and Rochelle A. Dicker. "Surgical Task-Shifting in a Low-Resource Setting: Outcomes after Major Surgery Performed by Nonphysician Clinicians in Tanzania." *World Journal of Surgery* 38, no. 6 (2014): 1398–1404. https://doi.org/10.1007/s00268-013-2446-2.
10. Ashley, Thomas, Hannah Ashley, Andreas Wladis et al. "Outcomes After Elective Inguinal Hernia Repair Performed by Associate Clinicians vs Medical Doctors in Sierra Leone: A Randomized Clinical Trial." *JAMA Network Open* 4, no. 1 (2021): e2032681. https://doi.org/10.1001/jamanetworkopen.2020.32681.
11. Ryan, Isabel, Keshav V. Shah, Carlos E. Barrero, Tjinjeka Uamunovandu, Andre Ilbawi, and Jordan Swanson. "Task Shifting and Task Sharing to Strengthen the Surgical Workforce in Sub-Saharan Africa: A Systematic Review of the Existing Literature." *World Journal of Surgery* 47, no. 12 (2023): 3070–3080. https://doi.org/10.1007/s00268-023-07197-w.
12. Bognini, Maeve S, Christian I. Oko, Meskerem A. Kebede et al. "Assessing the Impact of Anaesthetic and Surgical Task-Shifting Globally: A Systematic Literature Review." *Health Policy and Planning* 38, no. 8 (2023): 960–94. https://doi.org/10.1093/heapol/czad059.
13. van der Merwe, Freliza, Nicola J. Vickery, Hyla-Louise Kluyts et al. "Postoperative Outcomes Associated with Procedural Sedation Conducted by Physician and Nonphysician Anesthesia Providers: Findings from the Prospective, Observational African Surgical Outcomes Study." *Anesthesia & Analgesia* 135, no. 2 (2022): 250–63. https://doi.org/10.1213/ANE.0000000000005819.
14. Asemu, Yohannes Molla, Etienne Nsereko, Dan Ian McIsaac, and M. Dylan Bould. "Nonphysician Sedation Providers in Africa: What Counts and What Is Being Counted?" *Anesthesia & Analgesia* 135, no. 2 (2022): 246. https://doi.org/10.1213/ANE.0000000000006037.
15. Bolkan, Håkon Annfelt, Arjen van Duinen, Bram Waalewijn et al. "Safety, Productivity and Predicted Contribution of a Surgical Task-Sharing Programme in Sierra Leone." *British Journal of Surgery* 104, no. 10 (2017): 1315–26. https://doi.org/10.1002/bjs.10552.
16. World Health Organization. *WHO Recommendations: Optimizing Health Worker Roles to Improve Access to Key Maternal and Newborn Health Interventions through Task Shifting*. World Health Organization, 2012. https://www.who.int/publications/i/item/9789241504843.
17. Ryan, Imelda, Shah, Kavitha V., Barrero, Carlos Eduardo et al. "Task Shifting and Task Sharing to Strengthen the Surgical Workforce in Sub-Saharan Africa: A Systematic Review of the Existing Literature." *World Journal of Surgery* 47 (2023): 3070–3080. https://doi.org/10.1007/s00268-023-07197-w.

12. RESEARCH IN GLOBAL SURGERY

1. Bhakuni, Himani, and Seye Abimbola. "Epistemic Injustice in Academic Global Health." *The Lancet Global Health* 9, no. 10 (2021): e1465–70. https://doi.org/10.1016/S2214-109X(21)00301-6.
2. National Commission for the Protection of Human Subjects of Biomedical and Behavioral Research. *The Belmont Report: Ethical Principles and Guidelines for the Protection of Human Subjects of Research.* U.S. Department of Health, Education, and Welfare, April 18, 1979. https://www.hhs.gov/ohrp/sites/default/files/the-belmont-report-508c_FINAL.pdf.
3. NIHR Global Research Health Unit on Global Surgery. "Reducing Surgical Site Infections in Low-Income and Middle-Income Countries (FALCON): A Pragmatic, Multicentre, Stratified, Randomised Controlled Trial." *The Lancet* (London, England) 398, no. 10312 (2021): 1687–99. https://doi.org/10.1016/S0140-6736(21)01548-8.
4. Andoh, Aaron B., Abantanga Atindaana Francis, Abdulhafiz A. Abdulkarim et al. "Routine Sterile Glove and Instrument Change at the Time of Abdominal Wound Closure to Prevent Surgical Site Infection (ChEETAh): A Pragmatic, Cluster-Randomised Trial in Seven Low-Income and Middle-Income Countries." *The Lancet* 400, no. 10365 (2022): 1767–76. https://doi.org/10.1016/S0140-6736(22)01884-0.
5. Jumbam, Desmond T. "How (Not) to Write about Global Health." *BMJ Global Health* 5, no. 7 (2020). https://doi.org/10.1136/bmjgh-2020-003164.
6. Ravi, Krithi, Zineb Bentounsi, Aiman Tariq et al. "Systematic Analysis of Authorship Demographics in Global Surgery." *BMJ Global Health* 6, no. 10 (2021): e006672. https://doi.org/10.1136/bmjgh-2021-006672.

13. INNOVATION IN GLOBAL SURGERY

1. Tongaonkar, Ravindranath R., Brahma V. Reddy, Virendra K. Mehta, Ningthoujam Somorjit Singh, and Sanjay Shivade. "Preliminary Multicentric Trial of Cheap Indigenous Mosquito-Net Cloth for Tension-Free Hernia Repair." *Indian Journal of Surgery* (Medknow Publications on behalf of the Association of Surgeons of India), December 31, 2003. http://hdl.handle.net/1807/24057.
2. Ahmad, M H, S Pathak, K D Clement, and E H Aly. "Meta-Analysis of the Use of Sterilized Mosquito Net Mesh for Inguinal Hernia Repair in Less Economically Developed Countries." *BJS Open* 3, no. 4 (2019): 429–35. https://doi.org/10.1002/bjs5.50147.
3. Association of Rural Surgeons of India–Lancet Commission on Global Surgery Consensus Committee (ARSI-LCoGS Consensus Committee). "The Lancet Commission on Global Surgery–Association of Rural Surgeons of India Karad Consensus Statement on Surgical System Strengthening in Rural India." *Healthcare* (Amsterdam, Netherlands) 7, no. 2 (2019): 7–9. https://pubmed.ncbi.nlm.nih.gov/30709795/.
4. Aruparayil, N., J. Gnanaraj, A. Mishra et al. "Gasless Laparoscopy in Rural India-Registry Outcomes and Evaluation of the Learning Curve." *Surgical Endoscopy* 37, no. 11 (2023): 8227–35. https://doi.org/10.1007/s00464-023-10392-4.
5. Karki, B B, S Katuwal, J Walshaw, C Atkinson, S Satyal, and M Loubani. "How to Design a Low-Cost 3D Printed Laparoscopic Appendicectomy Simulation Model (LaApSi)?" *British Journal of Surgery* 110, no. Supplement_7 (2023): znad258.017. https://doi.org/10.1093/bjs/znad258.017.
6. Bolton, William S., Noel K. Aruparayil, Bonnie Cundill et al. "No Frugal Innovation without Frugal Evaluation: The Global IDEAL Sub-Framework." *BMJ Surgery, Interventions, & Health Technologies* 6, no. 1 (2024): e000248. https://doi.org/10.1136/bmjsit-2023-000248.
7. Association of Rural Surgeons of India–Lancet Commission on Global Surgery

Consensus Committee (ARSI-LCoGS Consensus Committee). "The Lancet Commission on Global Surgery–Association of Rural Surgeons of India Karad Consensus Statement on Surgical System Strengthening in Rural India." *Healthcare* (Amsterdam, Netherlands) 7, no. 2 (2019): 7–9. https://pubmed.ncbi.nlm.nih.gov/30709795/.

14. NATIONAL SURGICAL, OBSTETRIC AND ANAESTHESIA PLANS (NSOAPS)

1. World Health Organization. *Surgical Care Systems Strengthening: Developing National Surgical, Obstetric and Anaesthesia Plans.* World Health Organization, 2017. https://iris.who.int/bitstream/handle/10665/255566/9789241512244-eng.pdf. Licensed under CC BY-NC-SA 3.0 IGO.
2. Ibid.
3. Republic of Zambia, Ministry of Health. *National Surgical, Obstetric, and Anaesthesia Strategic Plan NSOASP Year 2017-2021.* Ministry of Health, May 2017. https://www.pgssc.org/_files/ugd/d9a674_70f6813fe4e74c4d99eb028336a38745.pdf.
4. Peters, Alexander W., Luis Roa, Emmanuel Rwamasirabo, Emmanuel Ameh, Marco M. Ulisubisya, Lubna Samad, Emmanuel M. Makasa, and John G. Meara. "National Surgical, Obstetric, and Anesthesia Plans Supporting the Vision of Universal Health Coverage." *Global Health: Science and Practice* 8, no. 1 (2020): 1–9. https://doi.org/10.9745/GHSP-D-19-00314.
5. Massenburg, Benjamin B., Saurabh Saluja, Hillary E. Jenny et al. "Assessing the Brazilian Surgical System with Six Surgical Indicators: A Descriptive and Modelling Study." *BMJ Global Health* 2, no. 2 (2017): e000226. https://doi.org/10.1136/bmjgh-2016-000226.
6. Royal Australasian College of Surgeons. *RACS Global Health Pacific Strategic Plan 2022–2027.* RACS, 2022. https://www.surgeons.org/-/media/Project/RACS/surgeons-org/files/Nick-Taylor/RACS_Global_Health_Pacific_Regional_Strat_Plan.pdf.
7. Guest, Glenn Douglas, Elizabeth McLeod, William R. G. Perry et al. "Collecting Data for Global Surgical Indicators: A Collaborative Approach in the Pacific Region." *BMJ Global Health* 2, no. 4 (2017). https://doi.org/10.1136/bmjgh-2017-000376.
8. Peters, Alexander W., Luis Roa, Emmanuel Rwamasirabo, Emmanuel Ameh, Marco M. Ulisubisya, Lubna Samad, Emmanuel M. Makasa, and John G. Meara. "National Surgical, Obstetric, and Anesthesia Plans Supporting the Vision of Universal Health Coverage." *Global Health: Science and Practice* 8, no. 1 (2020): 1–9. https://doi.org/10.9745/GHSP-D-19-00314.
9. Federal Ministry of Health, Nigeria. *Second National Strategic Health Development Plan (NSHDP II) 2018–2022: Ensuring Healthy Lives and Promoting the Wellbeing of Nigerian Populace at All Ages.* Federal Government of Nigeria, 2018. https://nipc.gov.ng/wp-content/uploads/2019/02/NSHDP-II-final-version-health-plan.pdf.
10. Peters, Alexander W., Lina Roa, Emile Rwamasirabo, Emmanuel Ameh, Mpoki M. Ulisubisya, Lubna Samad, Emmanuel M. Makasa, and John G. Meara. "National Surgical, Obstetric, and Anesthesia Plans Supporting the Vision of Universal Health Coverage." *Global Health: Science and Practice* 8, no. 1 (2020): 1–9. https://doi.org/10.9745/GHSP-D-19-00314.
11. Harvard Medical School and World Health Organization. *National Surgical, Obstetric and Anaesthesia Planning Manual.* 2020 Edition. United Nations Institute for Training and Research; Harvard Medical School Program in Global Surgery and Social Change; Global Surgery Foundation, 2020. ISBN 978-2-9701428-0-5. https://doi.org/10.5281/zenodo.3982869.
12. Kapologwe, Ntuli A., Anna Marwa, Joseph M. Kibusi et al. "Development and Upgrading of Public Primary Healthcare Facilities with Essential Surgical Services Infrastructure: A Strategy Towards Achieving Universal Health Coverage in Tanza-

nia." *BMC Health Services Research* 20, no. 1 (2020): 218. https://doi.org/10.1186/s12913-020-5057-2.

13. Ministry of Health, Community Development, Gender, Elderly and Children (Tanzania). *National Surgical, Obstetric and Anaesthesia Plan (NSOAP) 2018-2025*. 2018. https://docs.wixstatic.com/ugd/d9a674_4daa353b73064f70ab6a53a96bb84ace.pdf.
14. Cook, Kayleigh R., Zebenay B. Zeleke, Ephrem Gebrehana et al. "Quality and Sustainability of Ethiopia's National Surgical Indicators." *PLOS Global Public Health* 4, no. 3 (2024): e0002600. https://doi.org/10.1371/journal.pgph.0002600.
15. World Health Organization, Regional Office for the Western Pacific. *Action Framework for Safe and Affordable Surgery in the Western Pacific Region, 2021-2030*. World Health Organization, 2021. https://iris.who.int/bitstream/handle/10665/340914/9789290619345-eng.pdf.

15. HUMANITARIAN SURGERY — LESSONS FROM HAITI AND OTHER DISASTERS

1. Oxford English Dictionary, "Humanitarian (adj.), sense 2," March 2025, https://doi.org/10.1093/OED/1140141295.
2. Pan American Health Organization. *Health Response to the Earthquake in Haiti, January 2010: Lessons to be Learned for the Next Massive Sudden-Onset Disaster*. PAHO, 2011. https://www.paho.org/en/documents/health-response-earthquake-haiti.
3. Schuller, Mark. *Killing with Kindness: Haiti, International Aid, and NGOs*. Foreword by Paul Farmer. New Brunswick, Rutgers University Press, 2012.
4. Ayele, Sophia. "The Indian Ocean Tsunami, 10 Years On: Lessons from the Response and Ongoing Humanitarian Funding Challenges." *Oxfam Policy & Practice* (Research Report), December 2014. https://policy-practice.oxfam.org/resources/the-indian-ocean-tsunami-10-years-on-lessons-from-the-response-and-ongoing-huma-337007.
5. Pan American Health Organization. *Health Response to the Earthquake in Haiti, January 2010: Lessons to Be Learned for the Next Massive Sudden-Onset Disaster*. PAHO, 2011. https://www.paho.org/en/documents/health-response-earthquake-haiti.
6. World Health Organization, Regional Office for South-East Asia. *Nepal Earthquake 2015: An Insight into Risks - A Vision for Resilience*. WHO Regional Office for South-East Asia, 2016. https://www.who.int/publications/i/item/9789290225188.
7. Walter, Jonathan, ed. *World Disasters Report 2005: Focus on Information in Disasters*. Geneva: International Federation of Red Cross and Red Crescent Societies, 2005. https://archive.org/embed/worlddisastersre0000unse_o1z7.
8. United Nations General Assembly. "Strengthening of the Coordination of Humanitarian Emergency Assistance of the United Nations: Resolution / Adopted by the General Assembly." A/RES/46/182. United Nations, 1992. https://digitallibrary.un.org/record/135197/files/A_RES_46_182-EN.pdf.
9. World Health Organization. *Classification and Minimum Standards for Emergency Medical Teams*. World Health Organization, 2021. https://www.who.int/publications/i/item/9789240029330.
10. Randolph, Marilys G., Leonard Elbaum, Pey-Shan Wen et al. "Functional and Psychosocial Status of Haitians Who Became Users of Lower-Limb Prostheses as a Result of the 2010 Earthquake." *Journal of Prosthetics and Orthotics* 26, no. 4 (2014): 177. https://doi.org/10.1097/JPO.0000000000000039.

16. GLOBAL SURGERY ORGANISATIONS AND FUNDING SOURCES

1. "BBC News. "Oxfam: UK Halts Funding over New Sexual Exploitation Claims." April 8, 2021. https://www.bbc.com/news/health-56670162.
2. Polman, Linda. *War Games: The Story of Aid and War in Modern Times*. Viking, 2011.
3. Polman, Linda. *The Crisis Caravan: What's Wrong with Humanitarian Aid*. Picador, 2011.
4. Thomson, Andrew, Heidi Postlewait, and Kenneth Cain. *Emergency Sex (And Other Desperate Measures): True Stories from a War Zone*. Ebury Publishing, 2011.
5. World Health Organization. "How WHO Is Funded." World Health Organization. Accessed October 24, 2025. https://www.who.int/about/funding.
6. Debas, H. T., P. Donkor, A. Gawande, D. T. Jamison, M. E. Kruk, and C. N. Mock, editors. 2015. *Essential Surgery. Disease Control Priorities*, third edition, volume 1. World Bank. doi:10.1596/978-1-4648-0346-8. License: Creative Commons Attribution CC BY 3.0 IGO.
7. Dreher, Axel, Jan-Egbert Sturm, and James Raymond Vreeland. "Development Aid and International Politics: Does Membership on the UN Security Council Influence World Bank Decisions?" *Journal of Development Economics* 88, no. 1 (2009): 1–18. https://doi.org/10.1016/j.jdeveco.2008.02.003.
8. Sgard, Jérôme. *The Debt Crisis of the 1980s: Law and Political Economy*. Edward Elgar Publishing, 2023. https://www.sciencespo.fr/ceri/sites/sciencespo.fr.ceri/files/TheDebtCrisisOfThe1980s-Introduction.pdf.
9. International Monetary Fund, "Debt Relief Under the Heavily Indebted Poor Countries Initiative," last modified February 2, 2023, https://www.imf.org/en/About/Factsheets/Sheets/2023/Debt-relief-under-the-heavily-indebted-poor-countries-initiative-HIPC.
10. World Bank, "Heavily Indebted Poor Countries (HIPC) Initiative," last modified May 8, 2024, https://www.worldbank.org/en/topic/debt/brief/hipc.
11. World Bank. "Developing Countries Paid Record $1.4 Trillion on Foreign Debt in 2023." News release, December 3, 2024. https://www.worldbank.org/en/news/press-release/2024/12/03/developing-countries-paid-record-1-4-trillion-on-foreign-debt-in-2023.
12. Toussaint, Eric. "'Developing Countries' Are Trapped in a New Debt Crisis — World Bank: How Can This Be Explained?" CADTM (Comité pour l'Abolition des Dettes Illégitimes), December 18, 2023. https://www.cadtm.org/Developing-countries-are-trapped-in-a-new-debt-crisis-World-Bank.
13. Bill & Melinda Gates Foundation. *Global Health Program Overview*. Seattle, WA: Bill & Melinda Gates Foundation, 2010. https://docs.gatesfoundation.org/documents/global-health-program-overview.pdf
14. International Federation of Gynecology and Obstetrics (in collaboration with the Royal College of Obstetricians and Gynaecologists and the American College of Obstetricians and Gynecologists). *FIGO Statement – Childbirth: A Bill of Rights.* September 2021. https://www.figo.org/sites/default/files/2021-09/FIGO_Statement_Childbirth_Bill_of_Rights_0.pdf.
15. British Association of Urological Surgeons. "About Urolink." Accessed August 18, 2025. https://www.baus.org.uk/professionals/urolink/about_urolink_2017.aspx.
16. World Health Organization. *Sixty-eighth World Health Assembly: Resolution WHA68.15, Agenda Item 17.1, 26 May 2015. Strengthening Emergency and Essential Surgical Care and Anaesthesia as a Component of Universal Health Coverage.* Document A68/31. World Health Organization, 2015. https://apps.who.int/gb/ebwha/pdf_files/wha68/a68_r15-en.pdf.

17. FROM POLICY TO PRACTICE: MODES OF DELIVERY

1. Debas, H. T., P. Donkor, A. Gawande, D. T. Jamison, M. E. Kruk, and C. N. Mock, editors. 2015. *Essential Surgery. Disease Control Priorities*, third edition, volume 1. World Bank. doi:10.1596/978-1-4648-0346-8. License: Creative Commons Attribution CC BY 3.0 IGO.
2. Maine, Rebecca G., William Y. Hoffman, Jorge H. Palacios-Martinez, D. Scott Corlew, and George A. Gregory. "Comparison of Fistula Rates after Palatoplasty for International and Local Surgeons on Surgical Missions in Ecuador with Rates at a Craniofacial Center in the United States." *Plastic and Reconstructive Surgery* 129, no. 2 (2012): 319e–26. https://doi.org/10.1097/PRS.0b013e31823aea7e.
3. Farmer, Paul E., and Jim Y. Kim. "Surgery and Global Health: A View from Beyond the OR." *World Journal of Surgery* 32, no. 4 (2008): 533–36. https://doi.org/10.1007/s00268-008-9525-9.
4. Cancedda, Corrado, Phil Cotton, Joseph Shema et al. "Health Professional Training and Capacity Strengthening Through International Academic Partnerships: The First Five Years of the Human Resources for Health Program in Rwanda." *International Journal of Health Policy and Management* 7, no. 11 (2018): 1024–39. https://doi.org/10.15171/ijhpm.2018.61.
5. Cancedda, Corrado, Paul E. Farmer, Vanessa Kerry et al. "Maximizing the Impact of Training Initiatives for Health Professionals in Low-Income Countries: Frameworks, Challenges, and Best Practices." *PLoS Medicine* 12, no. 6 (2015): e1001840. https://doi.org/10.1371/journal.pmed.1001840.
6. Punchak, Maria A., Daksh Chauhan, Bethany J. Thach, Nathan A. Shlobin, and Gail Rosseau. "Application of Telemedicine in Global Surgery Partnerships between High-Income and Low- and Middle-Income Countries: A Scoping Review." *Global Surgical Education* 2, no. 1 (2023): 94. https://doi.org/10.1007/s44186-023-00169-7.
7. Hamlin, Catherine. *The Hospital by the River: A Story of Hope*. Monarch Books, 2018.

18. MOTIVES, SKILLS AND READINESS

1. Carlson, Matt. "Global Surgery on a Ship: Special On-Site Episode." Featuring guest Dr. Mark Shrime, hosted by Dr. Josh Wiedermann. *Headmirror Podcast*. August 2023. Podcast, audio. https://www.headmirror.com/podcast/mercy-ships.
2. Hardy, Mark A., and Beth R. Hochman, eds. *Global Surgery: How to Work and Teach in Low- and Middle-Income Countries*. Springer, 2023.
3. Nelson, Brett D., Jennifer Kasper, Patricia L. Hibberd, Donald M. Thea, and Julie M. Herlihy. "Developing a Career in Global Health: Considerations for Physicians-in-Training and Academic Mentors." *Journal of Graduate Medical Education* 4, no. 3 (2012): 301–6. https://doi.org/10.4300/JGME-D-11-00299.1.
4. Peregrin, Tony. "Opportunities for Global Volunteerism: How Two Practices in Michigan Make It Work." *Bulletin of the American College of Surgeons* 106, no. 7 (July 2, 2021). https://www.facs.org/for-medical-professionals/news-publications/news-and-articles/bulletin/2021/07/opportunities-for-global-volunteerism-how-two-practices-in-michigan-make-it-work/.

19. CHOOSING YOUR FIRST PROGRAMME

1. Peregrin, Tony. "Opportunities for Global Volunteerism: How Two Practices in Michigan Make It Work." *Bulletin of the American College of Surgeons* 106, no. 7 (July 2, 2021). https://www.facs.org/for-medical-professionals/news-publications/news-

and-articles/bulletin/2021/07/opportunities-for-global-volunteerism-how-two-practices-in-michigan-make-it-work/.
2. Hallard, Valentine. "Doing Good or Doing Harm? A Critical Examination of Voluntourism in a Globalized World." *Human Rights Research Center*, May 29, 2025. https://www.humanrightsresearch.org/post/doing-good-or-doing-harm-a-critical-examination-of-voluntourism-in-a-globalized-world.
3. Bolkan, Håkon A., Lars Hagander, Johan von Schreeb et al. "The Surgical Workforce and Surgical Provider Productivity in Sierra Leone: A Countrywide Inventory." *World Journal of Surgery* 40, no. 6 (2016): 1344–51. https://doi.org/10.1007/s00268-016-3417-1.
4. Kirkpatrick, James D., and Wendy Kayser Kirkpatrick. *Kirkpatrick's Four Levels of Training Evaluation*. ATD Press, 2016. ISBN 9781607280088.
5. Tiggelaar, Isabelle G., Erica W. M. Janszen, Marianne van Elteren et al. "Dutch Post-Graduate Training in Global Health and Tropical Medicine: A Qualitative Study on Graduates' Perspectives." *BMC Medical Education* 25, no. 1 (2025): 663. https://doi.org/10.1186/s12909-025-07126-6.

20. SELF-IMPROVEMENT

1. Brown, Colin, Fred Martineau, Emily Spry, and John S. Yudkin. "Postgraduate Training in Global Health: Ensuring UK Doctors Can Contribute to Health in Resource-Poor Countries." *Clinical Medicine* 11, no. 5 (2011): 456–60. https://doi.org/10.7861/clinmedicine.11-5-456.
2. Médecins Sans Frontières and International Development Committee of the Association of Surgeons of Great Britain and Ireland. *Issues in Professional Practice: How to Work as a Surgeon Overseas*. Association of Surgeons of Great Britain and Ireland, May 2011. https://www.asgbi.org.uk/userfiles/file/ipp/_iipp-how-to-work-as-a-surgeon-overseas-as-gone-to-press.pdf.

21. PRACTICAL MATTERS

1. Oosterhoff, Pauline, and Elise Wach. "Why It's Time We Talked about the Sex Lives of Humanitarians." Global Development Professionals Network, *The Guardian*, July 10, 2014. https://www.theguardian.com/global-development-professionals-network/2014/jul/10/humanitarian-workers-sex-global-development.
2. Dahlgren, Atti-La, Lisa Deroo, Jacqueline Avril, Gerard Bise, and Louis Loutan. "Health Risks and Risk-Taking Behaviors among International Committee of the Red Cross (ICRC) Expatriates Returning from Humanitarian Missions." *Journal of Travel Medicine* 16, no. 6 (2009): 382–90. https://doi.org/10.1111/j.1708-8305.2009.00350.x.
3. Cameron, Lily, Mary McCauley, Nynke van den Broek, and Hannah McCauley. "The Occurrence of and Factors Associated with Mental Ill-Health amongst Humanitarian Aid Workers: A Systematic Review and Meta-Analysis." *PloS One* 19, no. 5 (2024): e0292107. https://doi.org/10.1371/journal.pone.0292107.
4. Jachens, Liza, Jonathan Houdmont, and Roslyn Thomas. "Effort-Reward Imbalance and Heavy Alcohol Consumption Among Humanitarian Aid Workers." *Journal of Studies on Alcohol and Drugs* 77, no. 6 (2016): 904–13. https://doi.org/10.15288/jsad.2016.77.904.
5. Brennan, N., N. Langdon, T. Gale, N. Humphries, A. Knapton, and M. Bryce. "Exploring Recent Patterns of Migration of Doctors to the United Kingdom: A Mixed-Methods Study." *BMC Health Services Research* 23 (November 2023): 1204. https://doi.org/10.1186/s12913-023-10199-y.
6. Tull, Katharine. *Drug Expiry Standards in Developing Countries*. K4D Helpdesk Report. Institute of Development Studies, 2018. https://assets.publishing.service.gov.

uk/media/5b3b5c8ce5274a701490d855/Drug_expiry_standards_in_developing_countries.pdf.
7. Ridde, Valéry. “Per Diems Undermine Health Interventions, Systems and Research in Africa: Burying Our Heads in the Sand.” *Tropical Medicine & International Health* 15, no. 7 (2010): E1–4. https://doi.org/10.1111/tmi.2607.

22. POOR BEHAVIOUR — PRIMUM NON NOCERE

1. Hardy, Mark A., and Beth R. Hochman, eds. *Global Surgery: How to Work and Teach in Low- and Middle-Income Countries*. Springer, 2023.
2. Ng-Kamstra, Joshua S., Sarah L. M. Greenberg, Fizan Abdullah et al. “Global Surgery 2030: A Roadmap for High Income Country Actors.” *BMJ Global Health* 1, no. 1 (2016): e000011. https://doi.org/10.1136/bmjgh-2015-000011.
3. Parker, Ben. “EXCLUSIVE: Oxfam Sexual Exploiter in Haiti Caught Seven Years Earlier in Liberia.” *The New Humanitarian*, February 13, 2018. https://www.thenewhumanitarian.org/investigations/2018/02/13/exclusive-oxfam-sexual-exploiter-haiti-caught-seven-years-earlier-liberia.

INDEX

I

www.ingramcontent.com/pod-product-compliance
Ingram Content Group UK Ltd.
Pitfield, Milton Keynes, MK11 3LW, UK
UKHW022023041026
15591UKWH00012B/452

9 781919 328300